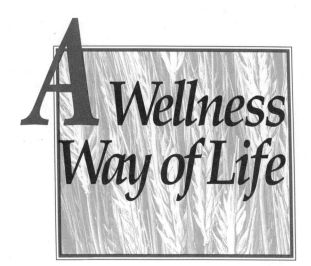

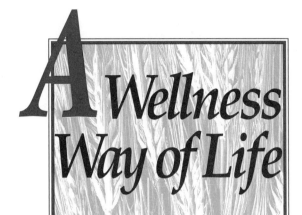

A Wellness Way of Life

Second Edition

Gwen Robbins
Debbie Powers   Sharon Burgess
Ball State University

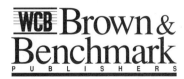

WCB Brown & Benchmark
P U B L I S H E R S

Madison, Wisconsin • Dubuque, Iowa • Indianapolis, Indiana
Melbourne, Australia • Oxford, England

Book Team

Editor *Scott Spoolman*
Production Editor *Diane Clemens*
Designer *Lu Ann Schrandt*
Photo Editor *Shirley Lanners*
Art Processor *Amy L. Ley*
Visuals/Design Developmental Consultant *Marilyn A. Phelps*
Publishing Services Specialist *Sherry Padden*
Marketing Manager *Pamela S. Cooper*
Advertising Manager *Jodi Rymer*

WCB Brown & Benchmark

A Division of Wm. C. Brown Communications, Inc.

Executive Vice President/General Manager *Thomas E. Doran*
Vice President/Editor in Chief *Edgar J. Laube*
Vice President/Sales and Marketing *Eric Ziegler*
Director of Production *Vickie Putman Caughron*
Director of Custom and Electronic Publishing *Chris Rogers*

Wm. C. Brown Communications, Inc.

President and Chief Executive Officer *G. Franklin Lewis*
Corporate Senior Vice President and Chief Financial Officer *Robert Chesterman*
Corporate Senior Vice President and President of Manufacturing *Roger Meyer*

Cover Photo © Jim Corwin/Allstock, Inc.

Photo Credits; Chapter 1: Pages 7, 10, 16, 19, 26, 30 (all): Brenda Lewis, Westminster, Colorado; **Chapter 2:** Page 39: Brenda Lewis, Westminster, Colorado; p. 42: Courtesy of Ball State University Photographic Services; figures 2.1, 2.2, p. 49: Brenda Lewis, Westminster, Colorado; p. 52: © Paul Troxell; **Chapter 4:** Figures 4.1, 4.2: Courtesy of Ball State University Photographic Services; 4.3, 4.4, 4.5, 4.6, 4.7, 4.8, 4.9, 4.10, 4.11, 4.12, 4.13, 4.14, 4.16, 4.17, 4.18, 4.19, 4.20: Brenda Lewis, Westminster, Colorado; **Chapter 5:** Pages 129, 140L-R, 141: Brenda Lewis, Westminster, Colorado; **Chapter 6:** Page 147: Gwen Robbins; p. 161: Courtesy of Ball State University Photographic Services; **Chapter 7:** Page 184: Brenda Lewis, Westminster, Colorado; figure 7.2: Brenda Lewis, Westminster, Colorado; **Chapter 8:** Pages 205, 220: Courtesy of Ball State University Photographic Services; p. 224: Brenda Lewis, Westminster, Colorado; **Chapter 9:** Pages 230, 236T: Brenda Lewis, Westminster, Colorado; **Chapter 10:** Page 271: Brenda Lewis, Westminster, Colorado; **Chapter 11:** Page 294: © Paul Troxell; **Chapter 12:** Page 327: Brenda Lewis, Westminster, Colorado; p. 343: ©Paul Troxell; **Chapter 13:** Page 348: Brenda Lewis, Westminster, Colorado; p. 364: © Paul Troxell; **Chapter 14:** Pages 370B, 372, 373, 374, 375, 380: Brenda Lewis, Westminster, Colorado.

A Times Mirror Company

Library of Congress Catalog Card Number: 92–76204

ISBN 0–697–12659–5

Printed in the United States of America by Wm. C. Brown Communications, Inc., 2460 Kerper Boulevard, Dubuque, IA 52001

10 9 8 7 6 5 4 3 2 1

Contents

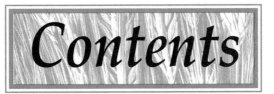

Chapter 1: Wellness

Chapter 2: Physical Fitness

Chapter 3: Strength and Flexibility

Chapter 4: Fitness Assessment

Chapter 5: Common Injuries and Care of the Lower Back

Chapter 6: Heart Health

Chapter 7: *Coping with Stress*

Chapter 8: Special Exercise Considerations

Chapter 9: Nutrition

Chapter 10: Weight Management

Chapter 11: Cancer Prevention and Personal Safety

Chapter 12: Substance Abuse

Chapter 13: Preventing Sexually Transmitted Disease

Chapter 14: Planning Wellness for a Lifetime

Preface

This book is about enjoying life—living it to your fullest potential. Its purpose is to help you pursue a wellness lifestyle. We wanted to provide a book that would present a body of knowledge that goes beyond fitness. This knowledge helps you make informed, responsible decisions affecting your wellness. However, we know it takes much more than knowledge. It takes personal commitment, self-management skills, and coping strategies to live such a lifestyle. Therefore, a primary focus in this book is identifying behavior changes that you can easily incorporate into your life. Our goal is not only to deliver fitness and health information, but to motivate and guide you toward making positive choices. This is a "how to" book that minimizes technical jargon. Detailed anatomical descriptions and physiological principles have not been included because we feel this knowledge is not necessary in order to understand and apply wellness principles.

This book was developed to meet the needs of a course that evolved from physical fitness into the broader scope of wellness. The ideas, concepts, and strategies presented represent our many years of experience in teaching this course. The topics addressed can easily accommodate a variety of college fitness, wellness, and health courses. It is a flexible book that especially fits nicely into a lecture/fitness activity format.

This book offers several internal learning aids you will find helpful: chapter objectives, terms, chapter summary, references, suggested readings, and resources. The appendix section contains additional learning tools, including Student Activities and information on specific activities for the development of fitness (aerobic dance, bicycling, fitness swimming, jogging, walking, water exercise/aqua aerobics).

Abraham Lincoln once said, "We are about as happy as we make up our minds to be." We believe that one secret to this happiness is having the competence and confidence to make informed decisions that affect your daily well-being. There is no better feeling than to know that you are doing something good for yourself! As you read each chapter, you will learn strategies for taking control of your life and discover the joy in traveling the wellness journey. This book will help you wade through the myriad of health and wellness information and ultimately make you an informed wellness consumer. The end result will be the undescribable joy in knowing that you are attaining your highest potential for well-being.

Acknowledgements

We would like to thank the reviewers of this edition for their time and assistance:

- John S. Carter
  The Citadel
- Denyce Stokes Ford
  Howard University
- Jean Martin Frazier
  East Tennessee State University

- Warren Hammer
  University of Richmond
- Cindy L. Hanawalt
  University of Iowa
- Patsy Livingston
  Point Loma Nazarene College

- Jeryl J. Neff
  *University of Wisconsin-
  Superior*
- Cynthia J. Petri
  *University of Alabama-
  Birmingham*

- Jacquie Rainey
  Ball State University
- Michael L. Teague
  University of Iowa
- Donna J. Terbizan
  North Dakota State University

We wish to express our gratitude to the following individuals for their assistance in the development of this book:

- Sam Minor II, *Department of Art,
  College of Fine Arts, Ball State
  University*, for the artwork;
- Brenda Lewis and Paul Troxell for
  the photographs;

- Evelyn Goss for secretarial
  assistance;
- Scott Spoolman for his guidance
  as editor.

A special thank you goes to Dr. John Reno and Dr. Duane Eddy for their continued support of the fitness/wellness program at Ball State University.

We dedicate this second edition to the devoted fitness/wellness faculty at Ball State. Their support and suggestions have been invaluable.

1
Wellness

Chapter Objectives

After reading this chapter, you will be able to:

1. Discriminate between health and wellness.
2. List seven of the ten health habits that, when practiced, can reduce the risk of health problems.
3. Identify the six dimensions of wellness, and give three examples within each dimension.
4. List and describe the four tools necessary for growth in wellness, as shown on the wellness wheel.
5. Explain how motivation and support affect wellness living.
6. Differentiate between self-management and willpower.
7. Identify and describe the five steps of a self-management strategy.
8. Explain the impact of antecedents (triggers) on behavior change.
9. Identify strategies that can be included in a wellness plan to influence a change in behavior.
10. Write a wellness contract.
11. Give four examples of ways society supports wellness, and four examples of ways society detracts from wellness.

Terms

- Behavioral antecedent
- Behavior chain
- Behavioral consequence
- Emotional dimension
- External locus of control
- Health

- Health promotion
- Intellectual dimension
- Internal locus of control
- Locus of control
- Occupational dimension
- Physical dimension

- Self-management
- Social dimension
- Societal norm
- Spiritual dimension
- Wellness

*"You, the individual, can do more for your health and
well-being than any doctor, any hospital, any drug, any
exotic medical device."*

Joseph A. Califano,
Former Secretary of Health, Education, and Welfare

A s Rob lay in the coronary care unit, his eyes surveyed various tubes and wires connected to his tired body. The nightmare of the last twenty-four hours was over, but the pain and confusion lingered.

"How can this be? I'm only forty-nine years old. How could I have had a heart attack? What if I die? What about my wife? My son? My daughter? I've just become a grandpa. I was given a big promotion at work. Why now?" Rob's mind drifted.

"But I'm an athlete! . . . Well, I *was* an athlete, back in high school. Once I started college there was no time for sports or exercise. . . . Started smoking, too. Figured I'd stop when the pressure was off, but the pressure never stopped. . . . Drank too much, too; partied a lot. Still like several drinks to end the day. . . . I always thought I'd lose those extra 30 pounds—always next year, always a New Year's resolution. Diet? Too busy. Vending machines, hot dog stands, snacks in front of the TV, fast food. . . . No time. . . . Too much to do . . . Money to make . . . A lot of stress . . . Can't stop now. There'll be time later."

Rob's mind drifted back to his room. He could hear his doctor's voice—

"Stop smoking. . . . Change in lifestyle. . . . Low-fat diet. . . . Start exercising . . . . Cholesterol is 280. . . . Break old habits." Rob thought, "How I wish I could turn back the clock!"

This scenario is all too common in the United States. In fact, more than half of all deaths in this country are attributed to coronary heart disease and stroke. Even though most heart attacks occur after middle age, many are a result of years of lifestyle abuse. One hundred years ago the leading causes of death were infectious diseases such as tuberculosis, polio, diphtheria, pneumonia, influenza, and various diseases of infancy. Advances in medicine, the discovery of antibiotics, and improved sanitation diminished these ravaging diseases, and increased the average life span. Through scientific discovery, technology, industrial growth, and automation, the entire American lifestyle has changed. We use remote controls to change television channels and to open garage doors. Appliances wash our clothes, dishes, and teeth. We ride vehicles to work, school, and even while playing golf! We allow ourselves to be bused and trucked, elevated, and escalated, and then wonder why we grow fat and are out of shape. This so-called "good life" has created sedentary living, changes in eating habits (fast foods, increased fats and sweets, processed foods), stress, alcohol and drug abuse, and obesity. The latest statistics released by the American Heart Association are startling. In a single year, diseases of the heart and blood vessels kill far more Americans than were killed in World Wars I and II, the Korean War, and the Vietnam War, *combined*. And those that survive a coronary incident are often faced with a restricted, less fulfilling life that causes an unnecessary, costly drain on the resources available for health care. Such horrendous figures should

The "good life"?

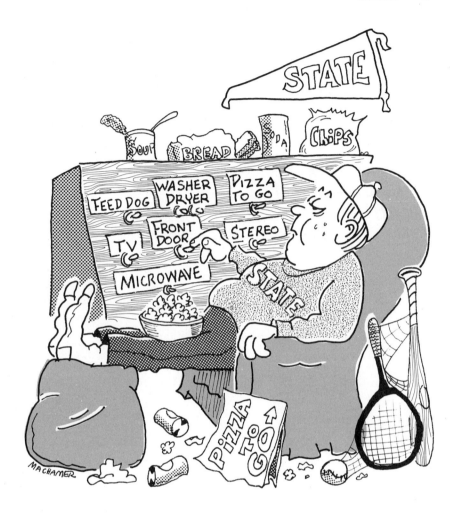

outrage the public and should cause a demand for reform, since carnage is normally the basis for alarm and legislation. Instead, it is disheartening to find that apathy is the general response of many, and that many of us do not even begin to worry about health until it is lost!

The harsh truth is that a high percentage of disease and disability affecting the American people is preventable; a consequence of unwise behavior and lifestyle choices. The decision to smoke, for instance, is responsible for one of every six deaths in America each year. Twenty-one percent of heart disease deaths, 87 percent of lung cancer deaths, and 30 percent of all cancer deaths are linked to smoking. Smoking costs our society over $52 billion annually.[1]

You may already possess some knowledge about these and other health topics. If you are like most, however, you generally underestimate your future risk of lifestyle diseases. This underestimation is of substantial concern, because action should be an outcome of knowledge! It is encouraging to know that the evidence is becoming more and more clear—health and longevity are not solely a result of genetics and luck but an outcome of personal behavior. This personal behavior involves responsible choices, self-discipline, and a commitment to excellence.

This chapter introduces the basic concept of health, the impact of lifestyle on well-being, and the dynamics of high-level wellness. It also explores the challenges and strategies involved in making self-managed behavior changes.

Basic Concepts of Health

The word health makes most people think of illness. After all, the sick are treated at a health center, the mentally ill go to a mental health facility, and doctors, nurses, and technicians are called health-care professionals. Traditionally, **health** has been viewed as the "lack of disease." If you show no signs or symptoms of illness, you are healthy. Health is seen as a state of being. You are either ill; or you are healthy. Some health-care facilities still reflect this simplistic view. Many insurance companies pay for treatments and hospitalization when sickness occurs but pay nothing for preventive checkups or procedures. Employers allow "sick days," yet personal days or vacation days must be used for pursuing health-promoting activities. What is currently prevalent in this country is a "sickness-care" system rather than a "health-care" system. And, with all of the medical procedures, drugs, and technologies presently available, many people are complacent about their health habits. They think they can be "bailed out" by medical science (at the cost of billions of dollars a year to society!).

What is evolving from this narrow concept is an expanded health strategy that encompasses medical care, disease prevention, and health promotion. Medical care begins with the sick and seeks to keep them alive, make them well, or minimize their disability. Disease prevention begins with a threat to health—a disease or environmental hazard—and seeks to protect as many people as possible from the harmful consequences of that threat. In other words, an effort is made to reduce the occurrence and severity of disease. **Health promotion** is "the science and art of helping people change their lifestyle to move toward a state of optimal health."[2] Health promotion involves the systematic efforts by an organization to create healthy policies and supportive environments, as well as reorienting health services beyond clinical and curative care. Examples of health promotion programs are weight loss workshops, smoking cessation clinics, and stress management seminars. More discussion of health promotion is found in chapter 14.

Another recent trend in health care is renewed emphasis on medical self-care. Medical self-care includes all actions taken by an individual with respect to a medical problem. It accounts for 85–95 percent of all medical care.[3] Medical self-care promotes self-sufficiency in diagnosis and requires decision making as to whether a physician's services are needed. It is usually used in minor illnesses or injuries such as colds, flu, cuts, and sprains. Individual decision making becomes the focus. Do I need a physician for this problem? What can I do for myself?

What can I expect from the health-care profession? Medical self-care goes beyond minor illness. Individuals with diabetes, asthma, and allergies have a major responsibility for their own care. Even emergency procedures such as cardiopulmonary resuscitation (CPR) and the Heimlich maneuver fall into the realm of medical self-care. No longer are thermometers the only diagnostic tool in home medicine cabinets. It is now common to find blood pressure kits, home pregnancy tests, colon-rectal cancer detection kits, and blood sugar self-tests. The purpose of self-care is not to replace the physician but to promote personal responsibility for health, rather than total dependence on physicians.

Lifestyle and Health

The preventive aspects of health have become increasingly clear. During the 1970s, much research was done to link lifestyle factors and health. Most revealing were Belloc and Breslow's five and a half-year study of the lifestyle habits of nearly 7,000 adults and the 1979 report from the Surgeon General's office entitled *Healthy People.*[4,5] These comprehensive studies showed that life expectancy and health are significantly related to ten distinctive health habits:

1. eating three meals a day at regular intervals instead of snacking
2. eating breakfast every day
3. engaging in moderate exercise two or three times a week
4. getting adequate sleep (7–8 hours) every night
5. not smoking
6. maintaining moderate weight
7. consuming little or no alcohol
8. reducing intake of excess calories, fat, salt, and sugar
9. undergoing periodic screenings (at intervals determined by age and sex) for major disorders such as high blood pressure and certain cancers
10. adhering to speed laws and using seat belts

For most individuals, these are only modest changes, yet they can substantially reduce the risk of several health problems. One physician has appropriately summarized the issue by stating

"One of my frustrations in medicine was having people come to me expecting way too much of me and not expecting anything of themselves."[6] To evaluate your personal lifestyle habits, look to "Healthy Lifestyle: A Self-Assessment," found in the activities section at the end of the book.

Healthy People 2000 A vigorous national crusade for health promotion and disease prevention was initiated in 1990 with the publication of *Healthy People 2000: National Health Promotion and Disease Prevention Objectives,* a document facilitated by the U.S. Public Health Service. *Healthy People 2000* is a statement of national opportunities, emphasizing individual control of our health destinies . . . "personal responsibility, which is to say responsible and enlightened behavior by each and every individual, truly is the key to good health."[7]

This document outlines specific health goals for the nation targeted for the year 2000 in 22 priority areas (physical activity, nutrition, tobacco use, family planning, cancer, alcohol and drug use, sexually transmitted diseases, and heart disease to name a few). Three broad goals are identified by the document as means of bringing about fuller human potential. These goals[8] are:

1. Increase the span of healthy life for Americans.

2. Reduce health disparities among Americans.

3. Achieve access to preventive services for all Americans.

In this way the Federal government is playing a leadership role in cultivating a culture of healthier, life-enhancing habits for all Americans, regardless of income, race, sex, or other status. If we do not act now, the cost of health care in this country will reach $1.5 trillion by the end of the decade.[9]

Understanding Risks

Often in this book we will talk about risks. In an effort to prevent disease and to promote health, it is important to identify the factors that cause disease and injury. From this, probabilities are determined as to the chances for occurrence. For example, consider the fact that half of all highway fatalities could be prevented by wearing seat belts. Once this risk factor is identified, changes in the environment can be initiated (in this case, seat belts as a manufacturer's requirement in all automobiles). Next is to persuade people to adjust their behavior (for example, convince them to buckle up, or pass a law requiring fastening of seat belts). Like placing a bet at a race track, identifying risks is a way of quoting the odds. No one can honestly promise you that doing something or refraining from something will keep you safe, or that doing one thing will positively kill you. You simply must draw your own conclusions from the evidence. Since there is no such thing as absolute safety, you can only choose to widen or to narrow your risk margins with your habits.

It is important also to realize that the media often reports health news with brevity and drama, which can be misleading and oversimplified. Many in audiences are looking for impossibly clear and simple answers. Is it safe to eat this? Drink that? Take that pill? Since risks are not absolute, some end up rejecting all information, and conclude "nothing is safe." Health risks are a highly individual matter, where extreme overgeneralizations should be avoided. Mark Twain's comment is one to ponder: "Be careful about reading health books; you may die of a misprint!"

One ongoing study has resulted in much of the information we know about the risk factors associated with coronary heart disease. The people of Framingham, Massachusetts, a community 18 miles west of Boston, have been studied and charted since 1950. The Framingham Study, as it has become known, has resulted in much that is known about how heredity, environment, medical care, and lifestyle factors affect heart disease and general well-being. A comprehensive longitudinal study such as this results in reputable data, in contrast to a short-term, isolated study involving very few people.

The typical American diet has become a serious health risk factor.

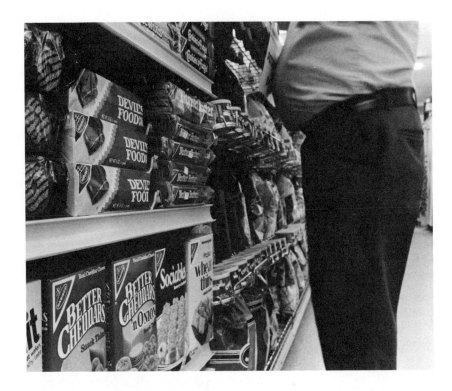

Heredity is Not Destiny For some, familial tendencies constitute a mental trap. If your father died young of a heart attack or your mother has diabetes, your chances for following in their footsteps are greater than someone whose parents are healthy at 75 years of age. This is only the case if your parents' health problems were an actual result of genetics rather than environment or lifestyle habits. If you have inherited a genetic liability, this knowledge should give you additional motivation to live in such a way as to fight this tendency. In the case of a family history of heart disease, your genetic odds are lowered significantly by controlling your blood pressure, blood cholesterol, weight, stress level, and getting regular exercise. On the other hand, having a father like Winston Churchill (who habitually smoked, drank, ate rich food, was obese, sedentary, and lived to 90) does not mean you are indestructible. Heredity is only one factor in the link to health and well-being. Even though our biological inheritance predisposes us to certain illnesses and protects us from others, it is the interaction of genetics, culture, environment, and habits that counts. Your environment and personal health habits can either magnify or inhibit the tendencies with which you were born. Of course, we hope you are thinking beyond mere "risk avoidance" to a life full of enrichment, self-fulfillment, and satisfaction. This dramatic shift in emphasis toward self-responsibility and an expanded quality of life has evolved into a concept called "wellness."

High-Level Wellness

It is reassuring to know that we have a considerable amount of control over our health destiny. However, what are the upper limits of health? What is the ultimate in health? Around 1958, Dr. Halbert L. Dunn, then the first director of the U.S. National Office of Vital Statistics, began describing and writing about a state of health that is so much more than the absence of disease. He talked about the interrelated and interdependent whole person, a positive energy and vitality for living, personal growth and satisfaction, and the importance of viewing and promoting health as an elevated state of superb well-being, or high-level wellness. He viewed wellness as something more than a flat, uninteresting area of unsickness—he viewed it as a fascinating, ever-changing lifelong adventure.[10] **Wellness** is defined as an integrated and dynamic level of functioning oriented toward maximizing potential, dependent upon self-responsibility. This is a lifestyle in which you strive to achieve your highest potential of well-being! This implies that high-level wellness is impossible to reach in an absolute sense. It is not a static state, but an ever-changing level of functioning. That is, wellness can be viewed as an expanded continuum of health functioning. A common continuum of health is seen in figure 1.1.

Figure 1.1

A common continuum of health.

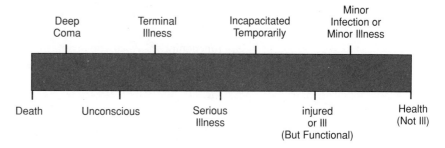

Wellness, on the contrary, has a range of full potential functioning. Inspired by Dr. Dunn's concept of wellness, Dr. John Travis pioneered the contemporary wellness movement in the mid-1970s. He became the first physician to offer wellness services. He conducted wellness seminars for the general public and health professionals and developed a Wellness Resource Center. His wellness continuum has become the most recognized model used in describing the dynamic state of wellness (fig. 1.2).

Not so long ago this country's medical care system functioned entirely left of center (treatment model). Now, however, wellness centers have begun to emerge. The rapid increase in community wellness programs is astounding. Schools, YMCAs, corporations, and hospitals are offering wellness programs and services to consumers. Wellness is recognized as a viable alternative to the neutral state of non-illness or "just getting by." Thus, thirty-five years after Dr. Dunn first introduced the concept, wellness is finally being given serious attention.

Naturally, high-level wellness is unique to age, resources, and circumstances. That is, it is applicable to all ages (old and young), all socioeconomic groups (poor and wealthy), and all types of people (able-bodied and disabled). It means

Figure 1.2

Illness/wellness continuum. Moving from the center to the left shows a progressively worsening state of health. Moving to the right of center indicates increasing levels of health and well-being. The treatment model can bring you to the neutral point, where the symptoms of disease have been alleviated. The wellness model, which can be utilized at any point, directs you beyond neutral, and encourages you to move as far to the right as possible. It is not meant to replace the treatment model on the left side of the continuum, but to work in harmony with it. If you are ill, treatment is important, but do not stop there.

Reprinted with permission of Publisher © 1981, 1988 by John W. Travis from The Wellness Workbook, *2nd edition, by John W. Travis, M.D. and Regina Sara Ryan. Published by Ten Speed Press, Berkeley, CA.*

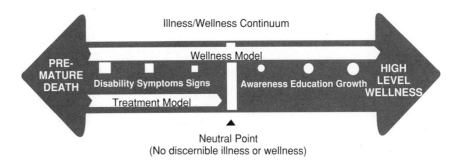

working toward becoming the best you can be without accepting "traditional" limitations (i.e., age, race, gender, genetics, etc.). Wellness is a way of living in which growth and improvement is sought in all areas. It involves a lifestyle of deliberate choices and self-responsibility, requiring conscientious management and planning. Living a wellness lifestyle is not by accident or luck. It is much more than curing sickness, preventing illness, or medical self-care. Rather, it is a continuous effort to reach full potential—a process of gaining control of yourself and your environment. It means approaching life with optimism, confidence, and energy. Rather than wishing to be someone else, a wellness-oriented person strives to develop within the realm of personal potential. Unlike sickness-care health, which involves treatment, wellness is a lifelong quest toward optimal functioning in which you take the reins. It involves accepting the changes in life while seeking the positive payoffs of change. This quest has rewards of high self-esteem, commitment to excellence, positive health, productivity, and a zest for living. Much like Maslow's self-actualizing person, individuals who strive for wellness have an exceptional openness to experience. Rather than fearing new experiences and different ideas, they welcome them as a way to grow. They do not allow prejudices or stereotypes to distort their perceptions. They are autonomous in thought and action. They take control of life. Life is faced with creativity and freshness. Living a wellness lifestyle has good potential for increasing longevity. However, this is not the main purpose of wellness living. Wellness advocate Donald Ardell agrees. He states, "The motive force behind wellness lifestyles is near-term, attractive payoffs and benefits. Living this way is considered a richer way to be alive."[11] Wellness should be a fun, satisfying existence.

The Dimensions of Wellness

The wellness lifestyle is a coordinated and integrated living pattern involving six dimensions: physical, intellectual, emotional, social, spiritual, and occupational. There is a strong interdependence between dimensions, even though they function separately. For example, joining an exercise class in your community most notably enhances your physical well-being. Can you determine in what ways participating in such a class positively affects the other dimensions? In each dimension there is opportunity for personal growth, and, due to their interrelationship, growth in one area often sparks interest in another. Balancing these dimensions, however, is an important factor in pursuing wellness. For example, being an avid reader, yet not being able to get along with anyone, is not an example of balanced wellness.

Physical Dimension   The **physical dimension** deals with the functional operation of the body; in other words, is your body the best machine possible? The physical dimension involves the health-related components of physical fitness—muscular strength, muscular endurance, cardiorespiratory endurance, flexibility, and body composition. Dietary habits have a significant effect on physical well-being. Your sexual, drinking, and drug behaviors also play a role in physical health. Do you smoke? Do you get an adequate amount of sleep? Do you catch many colds? These questions deal with physical health.

The physical dimension also includes medical self-care—regular self-tests, checkups, proper use of medications, taking necessary steps when you are ill, and appropriate use of the medical system. Managing your environment also affects physical well-being. For example, do you try to minimize your exposure to tobacco smoke and harmful pollutants? Obviously, positive health habits are critical to physical well-being.

Learning should continue throughout life.

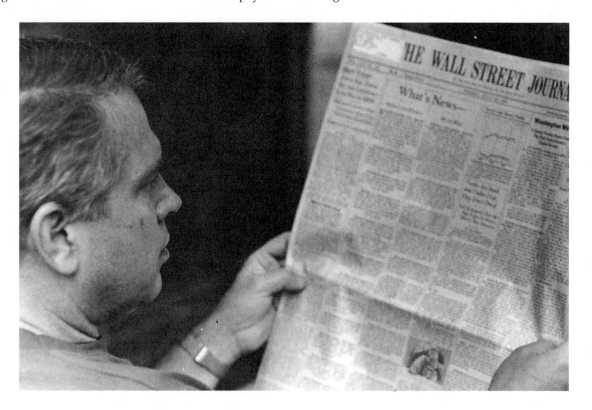

Intellectual Dimension   The **intellectual dimension** involves the use of your mind. Maintaining an active mind contributes to total well-being. Intellectual growth is not restricted to formal education, that is, school learning. It means a continuous acquisition of knowledge throughout life. It involves engaging your mind in creative and stimulating mental activities. Curiosity and learning should never stop. Reading, writing, and keeping abreast of current events are intellectual pursuits. Being able to think critically and apply knowledge are also associated with this dimension. The link between intellectual stimulation and healthy living is undeniable.

Emotional Dimension   Having a positive mental state is directly linked to wellness. Emotional wellness includes three areas: awareness, acceptance, and management. Emotional awareness involves recognizing your own feelings, as well as the feelings of others. Emotional acceptance means understanding the normality of human emotion, in addition to realistically assessing your own personal abilities and limitations. Emotional management means the ability to control or cope with personal feelings and knowing how to seek interpersonal support when necessary. The ability to maintain emotional stability at some midrange between the highs and the lows is essential. The abilities to laugh, to enjoy life, to adjust to change, to cope with stress, and to maintain intimate relationships are examples of the **emotional dimension** of wellness.

The six dimensions of wellness.

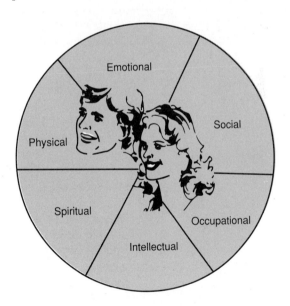

Social Dimension   Everyone, with the possible exception of a hermit, must interact with people. Social wellness involves the ability to get along with others, as well as appreciating the differences in people. It means exhibiting fairness, justice, and concern for the welfare of your community. The **social dimension** of wellness also includes concern for the environment and for mankind as a whole. Good friends, close family ties, and trusting relationships go hand in hand with high-level wellness.

Spiritual Dimension   Spiritual wellness is not always synonymous with religion. The **spiritual dimension** need not identify a creator, a god, or a theology. Instead, it involves the development of the inner self and one's soul. Spiritual wellness is a way of living that views life as purposeful and pleasurable, and seeks out life-sustaining and life-enriching options, which are freely chosen at every opportunity.[12] Spiritual wellness involves experiencing life and reflecting on that experience in order to discover a personal meaning and purpose in life. It involves the development of a clear and comfortable sense of right and wrong—a philosophy of life. Being able to identify the true sources of joy, pleasure, and fulfillment in your life is the spiritual clarification of personal values and beliefs.

Occupational Dimension   The **occupational dimension** involves deriving personal satisfaction from your vocation. Much of your life will be spent at work. Therefore, it is important that your chosen career provides the internal and external rewards you value. Do you want a job that allows for creativity, interaction with others, daily challenge, autonomy? Do you prefer opportunities for advancement, personal entrepreneurship, leadership, or helping others? How do you feel about mobility? Is salary your major motivation? Answering these questions may help you with career selection. Occupational wellness also involves maintaining a satisfying balance between work time and leisure time. It involves a work environment that minimizes stress and exposure to physical health hazards. A majority of your college life is spent analyzing and integrating your skills and interests with career choices. It is vital that your vocational choice is personally enriching and stimulating. If you are not happy with your occupation, you will find that your entire well-being suffers.

Wellness is a combination of all six dimensions. It means striving for growth in each dimension. Is there one dimension in which you are strongest? Which dimension is your weakest? Neglecting any dimension destroys the balance critical to high-level wellness. Certain dimensions may take on a greater importance at different times throughout your life. Nevertheless, striving for balance contributes to your wholeness. To evaluate your wellness in the six dimensions, you are encouraged to take the wellness assessment in the activities section at the end of the book.

Growth in Wellness

We have described wellness as a dynamic course of action based on self-responsibility. The goal is to assume greater responsibility for your quality of life by making positive lifestyle decisions. How do you begin making positive lifestyle choices? How do you know the options available to you? How do you grow in wellness? Table 1.1 gives examples of positive choices in each dimension of wellness to assist your growth.

Figure 1.3 depicts a multifaceted wheel for growth in wellness. The spokes of the wheel divide and identify five lifestyle areas that have enormous impact on our physical wellness: personal habits, stress management, nutrition and weight management, heart health, and physical fitness. The rim of the wheel describes

Figure 1.3

Wheel for growth in wellness.

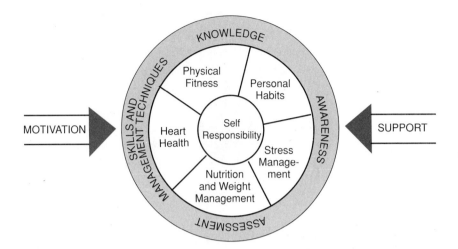

the tools necessary for growth in the lifestyle areas: awareness, assessment, knowledge, and skills and management techniques. The arrows pointing toward the wheel (motivation and support) strongly influence your wellness behavior.

Awareness   Before you can grow in wellness you must have an awareness of the wellness option. It is an exciting alternative! This chapter differentiates between the state of wellness and "treatment" health. You are now aware that your health, happiness, and quality of life are strongly affected by your willingness to make wellness choices. The increasing interest in wellness by the population has made it easier to adopt a wellness lifestyle, because wellness choices now are not only available, but valued.

Assessment   Once you are aware of the wellness option, you should assess your lifestyle. Assessment allows you to see how you are presently conducting your life and identifies where changes should occur. Assessments can be everything from medical tests (blood lipid profile, blood pressure, etc.) to physical fitness tests. They can be stress inventories, health risk appraisals, dietary logs, or even attitude questionnaires. Even personality assessments can help you understand your social and professional relationships. Assessments are an opportunity to begin the process of self-observation as you confront a wellness issue.

Knowledge   Having knowledge in the lifestyle areas helps you make decisions. For example, suppose from an assessment you learn you have a high blood cholesterol level. First of all, what number constitutes a high blood cholesterol? What does this mean? How do you go about reducing the fat in your diet? Knowledge can help you to understand your risk and can guide you in accomplishing your goal.

Skills and Management Techniques   Skills and management techniques help you try some of the options. Skills in goal-setting, behavior modification, and personal strategy-building enable you to make the necessary lifestyle changes.

Table 1.1

Positive Choices
in the Dimensions of Wellness

Source: Adapted from Jerry Lafferty, "A Credo for Wellness," Health Education, *Vol. 10, September/October 1979, p. 10–11. This article is reprinted with permission from* Health Education, *September/October, 1979, p. 10–11.* Health Education *is a publication of the American Alliance for Health, Physical Education, Recreation and Dance, 1900 Association Drive, Reston, VA 22041.*

Physical

1. *Eliminate* smoking.
2. Reduce consumption of cigarettes.
3. Eat a balanced diet.
4. Lose weight/gain weight.
5. Lower cholesterol/triglycerides in blood.
6. Increase rest or sleep time.
7. Decrease use of alcoholic beverages.
8. *Eliminate* alcoholic beverages.
9. Improve dental or personal hygiene.
10. *Eliminate* use of all drugs.
11. Improve cardiovascular fitness.
12. Improve muscle strength.

Intellectual

1. Improve reading skills (read a book a week).
2. Increase concentration while studying.
3. Attend special lectures and programs when available.
4. Decrease amount of time watching television.
5. Develop a routine for study or reading.
6. Add a vocabulary word every day.
7. Watch more educational or scientific programs on television.
8. Read the front page of the newspaper every day.

Emotional

1. Learn to recognize your feelings and express them.
2. Find an alternative to hurting others when you are angry.
3. Accept compliments or praise graciously.
4. Recognize and accept personal shortcomings.
5. Deal appropriately with feelings toward the opposite sex.
6. Seek professional help with serious adjustment problems.
7. Relieve tension and stress with appropriate relaxation and/or leisure activities.
8. Identify coping devices and ego defense mechanisms used in adapting to stress.

Spiritual

1. Set some time each day for meditation, thought, and/or prayer.
2. Enter a value-oriented, spiritual, or religious discussion.

Table 1.1—*Continued*

3. Attend a spiritual or religious meeting.
4. Read a spiritual book.
5. Join a group which is intended to expand consciousness.
6. Select a highly valued personal characteristic (such as patience, forgiveness, or compassion) and make a concerted effort to more fully develop that characteristic.
7. Identify your weakest personal characteristic and improve on it.
8. Assess your value system in an effort to become reacquainted with yourself.
9. Be willing to state your value judgments among others.
10. Be more accepting of values expressed by others that are inconsistent with your own.
11. Make an effort to identify your values regarding controversial contemporary issues.

Social

1. Display more affection toward loved ones.
2. Be less critical of friends or loved ones.
3. Express your feelings so that others will know how you feel.
4. Overcome a fear of talking with individuals of another race, opposite sex, or persons in authority.
5. Be more consistent in fulfilling responsibilities to others.
6. Communicate more efficiently with your family and close friends.

Occupational

1. Identify what it is that you really want to do, and what you do best.
2. Take classes to develop new skills for vocational enhancement.
3. Identify your weakest work-related skill, and work to improve it.
4. Take advantage of/or initiate a wellness program at your workplace (health screening, employee trip, softball team, picnic, stress management workshop, etc.).
5. Identify a wellness-"robbing" aspect of your work environment, and pursue a means to change it.
6. Get to know peer workers better. Plan a social get-together.
7. Compliment management/labor in some way, and offer your help to them.
8. Place a wellness-oriented sign, motto, poem at your work station.

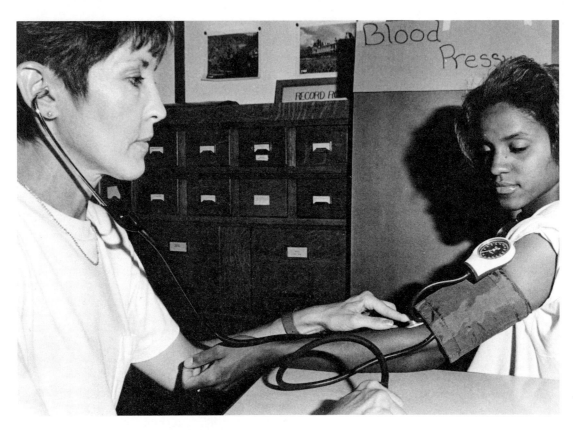

Having your blood pressure checked is an example of a wellness assessment.

How do I manage stress? Eat nutritiously in the dorm? Regulate my exercise intensity? Skills and management techniques help you to make wellness choices become lifetime habits.

Motivation   Motivation is a powerful force in the wellness lifestyle. Motivation gets you started and keeps you going as you strive for continued wellness growth. Motivation is personal and complex. It changes throughout life and is specific to each person. At age 19 you may want to lose weight to look better. The 65-year-old may want to lose weight to help reduce high blood pressure.

A powerful motivating factor underlying most actions is a strong sense of self-esteem. Self-esteem depends as much on the judgment of others as it does upon self-perception. For example, if you feel you are a poor conversationalist, it is probably a result of your own perception of your skill, in addition to your perception of how other people react to you during conversations. Self-esteem is increased if you tackle a difficult goal by starting with small, moderately easy steps, and move gradually to more difficult tasks. Self-esteem is also influenced by how realistic a goal is.

Another factor affecting motivation is how much you value what it is you wish to change. We usually value things we believe make life worth living or satisfying. Aristotle felt that happiness is the highest value, and that happiness is based on "reasoned action." Again, using our example of the poor conversationalist, you are motivated to enhance that skill if being a good conversationalist is important to you. Wellness growth takes place, then, when you take a class or you work to improve your conversation skills. Whether the goal is to lose weight, to manage stress, or to get along better with your parents, your self-esteem and personal values affect your ability to sustain motivation.

Support Maintaining positive lifestyle choices is best achieved when there is support and encouragement by the organizations and environments surrounding you. For example, suppose during one of your vacations you attend a smoking cessation class and quit smoking. You are starting your climb toward permanent behavior change. If you face returning to a roommate who smokes, or to a workplace where co-workers smoke, your chances of maintaining your new behavior are considerably lower. Your family, friends, and group affiliation have a strong influence on your behavior. In fact, it has been found that there are significant correlations among self-esteem, social support, and a healthy lifestyle.[13] Choosing a living or working environment where others strive for wellness can assist you in wellness growth. Do you feel your roommates, friends, and family are supportive of wellness? How about your campus? Why or why not?

Self-Responsibility At the center of wellness growth is self-responsibility. The goal is to assume greater responsibility for your quality of life by making positive lifestyle decisions. Understandably, for every decision to be made, there are alternatives and consequences. Your challenge is to make thoughtful decisions that direct you toward high-level wellness. It is a satisfying feeling to work toward being the best you can be. You are unique and should know your own needs and preferences. You know what you can and cannot control. Some circumstances are beyond your control. Part of self-responsibility is recognizing this and adjusting in order to continually strive toward full potential. Heredity is an example of something you cannot control. You had no voice in selecting your genetic tendencies. A physical disability is another uncontrollable life situation. Self-responsibility in wellness is making the best of the "hand you are dealt" regardless of your stage in life or your circumstances.

Self-responsibility in wellness means active involvement. It means understanding how choices affect the daily quality of your life, rather than looking at longevity as the primary payoff. The joy of wellness is the journey—the attempt to reach your potential in all six dimensions. In a pure sense, the state of high-level wellness can never be reached. Everyone has setbacks or weaknesses. For you it could be a quick temper, chocolate chip cookies, or impatience with your younger brother. We sometimes let our lives become unbalanced. Having realistic expectations, a sense of personal accountability, and a sense of humor will help you see wellness living as a joyful experience. Self-responsibility involves self-control as opposed to going along with the crowd or merely reacting to what seems to happen. Just because everyone else is eating a triple order of french fries does not mean you must, also. When everyone else is grumbling about the weather, why not find something positive about it?

If you are apprehensive about making changes or altering your lifestyle, understand that these changes do not need to be drastic. You are not doomed to a life without pleasure or to an existence full of rigid self-denial! It is not necessary that you jog 5 miles a day or become a vegetarian. On the contrary, the journey should be full of stimulation and satisfaction. It is exciting to realize that a few common-sense changes can make a big difference in the way you look and feel. With that in mind, how do you begin to assume responsibility and make changes? To make any permanent behavior change, it takes a distinct systematic plan of action.

Locus of Control   Your parents no longer influence what you eat and drink, when you sleep or study, or what you do with your free time. You are in charge of your own life. How easily you adopt wellness behaviors has a lot to do with your locus of control. **Locus of control** is your belief regarding major influences that affect your health status. If you have an **internal locus of control**, you feel that you are in control of your destiny and your health behaviors. You are more likely to seek and use information to make decisions, accept personal responsibility for health choices, and alter your behavior accordingly. If you have an **external locus of control**, you are more likely to view behavior as a result of fate, family, friends, chance, or luck. In other words, you'll say it is "out of my hands." You perceive that your well-being is dependent on doctors and other medical personnel. In this case, you are less likely to use wellness information to your benefit or engage in preventive health behaviors. Factors found to be associated with an internal locus of control include: (1) valuing good health, (2) achieving higher levels of education, (3) experiencing or being threatened by illness or disability, (4) having a positive self-image, and (5) feeling satisfied with life.[14] How would you categorize your locus of control?

Self-Management

Even though there is evidence linking lifestyle abuse and lack of well-being (and even premature death), some Americans still look to their physicians to keep them well. If we lump all the causes of death together, physicians can help approximately 10 percent of the time. The other 90 percent of those deaths are outside the control of physicians. They are the result of lifestyle abuse, heredity, and environment.[15] It is quite a paradox that in this technological age of instant transmission of scientific information, millions of people disregard the evidence that links lifestyle behavior and well-being. Many still smoke cigarettes, drink excessive amounts of alcohol and caffeine, burn out due to stress, eat vast amounts of high-fat foods, and refuse to fasten their seat belts. What a dilemma it is that . . . "information does not equal prevention, and even the most comprehensive public information campaigns have achieved rather limited success. Information is necessary but not sufficient for creating meaningful change."[16] Traditional educational messages devised to arouse

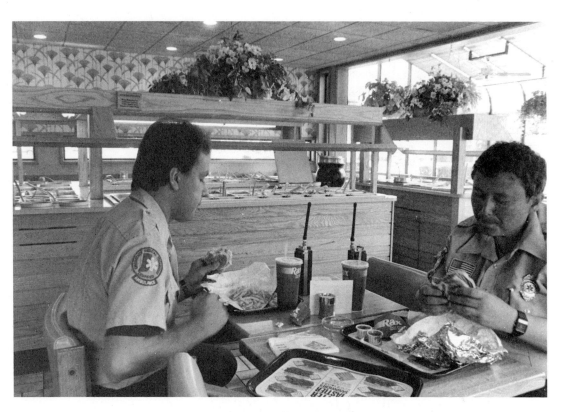

Do you make wise choices when eating out?

fear (antismoking brochures showing blackened lungs, seat-belt campaigns exhibiting crumpled cars, "this is your brain on drugs", etc.) have eliminated high risk behaviors in some people, but not for the majority of the population. Fear of a heart attack has not kept many Americans involved in an ongoing program of exercise and dietary change. Even when the information is positive or inspirational, many still have difficulty making lifestyle behavior changes. What is missing in the link between knowledge and action? . . . a systematic strategy called **self-management.**

More Than Willpower

Changing a behavior or breaking an unhealthy habit involves *learning new behavior.* Notice we used the word "learn." Just as in learning anything else, you must understand and practice the basic principles and techniques of self-management. Many people are already excellent managers of their lives. They can study when they need to, exercise regularly, turn down an offer of chocolate creme pie, and refuse a beer at a party. These are powerful choices, choices that are linked to wellness. What about good old willpower? Isn't that all it takes? Some say they have no willpower. "I want to lose weight, but I have no willpower." "I have some willpower, but could use more." Willpower is an ambiguous entity. For example, how can you stick to your goals in some situations, but not in others?

How can you have willpower when it comes to eating, but not when it comes to drinking alcohol? How can you have it some days, but not others? How do you get more of it? And what about desire? Some believe that merely *wanting* to change is enough. Certainly desire for change is important, but it has no strategy to follow through. This is the key to permanent change—have a plan. Self-management involves choosing goals and designing strategies to meet them. Self-management is actually a combination of specific skills where *knowledge* and *action* are linked for the purpose of controlling behavior.

A Self-Management Strategy

There are five crucial steps that can help you make positive lifestyle changes and achieve your behavior goals (fig. 1.4). The changes you choose to make can pertain to any dimension of wellness, anything from improving study skills to learning social assertiveness to losing weight to reducing stress. The five steps are:

1. Identify your goal.
2. Keep records.
3. Make a plan.
4. Build commitment.
5. Maintain the new behavior.

Figure 1.4
Self-management steps.

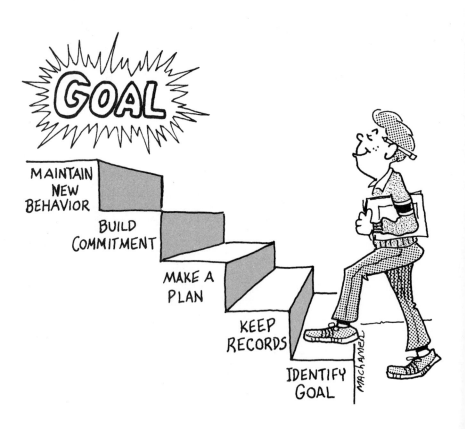

Identify Your Goal

Identifying a component in your lifestyle you wish to change in order to enhance your well-being is the first step. This identification has been preceded by an awareness of a lifestyle problem and an acceptance of its negative effect on you, as well as an integration of this information into your personal self-responsibility. For example: "I am aware that smoking is a harmful habit." "I accept the fact that since I smoke, I will be harmed by this habit." "I guess I could stop smoking." Certainly this process is preceded by acquiring knowledge about smoking. There are other points to remember in goal identification.

Prioritize Your Goals   Do not attempt to change everything at once. You may fail if you try all at once to lose weight, stop smoking, get along better with your mother-in-law, and make the Dean's List every semester. Start with only one goal.

Make Your Goal Realistic   For example, if your goal is to lose 30 pounds in three weeks, study every Friday night, go to church every Sunday, jog 4 miles every day, never lose your temper, or make straight As every semester, your plan is probably doomed!

Specify the Situation   Goal identification is easier if you can specify the situation in which the behavior occurs. For example, instead of saying, "I eat too much," you might say, "I can't resist desserts." Or, instead of saying, "I'm self-centered," you might say, "I talk about myself too much." When you are identifying a goal, it is important to be truthful with yourself. It is not a time for denial . . . "But I'm not a big eater!" (spoken as you devour an entire sausage pizza!)

Make Your Goal Specific, Measurable, and Have a Time Period   Not "lose some weight," but "lose 10 pounds in 12 weeks." Not "eat more nutritiously," but "eat 4 fruits/vegetables daily for 1 month." Not "smoke less," but "cut down to 3 cigarettes per day for 3 weeks." Not "get along with my roommate better," but "sincerely compliment my roommate in some way every day for 2 weeks." Not "study more," but "I will study every Monday, Tuesday, and Wednesday, from 7:00 to 10:00 P.M. for the remainder of the semester." Self-management strategies are more effective when goals are stated in behavioral terms and quantified. Also, try to express your goal in positive terms. If a goal is to start doing something that you are not presently doing (for example, fastening your seat belt), state the goal in terms of what you want to do and in what situation you will do it.

List Motivations   Be able to truthfully answer the question, "What's in it for me?" List the reasons why you want to change. Make a list of the pros and cons. Ask yourself how your life will be affected by your changed behavior. This helps you to assess the costs of changing, to face yourself, and to anticipate obstacles. Table 1.2 shows an example of a motivation list. To increase your motivation, you might talk to acquaintances who have successfully made the change you are attempting.

Table 1.2

Why I Should Increase My Study Time

Pros	Cons
■ Make better grades	■ Is a lot of work
■ Enjoy classes more	■ Professors and parents
■ Might learn something of	might keep expecting more
value	■ Less social/leisure time
■ Less stress/hassles	■ Friends might perceive me
■ Parents would be happier	as an "egghead," boring
■ Better career opportunities	■ Might become a workaholic,
■ Might be eligible for a	a perfectionist
scholarship	
■ Feel good about myself	
■ Better use of tuition money	

Keep Records

Before you can make a plan for behavior change, you must assess your current behavior. You do this by keeping a log of your behavior. This allows you to see when you are doing the unwanted behavior. This step is extremely important because most of us assume that we know our habits. However, careful self-monitoring almost always reveals some surprises. Knowing the truth about our behavior is essential before changes can be initiated. For this reason, accuracy is important. In the case of developing a new habit, a log helps you see when you could be doing the new behavior. Table 1.3 shows examples of behavior record-keeping. There is no set form for keeping records. Simplicity and honesty are essential.

By keeping records, you are able to identify the antecedent (trigger) of a behavior, as well as the consequences of the behavior. An **antecedent** is an event or situation that leads directly to the behavior. It triggers the behavior. The **consequence** of the behavior is the resultant feeling or situation that follows the behavior. Table 1.4 gives examples of antecedents (triggers), behaviors, and consequences. Once you identify the situations that cause a behavior, you are ready to plan your strategy.

Make a Plan

The heart of self-management lies in a plan of action. Having this plan is what differentiates between self-control and a fleeting New Year's resolution. Your strategy for behavior change revolves around the antecedent that causes the behavior. You can eliminate the antecedent, anticipate and prepare for the antecedent, substitute a different behavior for that particular antecedent, or break/scramble the behavior chain.

Eliminate the Antecedent   It is not possible in all situations, but sometimes you can eliminate the trigger altogether. For example, instead of walking past the bakery on your way home, take a different route.

Table 1.3
Behavior Record-Keeping

To assess drinking behavior:

Time	Count	Activity	Mood	Consequences
11:00 a.m.	2 drinks	waiting for friends to pick me up for football game	excited about being with friends and going to the game.	positive: felt "fired up" negative: upset stomach (no breakfast)
2:00 p.m.	4 drinks	post-game party	party mood	positive: felt socially accepted negative: getting drunk
6:00 p.m.	3 drinks	dinner with new date	anxious to get started on a good note	positive: felt less inhibited negative: felt sleepy

To assess study habits (time management):　　　　　　　　　When I Could Have Studied:

7:00 a.m.	woke and dressed	
7:30 a.m.	watched TV as I ate breakfast	
8:00 a.m.	talked to roommate	✓
8:30 a.m.	called boyfriend	✓
9:00 a.m.	class	
10:00 a.m.	cup of coffee with friend at student center	✓
11:00 a.m.	class	
12:00 noon	stopped by fraternity to chat with "big brother"	✓
1:00 p.m.	back home, snacked and watched MTV	✓
1:30 p.m.	went to library to start term paper	
3:00 p.m.	class	
4:00 p.m.	to gym to jog	
5:30 p.m.	home, relaxed, watched TV, talked to roommate	✓
6:30 p.m.	went to volleyball match	✓
8:30 p.m.	out for a pizza and beer	
10:00 p.m.	home, tired, to bed	

Table 1.4
Example of Antecedents, Behaviors, and Consequences

Antecedent	Behavior	Consequences
see pastries as walk past bakery	buy and eat donuts	feel guilty, full, gain weight
see philosophy professor	become argumentative and critical	continue unhappy relationship
go to aerobics class	exercise vigorously	feel good, energized
finish dinner	smoke a cigarette	calms nerves yet still short of breath
fraternity party	drink too much beer	get drunk, get sick
required speech for class	heart pounds, sweating	poor grade on speech
turn on TV	snack while watching	consume too many extra calories

There are many ways to avoid antecedents.

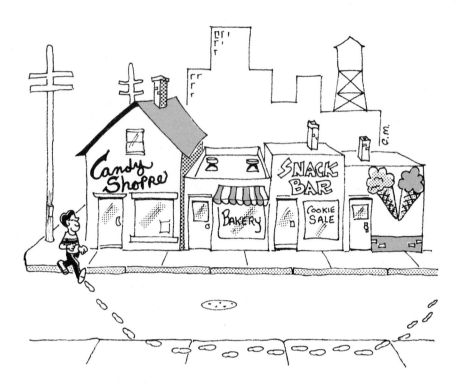

Anticipate and Prepare for the Antecedent   Suppose you are trying to lose weight and eat more nutritiously. You and your friends meet for lunch every day at a place where fast food and vending machines are the only source of food. Why not pack your own lunch of nutritious, desirable choices? This takes effort and planning, but the end result is a desirable response. You are setting yourself up for failure if you arrive at the lunch site starving and empty-handed, but with money in your pocket. In the case of shyness or stage fright, mentally rehearse the scene beforehand to over-prepare for the occasion. Planning ahead for a situation may even involve using mental imagery. Mentally rehearse the scene beforehand, just as an actor or speaker over-prepares before walking onto a stage. For example, avoiding alcohol at a party is easier if you have already planned to hold and sip a glass of soda, situating yourself as far as possible from the bar.

Substitute Behaviors   This strategy is used by many people trying to stop smoking. Rather than smoking as soon as dinner is finished, go for a walk, chew gum, play the piano, etc. Boredom or stress triggers snacking for many. If you can substitute enjoyable activities (play solitaire, listen to music, ride a bike, etc.), or necessary tasks (vacuum a room, write a thank-you note, balance the checkbook, etc.), the connection between the trigger and behavior could be broken over time. Substitute a new behavior for the old unwanted behavior, and do it immediately after the trigger.

Break or Scramble the Behavior Chain Many habits are a result of a **behavior chain**. A behavior chain is a series of habitual behaviors. A typical chain is much like this: Go home from class—go to the refrigerator—open a beer—watch TV—snack on chips—take a shower—go to bed. To alter this chain, you might try taking a shower as soon as you get home. This may give you time to reconsider your dinner menu. Before you can succeed at chainbreaking, you must be able to identify this habitual chain. Chapter 10 gives additional behavior modification tips helpful in changing behavior related to weight management.

Other Helpful Strategies Build in rewards for your successes (but not a hot fudge sundae for losing 3 pounds!). Buy something new; go to a movie. Make some rewards immediate. Plan small steps and chart your progress. Ask for support from those close to you; tell them your plan. Observe someone who is successful at what you are trying to accomplish. Modeling is one of the basic processes by which we learn—from racquetball to social manners. List barriers or obstacles that are a threat to your plan (Mom and Dad smoke, it is too cold to run, roommate is addicted to TV, etc.). Plan your coping strategies to counteract these difficulties.

Build Commitment

Did you know that nearly three-fourths of the people who own home exercise equipment don't use it? In addition, nearly half of those who join health clubs don't use their memberships as often as they planned.[17] It seems good intentions, not actions, are keeping sales of some fitness products quite healthy!

Commitment is not automatic. It is a set of behaviors in itself. "Commitment is not something you have, it is something you do."[18] The wellness lifestyle should focus on the positive consequences of choices. There will be temptations to quit; you may tire of the effort involved in changing. This is why it is important to review your goals and to continually view the change as positive rather than self-deprivating. It is helpful to review unexpected benefits that arise as a result of new behaviors, such as making new friends, or discovering a new pleasurable activity. The former smoker struggling to avoid cigarettes is tempted by the thought of the taste of a cigarette. For an instant, she feels deprived. This person should immediately switch her thoughts to the positive consequences of not smoking—fresher breath, more money to spend on other things, cleaner teeth, less coughing, cleaner lungs, etc. Part of your planning should involve identifying obstacles and saboteurs, as well as contingencies and reinforcers.

Suggestions for Building Commitment There are many ways to build commitment. You may want to try several of them. Post reminders and motivational pictures/slogans in prominent places. Keep a log and mark milestones. Make a monetary investment (health club membership, stationary bike, etc.). Join a class. Involve another family member or a friend. Make a pact with someone. A supportive environment of associates can help you maintain a commitment to wellness behaviors.

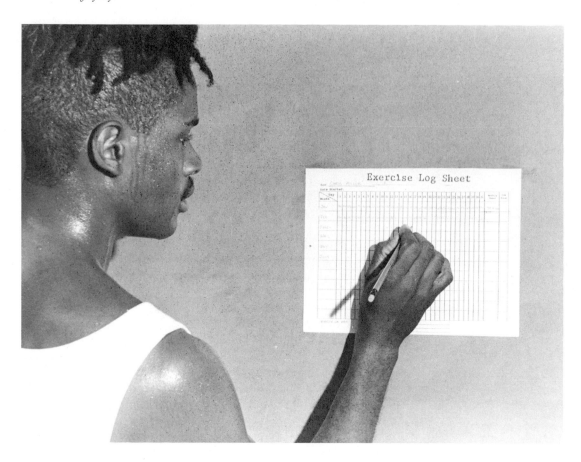

Keeping an exercise log helps you stick with your program.

Maintain the New Behavior

The goal is to enhance your well-being, to pursue high-level wellness. Often we get so hung up on making a change in our lifestyle that it interrupts our whole life rather than enhances it. The emphasis should be on the positive. Value your successes and your worth as a human being. Most of us do not realize that the majority of our supportive messages come from our own internal thought processes rather than from external sources. We carry on conversations with ourselves each day.[19] Called "self-talk," our inner voice can be a positive source of motivation. Self-talk that encourages us and reminds us of our achievements helps increase our self-esteem. Self-talk can also be negative, and, as a result, a source of discouragement. Suppose your goal is to become less verbally critical of your mother. For ten days you successfully avoid any confrontation. On the eleventh day, while riding with her in a car, you find yourself sharply criticizing her driving. An example of negative self-talk would be: "I am so awful. I have failed miserably in my goal. This just proves again what a rotten daughter I am." In contrast, a positive self-talk statement would be: "I didn't handle this situation very well. What can I learn from this so I'll do better next time?" Setbacks are common when you are trying to change a behavior. Instead of throwing in the towel, try to learn from these experiences. Maintaining your plan will require flexibility, particularly if it is not working properly, if unexpected obstacles arise, or if a support system is failing. Reevaluation is a necessary component in making a permanent lifestyle change.

One specific way to assume self-responsibility and commitment to a lifestyle change is to write a personal wellness contract incorporating the steps we have suggested for making change. A written contract makes you think out your plan in its entirety, rather than letting things happen as they may. It specifies the *details* for carrying out your plan. Table 1.5 shows a sample wellness contract. Every wellness contract is different and depends on the complexity of your goal. The most important outcomes in writing a contract are the self-evaluating and planning involved. A blank wellness contract is provided in the activities section at the end of the book for your use.

Remember that high-level wellness is a process involving growth and pursuit toward a fuller life. The process of self-managing behavior means reassessing goals, monitoring behavior, reviewing strategies, learning from setbacks, and acknowledging the joy in the effort of being the best you can be. As you become the *cause*, rather than the *effect*, of actions, your confidence and self-esteem are enhanced. Thus, your chances of personal success and ability to influence others increases. In this way, you continue to discover ways to expand your unending wellness growth.

As you travel this wellness path, you will probably become more aware of how society can help and hinder your trip.

Societal Norms

One challenge we all face in attempting to pursue a wellness lifestyle is societal norms. We are constantly bombarded by subtle, yet extremely powerful messages that are often obstacles to wellness. Our behavioral choices are strongly affected by unwritten codes that permeate our daily life, actually contradict, and can sabotage a wellness lifestyle. **Societal norms** are those behaviors or practices that are considered appropriate or acceptable. These unwritten rules are carried on from generation to generation. Table 1.6 contains circumstances and norms you have probably grown up with. As you look at them, consider the message they give. Do they promote wellness as you know it? You can probably think of more examples than those listed. Do you ever wonder why it is considered inappropriate for a woman to reapply her lipstick after dinner while sitting at a restaurant table? Discourteous, you say? Yet it is acceptable for her to pull a cigarette from her purse, light it, inhale, and then blow carcinogens into your air? And you politely hand her an ashtray!

Many of our norms encourage a sedentary lifestyle. Somehow we've absorbed the notion that minimal exertion is better. Heaven forbid if, when operating your car, you have to roll down your own windows, walk around the car to unlock the doors, or keep constant pressure on the accelerator while driving on the interstate! Do you realize that you can go to the bank, a fast food restaurant, a

Table 1.5

Wellness contract.

WELLNESS CONTRACT

1. Goal: To become a better listener (spend less than 50% of the time talking during all conversations)

2. Motivation (What's in it for me): I hope to enhance my personal relationships and build stronger friendship bonds.

3. Observations of present behavior related to the goal:
   (Over the past week, I noticed that ...)
   1. I interrupt too much.
   2. I have a tendency to think about what I'm going to say next rather than what others are saying.
   3. I do not maintain eye contact.
   4. I talk more than 50% of the time, even in 3- and 4-way conversations.

4. 3-4 obstacles/saboteurs:
   1. I am usually in a hurry and lack patience with others, especially slow talkers.
   2. I let my mind wander and think of my own plans and self a lot of the time.
   3. I am highly opinionated and have a tendency to ~~judge~~, criticize, and
5. Plan/strategies: advise when talking with others.
   (Give at least 3-5 steps, including how to overcome the obstacles noted above)
   1. Allot myself time during the day for friendly conversations.
   2. Work toward talking less than 50% of the time.
   3. Maintain eye contact — constantly
   4. Ask at least one question of the conversationalist/or ask for a clarification of a point/or summarize what they are saying.
   5. Sincerely compliment the conversationalist in some way.

6. Building commitment:
   (List at least 1 tangible reward and 1 source of support to encourage goal maintenance)
   1. Tell my roommate of my plan.
   2. Keep a log/diary of my talking time percentage, and successes/failures.
   3. Enroll in the community education class — "How to be a Good Conversationalist".
   4. Reward myself every Saturday for a successful week = see a movie, eat out, buy fresh flowers.
7. Evaluation – I know I have reached my goal when:
   1. I feel more special friendship bonds developing.
   2. People seek my company and regularly want to talk to me.

This action will be completed by __February 15__ .
                                              (Date)

__Amy L. Ley__   _____
My signature   Witness (optional)

Table 1.6

Societal Norms That Promote "Unwellness"

- The idea that everyone must be extremely thin
- The assumption that alcohol abuse is an acceptable rite of passage into college
- The media's portrayal of sex as being glamorous, without commitment or consequences
- Social events, parties, celebrations where alcohol and food abuse is expected (New Year's Eve, wedding receptions, Super Bowl parties, etc.)
- Halloween, Easter, Christmas, and Valentine's Day, and the multitude of high-sugar "gifts" associated with them
- Tanned skin being equated with beauty, wealth, power, and sex appeal (thus, the emergence of thousands of tanning salons)
- Ashtrays and salt shakers on all restaurant tables
- Miles and miles of roads built, *without* sidewalks
- The elimination of daily physical education in the schools, yet the parental push for private sports lessons and competitive Little League football, baseball, soccer, etc. (many times run by unqualified coaches)
- Access to television 24 hours a day, with a choice of 100 cable stations—all changed by remote control!
- Meals built around a red meat entree
- The notion that as you grow older it is okay to be inactive and fat

the interstate! Do you realize that you can go to the bank, a fast food restaurant, a dry cleaners, and a milk store without ever leaving the comfort of your car? What kind of message is this sending?

The advertising industry is especially effective at mesmerizing us with messages. After all, we are told, "It's doctor recommended." We see former athletes guzzling beer that is "less filling." Every Saturday morning high-sugar snacks that are fun to eat and that "your mother trusts" are displayed on television. If the thin, attractive models on billboards enjoy smoking, perhaps you will, too!

In traveling the road to optimum well-being, be aware of these pitfalls and obstacles our culture displays. Remember, it is you who will make the daily choices as to how to live your life. Self-responsibility is the key.

Changing Times: Making Wellness the Norm

Now that the wellness concept has begun to invade the health-care profession and into society as a whole, we can see some norms already changing. Fifteen years ago the only people you saw jogging were athletes in training or fitness "nuts." Now no one takes a second look even at little old ladies trudging along roads. Businessmen pack their workout gear next to their business reports.

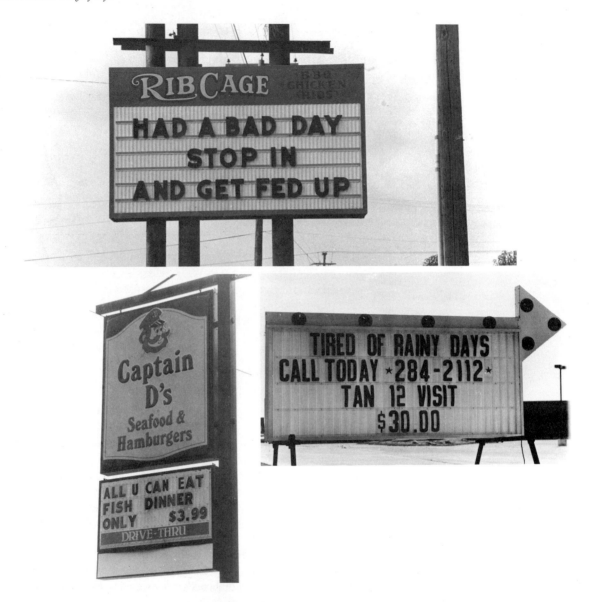

RIB CAGE · BBQ CHICKEN RIBS

HAD A BAD DAY
STOP IN
AND GET FED UP

Captain D's
Seafood &
Hamburgers

ALL U CAN EAT
FISH DINNER
ONLY $3.99
DRIVE-THRU

TIRED OF RAINY DAYS
CALL TODAY ★284-2112★
TAN 12 VISIT
$30.00

Are these messages in your best interest?

Hotels hand out jogging maps to guests. Stress management, parenting, addictive behavior, smoking cessation, and a multitude of other wellness topics are offered in community classes and workshops. As wellness permeates our society, there are more and more resources that support this lifestyle. There are positive choices available in grocery stores—more whole wheat breads and cereals, low-sugar and low-salt products, low-fat dairy items, even take-out salad and fruit bars. Restaurants are also responding to the consumer demand for more nutritious food selections. These are just a few of the positive changes that reflect wellness awareness. Only by drawing together all available resources (individual, community, media, schools, corporations, government) will current health problems be fixed. This multi-level approach is necessary to bring about changes in societal norms.

Beyond the physical, health-related factors of wellness, it is important to change peoples' attitudes. It should not be considered bizarre for people to arrive at work or at a class full of enthusiasm, rather than full of complaints. It is also not weird to take a few moments to stretch or close your eyes to relax during the day, congratulate another person for doing well on an exam, adhere to the speed limit, have a soft drink rather than a beer at a party, give someone a hug, or have fun in life. These are behaviors that reflect wellness and are brought about by awareness, education, and growth in wellness.

As we know, not everyone has responded to this trend of positive lifestyle choices. It will take time. You can do your part by encouraging those around you to make wellness a lifetime pursuit. Pass these attitudes and behaviors on to your children. Help continue to make wellness and self-responsibility society's norm.

Summary

Many adults in the United States die prematurely from diseases that are primarily a result of lifestyle abuse. Health promoters stress the importance of healthy behaviors in deterring the ravaging effects of these "diseases of choice." With the cost of health care increasing so rapidly, *Healthy People 2000* was published by the federal government in an effort to spark a national commitment to self-responsibility for well-being and acknowledge the need for support systems to help those pursuing a wellness lifestyle. Whereas health is often viewed as a neutral state of nonsickness, high-level wellness is a dynamic level of functioning that is oriented toward maximizing potential. It is an integrated living pattern involving six dimensions—physical, intellectual, emotional, social, spiritual, and occupational. It is a lifelong journey that involves a conscientious effort to reach full potential. The cornerstone of wellness living is self-responsibility. Wellness growth involves a multifaceted approach of awareness, assessment, knowledge, and self-management skills. It includes intelligent deciphering of societal norms, recognizing your own power, making choices, interpreting risks, seeking support, and understanding personal limitations.

Self-management is the use of a conscious, systematic plan for making a permanent change in behavior. To successfully change a behavior takes more than mere willpower. Self-management involves five steps: (1) identify your goal; (2) keep records; (3) make a plan; (4) build commitment; and (5) maintain the new behavior.

The objective of wellness is to pursue a richer, satisfying life. Wellness is an attitude, and not an end in itself. Our time on this earth is too short to be drawn toward complacency and futility. We should all consider and absorb the wisdom of W. Mitchell, Mayor of Crested Butte, Colorado, who, though paralyzed from an airplane crash, maintains an active schedule. He writes, "The way I look at it, before I was paralyzed, there were ten thousand things I could do; ten thousand things I was capable of doing. Now there are nine thousand. I can dwell on the one thousand, or concentrate on the nine thousand I have left. And, of course, the joke is that none of us in our lifetime is going to do more than two or three thousand of these things in any event."[20]

References

1. Sullivan, Louis W., M.D. "Creating a National Culture of Character: Personal Responsibility and Public Health." *Vital Speeches* 57 (January 15, 1991): 202–205.

2. O'Donnell, Michael P. "Definition of Health Promotion: Part III: Expanding the Definition." *American Journal of Health Promotion* 3 (Winter 1989): 5.

3. Vickery, Donald M., M.D. "Medical Self-Care: A Review of the Concept and Program Models." *American Journal of Health Promotion* 1 (Summer 1986): 23–28.

4. Belloc, Nedra, and Lester Breslow. "Relationship of Physical Health Status and Health Practices." *Preventive Medicine* 1 (August 1972): 409–21.

5. U.S. Department of Health and Human Services, Public Health Service. *Healthy People.* Washington, DC: Government Printing Office, 1979.

6. Hettler, Bill, M.D. "Presenting the Wellness Concept to the Uninitiated." *Wellness Promotion Strategies.* Selected Proceedings of the Eighth Annual National Wellness Conference, edited by Joseph P. Opatz: 28–38. Dubuque, IA: Kendall/Hunt Publishing Co., 1984.

7. Department of Health and Human Services, Public Health Service. *Healthy People 2000: National Health Promotion and Disease Prevention Objectives.* Washington, DC: Department of Health and Human Services, 1990.

8. *Healthy People 2000.*

9. Sullivan, Louis W., M.D. "Sounding Board: Healthy People 2000." *The New England Journal of Medicine* 323 (October 11, 1990): 1065–67.

10. Dunn, Halbert L. "High-Level Wellness for Man and Society." *American Journal of Public Health* 49 (June 1959): 786–92.

11. Ardell, Donald B. *The History and Future of Wellness.* Dubuque, IA: Kendall/Hunt Publishing Co., 1985.

12. Pilch, John J. "Wellness Spirituality." *Health Values* 12 (May/June 1988): 28–31.

13. Muhlenkamp, A. F., and J. A. Sayles. "Self-Esteem, Social Support, and Positive Health Practices." *Nursing Research* 35 (1986): 334–38.

14. Kist-Kline, Gail, and Susan Cross Lipnickey. "Health Locus of Control: Implications for the Health Professional." *Health Values* 13 (September/October 1989): 38–47.

15. Hettler. "Presenting the Wellness Concept."

16. Atkin, Charles, and Lawrence Wallack (eds.). *Mass Communication and Public Health.* Newbury Park, CA: Sage Publications, 1990.

17. "Good Intentions Hold Up Fitness Sales." *The Wall Street Journal* (October 31, 1989): B-1.

18. Hafen, Brent Q., Alton L. Thygerson, and Kathryn J. Frandsen. *Behavioral Guidelines for Health and Wellness.* Englewood, CO: Morton Publishing Co., 1988.

19. Brammer, Lawrence M. *How To Cope With Life Transitions: The Challenge of Personal Change.* New York, NY: Hemisphere Publishing Corporation, 1991.

20. Corbet, Barry. *Options: Spinal Cord Injury and the Future.* Denver: A. B. Hirschfeld Press, 1980.

Suggested Readings

Ardell, Donald B. 1985. *The History and Future of Wellness.* Dubuque, IA: Kendall/Hunt Publishing Co.

Atkin, Charles, and Lawrence Wallack (eds.). 1990. *Mass Communication and Public Health.* Newbury Park, CA: Sage Publications.

Beasley, Joseph D., M.D. 1991. *The Betrayal of Health: The Impact of Nutrition, Environment, and Life-style on Illness in America.* New York, NY: Times Books.

Bellingham, Richard, Barry Cohen, Todd James, and Leroy Spaniol. "Connectedness: Some Skills for Spiritual Health." *American Journal of Health Promotion* 1 (September/October 1989): 18–24, 31.

Brammer, Lawrence M. 1991. *How To Cope With Life Transitions: The Challenge of Personal Change.* New York, NY: Hemisphere Publishing Corporation.

Brandon, Jeffrey E., Jeffrey Oescher, and J. Mark Loftin. "The Self-Control Questionnaire: An Assessment." *Health Values* 14 (May/June 1990): 3–9.

Bricklin, Mark, Mark Golin, Deborah Grandinetti, and Alexis Lieberman. 1990. *Positive Living and Health.* Emmaus, PA: Rodale Press.

Brownell, Kelly D., G. Alan Marlatt, Edward Lichtenstein, and G. Terence Wilson. "Understanding and Preventing Relapse." *American Psychologist* 41 (July 1986): 765–82.

Dawber, Thomas Royle. 1980. *The Framingham Study: The Epidemiology of Atherosclerotic Disease.* Cambridge, MA: Harvard University Press.

Department of Health and Human Services, Public Health Service. *Healthy People 2000: National Health Promotion and Disease Prevention Objectives.* Washington, DC: Department of Health and Human Services, 1990.

Dickman, Sherman R. 1988. *Pathways to Wellness.* Champaign, IL: Human Kinetics Publishers, Inc.

Friedman, Myles I., and George H. Lackey, Jr. 1991. *The Psychology of Human Control: A General Theory of Purposeful Behavior.* New York, NY: Praeger Publishers.

Glanz, Karen, Francis Marcus Lewis, and Barbara K. Riner (eds.). 1990. *Health Behavior and Health Education.* San Francisco: Jossey-Bass Publishers.

Green, Judith, and Robert Shellenberger. 1991. *The Dynamics of Health and Wellness: A Biopsychosocial Approach.* Fort Worth, TX: Holt, Rinehart and Winston, Inc.

Hafen, Brent Q., Alton L. Thygerson, and Kathryn J. Frandsen. 1988. *Behavioral Guidelines for Health and Wellness.* Englewood, CO: Morton Publishing Co.

Johnson, Jerry A. 1986. *New Dimensions in Wellness: A Context for Living.* Thorofare, NJ: SLACK Incorporated.

Klaidman, Stephen. "How Well the Media Report Health Risk." *Daedalus* 119 (Fall 1990): 119–32.

Lau, Richard R., Marilyn Jacobs Quadrel, and Karen A. Hartman. "Development and Change of Young Adults' Preventive Health Beliefs and Behavior: Influence from Parents and Peers." *Journal of Health and Social Behavior* 31 (September 1990): 240–59.

Ryan, Regina Sara, and John W. Travis. 1991. *Wellness: Small Changes You Use to Make a Big Difference.* Berkeley, CA: Ten Speed Press.

Shumaker, Sally A., Eleanor B. Schron, and Judith K. Ockene (eds.). 1990. *The Handbook of Health Behavior Change.* New York: Springer.

Sweeting, Roger L. 1990. *A Values Approach to Health Behavior.* Champaign, IL: Human Kinetics Publishers, Inc.

Taylor, Robert L. 1990. *Health Fact, Health Fiction.* Dallas: Taylor Publishing Co.

Tkac, Debora (ed.). 1990. *Lifespan-Plus: 900 Natural Techniques to Live Longer.* Emmaus, PA: Rodale Press.

Travis, John W., and Regina Sara Ryan. 1988. *The Wellness Workbook.* 2nd ed. Berkeley, CA: Ten Speed Press.

University of California, Berkeley. 1990. *The Wellness Encyclopedia: The Comprehensive Resource to Safeguarding Health and Preventing Illness.* Boston: Houghton-Mifflin Co.

Wallston, Kenneth A., Barbara Strudler Wallston, and Robert DeVellis. "Development of the Multidimensional Health Locus of Control (MHLC) Scales." *Health Education Monographs* 6 (Spring 1978): 160–70.

Watson, David L., and Roland G. Tharp. 1989. *Self-Directed Behavior.* 5th ed. Pacific Grove, CA: Brooks/Cole Publishing Co.

Williams, Robert L., and James D. Long. 1991. *Manage Your Life.* Boston: Houghton-Mifflin.

2
Physical Fitness

Chapter Objectives

After reading this chapter, you will be able to:

1. Define physical fitness.
2. Identify and define the five health-related fitness components.
3. Identify five benefits of fitness.
4. Define and apply the FITT prescription factors for developing physical fitness.
5. Calculate training heart rate using the Karvonen formula.
6. Explain how to use the Rate of Perceived Exertion scale.
7. Identify the amount of time necessary for the results of a fitness program to become apparent.
8. Describe the purpose, content, and time of the three parts of a workout.
9. Define and correctly apply the principle of overload.
10. Identify the principle of specificity.
11. Discriminate between aerobic and anaerobic exercise.
12. Define cross training.

Terms

- Aerobic
- Anaerobic
- Atrophy
- Ballistic stretch
- Body composition
- Cardiorespiratory endurance
- Conditioning bout
- Cool-down
- Cross training
- FITT prescription factors

- Flexibility
- Hypertrophy
- Hypokinetic disease
- Karvonen Equation
- Maximal heart rate
- Maximal oxygen uptake (max VO$_2$)
- Muscular endurance
- Muscular strength
- Physical fitness

- Principle of overload
- Principle of specificity
- Rate of Perceived Exertion (RPE)
- Static stretch
- Target heart rate range
- Task specific activity
- Three-segment workout
- Training effect
- Warm-up

*T*o live a wellness lifestyle, you must be physically active. Even moderate levels of activity produce improvements in health and well-being. Physical fitness, though, requires a higher level of activity and produces life-enhancing benefits at an accelerated rate. As you will discover in this chapter, physical fitness is possibly the most important spoke in the wellness wheel. It is the foundation upon which the other wellness spokes are developed. Remember, also, that the mind and body are a whole; they cannot be separated to act independently. What affects one, ultimately affects the other. Unless the body is in good physical condition, the mind, in addition to other aspects of wellness, will be adversely affected. This is not to say that physical fitness is the simple answer to living well in a complex world, but it is certainly a major step in the right direction.

So, you want to become more physically fit. How do you begin? This chapter will provide all the information you need to begin a fitness program—one you can live with!

Importance of Exercise

Human beings were designed for physical activity. The sedentary lifestyle produced by most occupations does not provide adequate physical labor. The homemaker, secretary, teacher, salesman, and attorney have hectic, stressful lives but lack the vigorous activity needed to be physically fit. Regular physical activity is a positive health habit and is vital to the overall wellness of the individual. We must learn to make intelligent decisions about lifetime health and physical fitness that include planning for daily vigorous exercise.

The decrease in the amount of physical labor required for survival has not reduced the body's need for physical activity. On the contrary, it has increased the need to obtain it from other sources. Yet, Americans desperately lack adequate physical fitness and suffer from lifestyle diseases called **hypokinetic diseases.** These are conditions caused by underactivity such as coronary heart disease, cancer, osteoporosis, diabetes, and obesity. The college student shows early symptoms of hypokinetic disease through low levels of energy, creeping obesity, and signs of heart disease. Can you relate to any of these warning signs? It is known that you reach the peak of your natural fitness during the late teens to early twenties, and unless you maintain physical activity, the body deteriorates and ages even more quickly.

Some surveys claim that 60 percent to 70 percent of American adults participate in some form of regular exercise. These studies, in reality, show that these adults did not understand what was meant by the term "regular exercise." The findings of the U.S. Public Health Service (USPHS) are much less optimistic and underscore the lack of exercise of most Americans. The USPHS concluded that fewer than 20 percent of adults get enough regular exercise to have a positive impact on cardiovascular health. Forty percent exercise intermittently, and 40 percent are entirely sedentary.[1] Even more appalling, ongoing research shows there is a youth fitness crisis. Our nation's children have increased risk of heart disease—too much body fat, elevated blood pressure, high cholesterol, and poor fitness—caused by lack of exercise. Several studies have shown that a full third of our nation's youth are not physically active enough for aerobic benefit.[2, 3] They

We have become a nation of spectators.

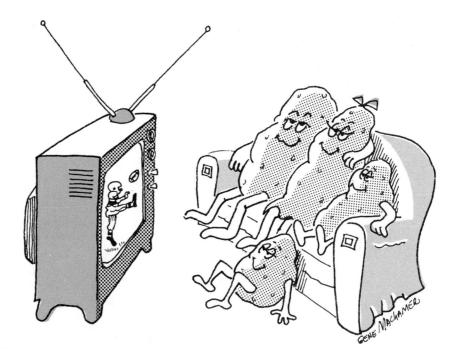

also weigh more and have more body fat than twenty years ago.[4,5] The implication is that our children are going soft. If things don't change, our children will likely contribute to America's future heart disease and cancer statistics. American parents are surprised, and often apathetic, about the state of our children's health. We have become a nation accustomed to olympic dominance, professional sports superiority, and college athletic prominence. Other studies indicate that current school programs do little to promote lifetime fitness. To make matters worse, many physical education programs face elimination because they are considered a "frill" when educational budgets are crunched. How sad! Youngsters are losing the use of their arms and legs, for little opportunity exists today for running, throwing, and climbing. Play, nowadays, consists of low exercise activities such as video games or sports lessons, where standing, sitting, or listening consumes the major portion of the time. This type of play does not promote fitness since it does not involve regular participation in vigorous heart-stimulating activities. Americans, children, *and* adults must "get off their duffs" and start moving. The old saying—"Use it or lose it"—has never been more true.

What Is Physical Fitness?

While there is no universally accepted definition, most experts in the field of exercise would agree that **physical fitness** is the ability of the body to function at optimal efficiency. The fit individual is able to complete the normal routine for the day and still have ample reserve energy to meet the other demands of daily life—recreational sports, rewarding relationships, and other leisure activities. Plus, the fit have adequate energy to handle life's emergency or crisis situations

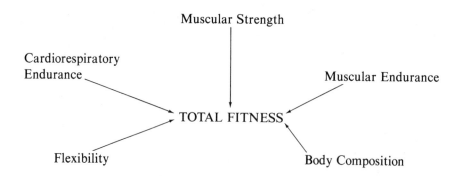

whenever they arise. Physical fitness is multifaceted and involves skill-related and health-related components. The skill-related components of fitness include speed, power, agility, balance, reaction time, and coordination. These are primarily important to achieving success in athletics and are not as crucial to the development of better health. The five health-related components of fitness include: cardiorespiratory endurance, muscular strength, muscular endurance, flexibility, and body composition.

Cardiorespiratory Endurance

Probably the most important fitness component is **cardiorespiratory endurance.** It is the ability to deliver essential nutrients, especially oxygen, to the working muscles of the body and to remove waste products during prolonged physical exertion. It involves the efficient functioning of the heart, blood vessels, and lungs. Cardiorespiratory endurance is often expressed in terms of your **maximal oxygen uptake** (max VO_2), which is the greatest amount of oxygen that can be utilized by the body during intense exercise. Vigorous exercise improves the functioning of the cardiorespiratory system and is directly related to reduced coronary risk. The American Medical Association states that exercise is the most significant factor contributing to the health of the individual.[6] This does not imply that if you exercise you will not have a heart attack. Other genetic and lifestyle factors may be involved. The heart attack death of Jim Fixx, marathon runner and author of *The Complete Book of Running,* in 1984 at age 52, is a case in point. Before he wrote *The Complete Book of Running* he weighed over 200 pounds, smoked three packs of cigarettes a day, and had a brother who died at an early age from a heart attack. Even though he changed his lifestyle, the accumulation of risk factors took its toll. If you smoke cigarettes, have high blood pressure, or other coronary risk factors, you may still be at risk of coronary accident even though you exercise.

Muscular Strength and Muscular Endurance

Muscular strength is the ability of a muscle to exert one maximal force against resistance. It is characterized by activities of short duration at high intensity. Lifting a heavy object such as a suitcase or 100-pound weight one time are examples. **Muscular endurance** is the ability of the muscle to exert repeated force

It's more fun to be a participant than a spectator.

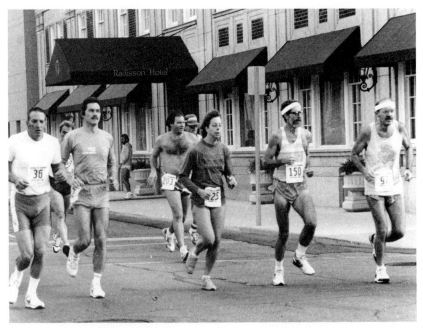

against resistance or to sustain muscular contraction. It is characterized by activities of long duration but low intensity. Examples of muscular endurance are performing repetitions of push-ups, sit-ups, or chin-ups. Strength and endurance are essential in everyday activities such as housework, yard work, and recreational sports. Increase in muscle size is called **hypertrophy** and is due to an enlargement of the existing muscle fibers. The actual number of fibers does not increase. The number of fibers is an inherited characteristic. Muscles hypertrophy when exercised and look firm and toned. Lower levels of the male hormone (testosterone) in females prevent their muscles from becoming bulky. **Atrophy** is the opposite condition, when muscle size and strength have diminished through lack of use (i.e., an arm or leg immobilized in a cast, not working out for a couple of years). Muscular strength and endurance tend to decline with age. This loss can be delayed and strength maintained by participating in a strength program. Many people have joined health clubs and are enjoying the benefits of using weight equipment such as Universal, Nautilus, and Cybex. The result is a better physical appearance and greater efficiency in both everyday activities and sudden emergencies. For more information about muscular strength and endurance see chapter 3.

Flexibility

Flexibility refers to the movement of a joint through a full range of motion. Flexibility is essential to smooth, efficient movement and may help prevent injuries to ligaments and joints. Being able to sit and touch your toes without bending your knees is an example of hamstring flexibility. You need arm and shoulder flexibility to scratch your back. Women usually have more joint flexibility than men because men have bulkier skeletal muscles. Older adults may have trouble performing routine tasks such as getting in and out of an automobile, turning to watch traffic while driving, and dressing when clothes fasten at the back since flexibility diminishes with age. This loss can be countered if stretching is part of your lifetime exercise program. Chapter 3 has more information about flexibility.

Body Composition

Body Composition refers to the amount of body fat in proportion to fat-free weight. The ratio between body fat and fat-free weight is a better gauge of fatness than body weight. There are various ways to measure body composition (Body Mass Index—See chapter 10, skinfold calipers, bioelectrical impedance, hydrostatic underwater weighing technique), and all are superior to the height/weight chart method. For instance, a height/weight chart may label a 6 foot, 210-pound football player as overweight, when in reality he has only 10 percent body fat, as measured with skinfold calipers. On the other hand, a coed may look good in her size 8 jeans, but when her body composition is analyzed, it is calculated to be 32 percent body fat! The best advice is to have your body composition analyzed by a professional. Obesity is not only unhealthy and uncomfortable, it is associated with increased risk for heart disease, diabetes, high blood pressure, and joint and lower back problems.

No single activity or sport develops all five fitness components. For example, joggers develop high levels of cardiorespiratory endurance but often have low levels of flexibility and upper body strength. For this reason, cross training has become a popular conditioning method that emphasizes the development of balanced fitness. You can read more about cross training later in this chapter.

Physical Fitness and Wellness

Becoming physically fit is a positive health habit that has a major impact on your wellness. It is one area where you can assume control of your lifestyle. It is the golden thread that penetrates all the dimensions of wellness (table 2.1).

There now is strong scientific evidence linking fitness not only to better health but also to decreased medical costs and to improved job productivity. Do you want an edge on the future job market? Employers who must absorb medical care costs of their employees are fast realizing it costs less to keep an employee healthy than to treat workers once sick. Many are now looking to hire the "fit employee," one who has already adopted a wellness lifestyle. This further reduces dollars they will need to invest in company wellness programs. Decide now to be more than half-well. Climb up the wellness ladder to become more physically fit and exert greater control over your wellness destiny.

Benefits of Physical Fitness

The number one reason people begin exercising is they want to improve their physical appearance. Physical appearance is enhanced because of decreased body fat and firmer, well-toned muscles. These are not the only benefits. There

Table 2.1

Benefits of Physical Fitness on
Wellness Dimensions

Dimensions	
Physical	Slows down the aging process; increases energy; improves posture and physical appearance; helps in weight control; improves flexibility; improves muscular strength and endurance; strengthens bones, reducing osteoporosis; reduces risk for coronary heart disease.
Emotional	Relieves tension; aids in stress management; improves self-image; evens out emotional swings; provides time for adult play.
Social	Enhances relationships with family and friends; increases opportunity for social contacts.
Intellectual	Develops concepts of mind and body oneness; increases alertness; enhances concentration; motivates toward improved personal habits (smoking cessation, reducing drug and alcohol use, better nutrition); stimulates creative thoughts.
Occupational	Less absenteeism; more productivity; decrease in disability days; lower medical care costs; lower job turnover rate; increases networking possibilities.
Spiritual	Appreciation of body and self; appreciation for healthy environment; builds compassion for those less able.

are a number of physiological (cardiorespiratory, body composition, and metabolic) and psychological (mental and emotional) health benefits. Exercise has both short- and long-term effects. The immediate effects of vigorous exercise, regardless of the fitness level, are an increase in the respiration rate, an increase in the heart rate, and some sweating. After a few weeks of regular, vigorous exercise, the body begins to adapt. It becomes better suited to meeting the demands of regular exercise. These physiological adaptations (the total beneficial changes) are called the **training effect.**

Cardiorespiratory benefits:

1. slow and consistent reduction in resting heart rate
2. increase in stroke volume (the amount of blood pumped out of the heart with each beat),

improving heart efficiency

3. increased rest for the heart between beats due to slower resting heart rate and increased stroke volume

4. increased oxygen-carrying capacity of the blood, due to the greater supply of red blood cells and hemoglobin; greater endurance in exercising muscles due to increased energy and improved elimination of waste products
5. improved exercise performance on timed tests (due to more efficient utilization of oxygen)
6. possible reduction in blood pressure
7. improved blood lipid profile by increasing the number of protective high-density lipoproteins
8. quicker recovery to resting heart rate after vigorous exercise due to improved cardiac efficiency
9. possible regression of atherosclerosis
10. fewer illnesses and deaths due to coronary heart disease

Everybody benefits from physical activity.

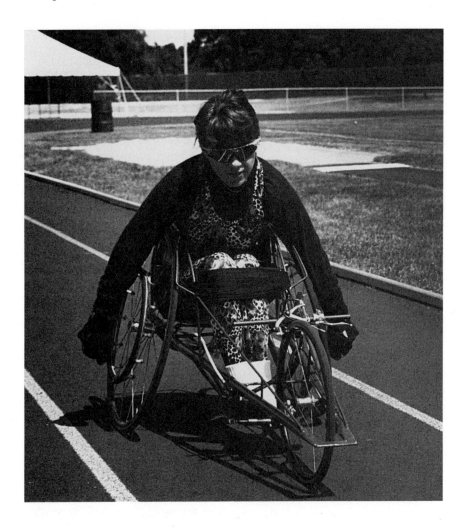

Body composition/physical appearance benefits:

1. reduced body fat percentage
2. increased lean body mass
3. firmer, more toned muscles

Psychological benefits:

1. enhanced sense of well-being and self-esteem, resulting in increased energy, alertness, and vitality.
2. increased sense of self-discipline due to the determination needed to stick to an exercise program.
3. reduced state of anxiety and mental tension, thereby increasing stress coping ability.
4. improved quality of sleep, resulting in the ability to fall asleep faster and with less tossing and turning during sleeping time.
5. decreased level of mild to moderate depression.
6. increased release of endorphins (brain chemicals) producing a relaxed state.

The psychological benefits are the most rewarding and are often the main reason people keep exercising. These mental and emotional benefits are real and can be measured.[7] Fitness produces other benefits that are also important to your health and well-being. You burn extra calories while exercising, which helps to promote weight loss and reverse obesity. Exercise and weight management helps prevent and manage diabetes.[8, 9] Fit people can exercise longer at the same level of intensity, and their perception of how hard they are working decreases. This is due to increased muscular strength and endurance. Tendons, ligaments, and joints may also be strengthened through exercise. Additionally, exercise stimulates bone strengthening and may help counteract and reverse osteoporosis.[10]

The FITT Prescription for Fitness

Many studies have been conducted in exercise physiology laboratories to determine the best prescription for developing physical fitness. These studies confirm that fitness development involves four **prescription factors:** Frequency, Intensity, and Time and Type of exercise (FITT).

F I T T =

| **FREQUENCY** | **INTENSITY** | **TIME** | **TYPE OF EXERCISE** |

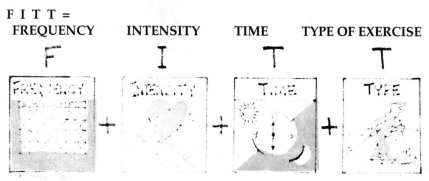

| **3–5 times/wk.** | **60–75% MHRR*** | **20–30 min.** | **continuous and rhythmic** |

*MHRR= Maximal Heart Rate Reserve

"F" Equals Frequency

How often should you exercise? Exercise three to five times per week with no more than 48 hours between workouts. After 48 hours, the body starts to decondition or lose some of the benefits gained in the last workout. It is not necessary to exercise every day of the week in order to develop fitness, although five-days-a-week programs produce greater improvements than do three-days-a-week programs. Since fitness exercise is vigorous, time for recovery is necessary. This is especially true if you are just beginning a fitness program. The body needs time to adapt to this new activity. So start slowly at first, working out three days per week, every other day, gradually increasing the frequency as your body can handle it.

"I" Equals Intensity

How hard should you exercise? The level of intensity of the workout needs to be between 60 percent and 75 percent of the maximal heart rate reserve. This allows for a range of intensity that assures adequate stimulation of the cardiorespiratory system (providing training effect benefits), yet is not so strenuous that symptoms of overtraining develop (see table 2.2).

Table 2.2

Symptoms of Overtraining, Overstress, Overuse, and Chronic Fatigue

1. Persistent soreness and stiffness in joints, tendons, or muscles
2. Increases of 6–8 beats per minute in resting pulse, checked regularly, first thing in the morning
3. Labored breathing during a workout of normal intensity, or a sudden drop in performance, or inability to finish a workout
4. Persistent lethargy, fatigue, and disinterest in exercise when normally you look forward to it
5. Lowered general resistance: frequent mild colds, sniffles, cold sores
6. Lack of enthusiasm, depression, inability to relax, irritability
7. Poor coordination (general clumsiness, tripping, poor auto driving)
8. Difficulty in getting to sleep or staying asleep
9. Swelling or aching lymph glands in the neck, underarm, or groin area
10. Skin eruptions in nonadolescents
11. Loss of appetite
12. Chronic thirst
13. Morning weight is 3% less than normal
14. Sudden case of diarrhea or constipation
15. Anemia or amenorrhea (in women)

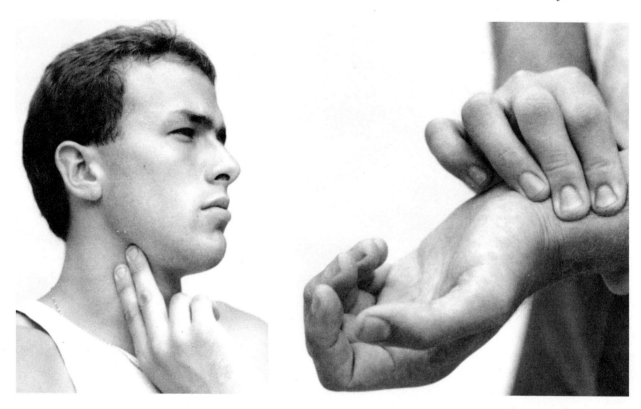

Figure 2.1
(left) Pulse at carotid artery.

Figure 2.2
(right) Pulse at the thumb side of wrist.

Karvonen Equation To determine the **target heart rate range** (THR) for exercise we will use a formula that takes into account your current fitness level based on your resting heart rate (RHR). It is called the **Karvonen Equation** (table 2.3). Karvonen, a Finnish researcher, discovered in 1957 that the heart rate during exercise must be raised by at least 60 percent of the difference between resting and maximal heart rates (called the Maximal Heart Rate Reserve) to gain cardiorespiratory fitness.[11] Subsequent research has revealed that an adequate upper intensity level is 75 percent of the difference between resting and maximal heart rate.

It is necessary to know your **maximal heart rate** in order to calculate your target heart rate range. The Maximal Heart Rate (Max.HR) is your highest possible heart rate. It can be determined during a treadmill exercise tolerance test in a laboratory or hospital while you exercise to exhaustion. The maximal heart rate ranges from 180–200 beats per minute (bpm) in young people and decreases with age. For most people it is easier and safer to estimate their Max.HR by subtracting their age from 220. For example, if you are 21 years old, your estimated Max.HR is 199 (220 – 21 = 199).

Next, you will need to know your resting heart rate (RHR) for one minute. Check it now, using a stop watch or a watch with a second hand. You can find the pulse with your finger tips (not the thumb) over the heart, at the carotid artery in the neck, or on the thumb side of the wrist (figs. 2.1 and 2.2). Count the number of beats for 30 seconds and multiply by two to calculate your one-minute pulse.

Table 2.3

Calculating the Target Heart Rate
Range Using the Karvonen Formula

THR =
[Maximal Heart Rate – Resting Heart Rate]
× Intensity Factor + Resting Heart Rate

This example shows a 22-year-old with a resting heart rate of
78 bpm.

Estimation of Maximal Heart Rate = 220 minus age 22
Resting Heart Rate = pulse at complete rest
Intensity = range of 60% to 75%

$$
\begin{aligned}
\text{THR at 60\%} &= [(220 - 22) - 78] \times .60 + 78 \\
&= [198 - 78] \times .60 + 78 \\
&= 120 \times .60 + 78 \\
&= 72 + 78 \\
&= 150 \\
\text{THR at 75\%} &= [(220 - 22) - 78] \times .75 + 78 \\
&= [198 - 78] \times .75 + 78 \\
&= 120 \times .75 + 78 \\
&= 90 + 78 \\
&= 168
\end{aligned}
$$

Target Heart Rate Range = 150 to 168

By using your age and your own RHR, you can calculate your personalized target heart rate range (table 2.3 and target heart rate worksheet in the activities section).

Now that you know your target heart rate range, you will be able to measure the intensity of every workout. Count your pulse during exercise and immediately upon finishing the conditioning bout. Rather than counting your pulse for a full minute, you may find it easier to count for 6 or 10 seconds only. It will take some practice, but in time you will become accurate at checking your heart rate.

Examining the chart for the Target Heart Rate Range, you can see that exercise heart rates differ by age (table 2.4). If your exercise heart rate is above the upper range (higher than 75 percent MHRR), you may be exercising more intensely than is necessary for fitness. The American College of Sports Medicine (ACSM) recommends an exercise intensity range of 60 percent to 90 percent during exercise. Ninety percent may be too intense for many exercisers, especially on a regular basis. A general rule of thumb is to apply the *talk test*. You should be able to comfortably carry on a conversation with a companion while exercising. If you are too breathless to talk, you are exercising too hard.

Use caution when using your running or walking THR to measure the intensity of your exercise when you swim or bike. Weight bearing-activities, such as running and walking, use more oxygen and make your heart beat faster than when you work out by cycling or swimming—at the same perceived level of

Table 2.4

Estimated Target Heart Rate Range
(based on RHR of 72 bpm)

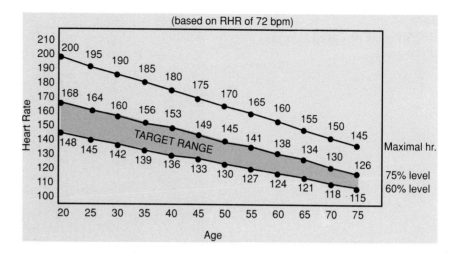

effort.[12] If you try to reach your running/walking THR during nonweight-bearing activities, you may feel uncomfortably stressed and more importantly, risk injury by working out too hard. As a general rule of thumb, reduce cycling THR by 5% and swimming THR by 10%. Also, remember to set different heart rate goals for cross training.

Rate of Perceived Exertion (RPE)   Since many people do not check their heart rate during exercise, an alternate method of assessing intensity of exercise has become popular in recent years. This method uses a **rate of perceived exertion (RPE)** scale developed by Gunnar Borg (see table 2.5). Borg discovered that exercisers are able to "sense" (or perceive) their own exercise intensity levels. He found that the RPE scale correlated very highly with heartrate, ventilation, oxygen consumption and blood lactate concentrates.[13] These items are commonly assessed in a laboratory setting to measure exercise intensity. Borg found that the descriptive words in the right column closely paralleled the actual heartrate of the exerciser, which is illustrated by the numbers in the left column.

Most exercisers should be working in the "Somewhat hard" to "Hard" zone, "Very, very light" describes feelings of exertion at rest, and "Very, very hard" describes feelings just before collapsing from exhaustion. Notice descriptors used for warm-up and cool-down zone. (table 2.5)

It is important to cross-check your heart rate with your perceived rating when first beginning to use this method. After several weeks, you should be able to predict your exercise heart rate by your own perceived exertion of the exercise session. When exercising ask "How do I feel?" Describe how you feel using the descriptors on the Borg scale. Adjust the intensity of your workout accordingly. This is a safe and accurate way to monitor exercise intensity anywhere, anytime without using a stopwatch or pace clock.

Whether you monitor the intensity of exercise by checking your pulse or through rate of perceived exertion, listen to your body and make adjustments in the intensity of your exercise when necessary.

Table 2.5

Borg's Rate of Perceived Exertion (RPE)

Borg's Rate of Perceived Exertion (RPE)		
(RPE) Chart		
6		
7	Very, very light	
8		Warm-up/cool-down zone
9	Very light	
10		
11	Fairly light	
12		
13	Somewhat hard	Target zone
14		
15	Hard	
16		
17	Very hard	
18		Working too hard zone
19	Very, very hard	
20		

"T" Equals Time

How long should each workout be? Research points out that the conditioning bout should be 20 or (preferably) 30 minutes in duration to provide the desired training effects. This does not include the warm-up and cool-down segments, but refers only to the actual conditioning bout when the intensity level is sustained at 60 percent to 75 percent maximal heart rate reserve. The time duration recommended by the ACSM is 20 minutes to 60 minutes. If time permits and the exercise session is enjoyable, or if you are training for a long distance event (i.e., mini-marathon, etc.), exercising for longer than 30 minutes is permissable, but not necessary for basic fitness. A typical workout would be as follows:

When beginning a fitness program, it is best to limit your conditioning periods to 20 minutes or less, then progress slowly until you can comfortably work out for 20–30 minutes in your target heart rate range.

warm-up **5–15 min.**	**conditioning bout** **20–30 min.**	**cool-down** **5–15 min.**

"T" Equals Type

What type of exercise promotes aerobic fitness? The activity should be vigorous, rhythmic, and continuous. This includes activities that accelerate respiration and maintain a heart rate in the target range. Aerobic dance, lap swimming, bicycling, cross-country skiing, jogging, and fitness walking are activities that come to mind. However, riding a bike across campus does not get the job done. This is not fitness riding. Ask yourself, "Did my heart rate reach the prescribed target

Recording workouts helps you see progress.

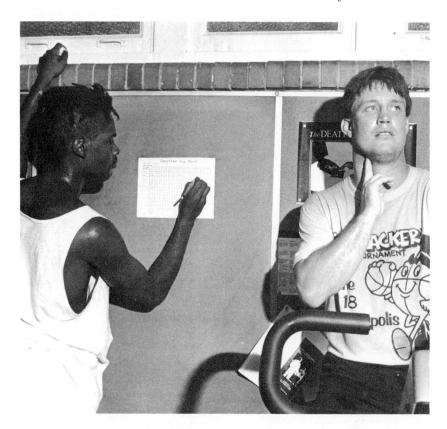

heart rate range? Did I keep my heart rate in that range for 20 to 30 minutes or more?" On the other hand, rope jumping or even stair climbing can be an aerobic activity, providing the FITT prescription factors are met. Tennis, bowling, golf, weight training, and softball, although enjoyable and worthwhile activities, are not considered to be aerobic. Can you name other sports or activities that meet the FITT prescription?

How Long Before Results Become Apparent?

How long before results become apparent? It varies with the individual, but results can occur within 8 to 12 weeks. The key is staying with the exercise program. Studies indicate over 50 percent of all adults who start an exercise program quit within a short time.[14] So how do you stay with an exercise program long enough to experience the benefits of the training effect?

Make up a contract. People who sign a contract for a definite period of time are more likely to reach their goals.[15] A contract for 12 weeks is ideal. At the end of the contract, reward yourself—you've earned it! Immediately, renegotiate your contract for another 12-week period.

Make exercise social and fun. Exercising with a partner or group of friends is more fun than working out alone. Friends rely on each other for moral support and help each other stay committed to their fitness program.

You may also enjoy taking lessons. Join an aerobic dance class or a health club. Try different activities until you find one you enjoy. Start slowly and progress gradually to avoid injuries. If exercise is too difficult or too intense, you are not likely to want to stay on your program. Treat exercise like an appointment. Schedule a time that works best for you; whether that be morning, noon, or evening, table 2.6 gives advantages and disadvantages of various times. Keep a chart to monitor your progress. It's rewarding to see how much you have progressed. Finally, *don't stop!* It's difficult to get going again. Remember to plan for changes in your schedule (for example, pack your exercise equipment when you travel). However, don't feel guilty if you miss an exercise session. Consider this a lifetime commitment, and resume exercising as soon as possible..

Three-Segment Workout

Warm-Up

The **warm-up** is an important beginning to a workout session. Two important physiological changes occur during the warm-up. The internal temperature of the muscles increases, enhancing their elasticity. Heart rate and respiration increase, thus providing greater blood flow to the exercising muscles. The warm-up prepares the body physically and mentally for the conditioning bout and may reduce the chance of injury while exercising. There is no set length of time for the warm-up, although 5–15 minutes is adequate. On cold days, or times when you feel sluggish, the warm-up may take longer. When you're feeling energetic or when the temperature is warm, the warm-up period may be shorter. A good method of gauging whether you have had an adequate warm-up is to pay attention to how you feel. Do you feel ready to exercise vigorously? If you still feel stiff and sluggish, you need a longer warm-up. A slight sweat is a good indication of an adequate warm-up.

Three activities may be included in the warm-up. They are simple calisthenics (like jumping jacks), mild stretching exercises, and a short period of **task specific activity.** The task specific activity is an exercise using the same muscles that will be used in the conditioning bout. It specifically prepares those muscles that will be used. **Static stretching,** in which a stretch is held for 15–30 seconds, is recommended. **Ballistic stretching,** with jerking and bouncing movements, is *not* recommended. Stretching during warm-up is mainly preparation for the activity, not for flexibility. Most experts agree that the best time to stretch for flexibility is during the cool-down phase because the muscles are warmer and more elastic.

The final portion of the warm-up should lead into the actual activity you will be doing in the conditioning bout but at a lowered intensity level (lower heart rate). For example, joggers should include a short period of walking or slow jogging before beginning the intensity of the conditioning bout. Aerobic dancers should do routines of lowered intensity before proceeding into the main body of the workout (conditioning bout) where the heart rate should reach target heart rate intensity. See chapter 3 for exercises that can be used for warm-up and cool-down.

Table 2.6
Best Time to
Exercise

Time	Advantage	Disadvamtage
Morning	■ Less chance for other activities to conflict with exercise. ■ Wakes you up and energizes you for the day's activities. ■ Usually cooler during hot summer days. ■ Fewer problems with ozone and other air pollutants. ■ Gets your showering over for the day. ■ Good time to organize a "to do" list for the day.	■ Some people like to "sleep in." ■ Energy reserves may be low because of the long span of time between the evening meal and breakfast. ■ May need longer warm-up because muscles are colder and stiffer than later in the day. ■ May be colder during winter months. ■ May rush you to be on time for work or school. ■ Dangerous to exercise outside before daylight.
Noon	■ Allows for a refreshing tension-relieving break during the middle of the day. ■ Can help curb lunch appetite. ■ Energizes you for the remainder of the day. ■ Generally, more people are around to share the workout. ■ Good time to "network" and make business and social contacts. ■ May be warmest time of the day during cold months.	■ Only possible if time, exercise facilities, and shower are available. ■ Easy to postpone due to commitments, redoing hair and makeup, etc. ■ Difficult if you have frequent business lunches. ■ May be too hot during warm months. ■ May feel rushed to combine workout with lunch.
Evening	■ Works off the accumulated stress of the day. ■ May help you sleep more soundly. ■ Can help curb dinner appetite. ■ A "pick-me-up" for the rest of the evening (if you plan to study late or have other activities). ■ May be cooler than midday during summer. ■ Exercising at a fitness facility on the way home from school or work is convenient.	■ Easy to postpone exercise due to other activities, coming home late, feeling too tired, etc. ■ Easy to say "I'll get up early tomorrow and work out." ■ May stimulate you too much so that falling asleep is difficult. ■ It is recommended that you wait an hour or two before exercising after a heavy meal.

There is no perfect time of day for exercise. What works best for one individual may not fit the life of another. Find the time that works best for your individual needs, preferences, and schedule. You may want to experiment with several exercise times before you are able to determine what "feels" best for you. The key is to commit to a lifestyle that includes a definite time for daily physical activity, and to stick with this commitment for life.

Flexibility gains are greatest during cool-down stretching.

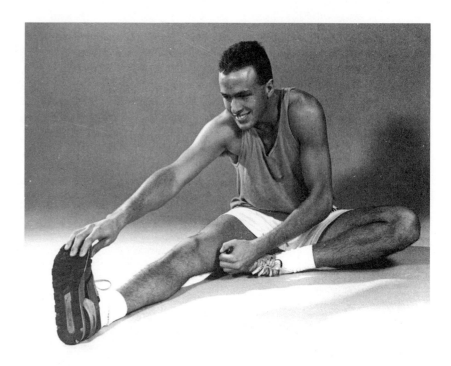

Conditioning Bout

The **conditioning bout** contains vigorous aerobic exercise that stimulates the cardiorespiratory system. It should follow the FITT formula. Progress slowly and listen to your body. Gradually increase the intensity and frequency of your workouts. You do not want to be sidelined by illness or injury because of overtraining. Your goal is a lifetime of exercise. Select an aerobic activity you will enjoy; do not be influenced into participating in an activity simply because it is in vogue. Depending on your age, current fitness level, or physical limitations, enjoy walking, jogging, aerobic dance, water exercise, fitness swimming, bicycling, cross-country skiing, or any other vigorous activity you like.

Cool-Down

The **cool-down** is the final segment of the workout. The purpose of the cool-down is to safely ease your body back to its resting state. You should gradually reduce the intensity of exercise to enhance your recovery. Failure to cool-down may allow the muscles to further tighten, potentially causing pain, soreness, and stiffness. Another problem with inadequate cool-down is the possibility of blood pooling in the lower extremities, resulting in faintness and dizziness. This is called venous pooling. Again, there is no set length of time for a cool-down period, but it will usually take 5-15 minutes. It should begin with the same activity performed in the conditioning bout, but at a lowered intensity. For example, if you jog, reduce the pace and end with a period of walking. Likewise, the aerobic dancer should reduce dance intensity. Cool-down should continue until the heart rate is approximately 100–110 beats per minute or less. In the cool-down, spend a few minutes stretching while the muscles are thoroughly warm and elastic. Use the stretching exercises illustrated in chapter 3. Greater flexibility is achieved when stretching occurs in the cool-down segment of the workout.

Principle of Overload

Overload is a gradual increase in physical activity, stressing a muscle group or body system beyond accustomed levels. The muscle group or system, such as the cardiorespiratory system, gradually adapts, resulting in improved physiological functioning. In addition, a decrease in the severity and a delay in the onset of fatigue occur. The overload doesn't have to be punishing or exhaustive for cardiorespiratory training effects to occur. The key to gradual overloading is to follow the FITT formula, but in the order of FTI (i.e., Frequency, Time, Intensity).

First, there should be a gradual increase in the *frequency* of workouts, starting with 3 and progressing to 5 workouts per week. Second, *time* or (duration) should be introduced. Start with workouts of 20 minutes (or less, if you are in poor condition) and gradually lengthen the workouts to 30 minutes each. The rate of increase should be no more than 10 percent per week. For example, if the conditioning bout is 20 minutes each, the next week's workouts can be 22 minutes. The third factor in the correct order of overloading is *intensity*. Workouts should begin at 60 percent intensity and progress to the 75 percent range. By following the FTI order of overloading, normal activity becomes a physiological "push-over," since the individual has trained to perform beyond normal levels.

The old saying, "No pain—no gain!" is inappropriate advice. Simply follow the prescription factors in the correct order and listen to your own body. Check your heart rate and stay within your target heart rate range. Watch for any signs of overtraining (shown in table 2.2).

Principle of Specificity

The **principle of specificity** means that only the muscles or body systems being exercised will show beneficial changes. To improve the cardiorespiratory system, exercise the heart and lungs through aerobic activities; to improve flexibility, do stretching exercises; and to improve muscular strength, lift weights.

You cannot strengthen the muscles of the arms by jogging, nor can you increase cardiorespiratory fitness by doing yoga. This principle also helps to explain why you are "wiped out" after a fitness swim workout when your usual mode of training is jogging!

Aerobic and Anaerobic

The term **aerobic** literally means "with oxygen." Aerobic activities are those that demand large amounts of oxygen and follow the FITT prescription. They are vigorous, continuous, and rhythmic. The outcome of aerobic exercise is improved cardiorespiratory endurance, which produces the many physiological and psychological benefits that come from improved fitness.

Anaerobic exercise means "without oxygen." Anaerobic activities are start and stop, such as sprinting, where the heart rate is not kept at a rhythmic, continuous level. Anaerobic exercise is high-intensity effort of short duration. This type of activity demands more oxygen than the body can supply while exercising, causing an oxygen debt. Anaerobic exercise causes waste products (lactic acid) to accumulate in muscles, which, along with the depletion of stored energy, leads to exhaustion. Many activities—tennis, baseball, basketball, and weight training—are anaerobic. They aid in the development of agility, eye-hand coordination, and muscular strength and endurance, as well as flexibility, but they are not aerobic.

Cross Training

Cross training involves developing all five health-related components of fitness. It is a method of exercise programming that achieves balanced fitness by emphasizing comprehensive conditioning in major muscle groups. Traditionally, cardiorespiratory endurance has been the fitness component receiving the most emphasis. Certainly, this component is essential to high-level health, but the other four health-related components are also important. No single type of exercise can offer complete conditioning for all parts of the body.

Originally, cross training referred to a conditioning regimen used by triathletes to train in three events—running, biking, and swimming. In the strictest sense, training for a triathlon is not cross training. It is triple task-specific training, where the athlete trains for three separate events in which the main emphasis is cardiorespiratory endurance. The purpose of cross training is to enhance several fitness components, not athletic performance, although performance may improve due to increased strength, flexibility, etc. An example of cross training (for a 20-year-old) would be to add one swimming session and two weight training workouts to a three-time-per-week jogging program. Add some stretching exercises after each workout and you have a balanced fitness program. (See table 2.7 for other cross training activities.)

It's not only the elite athlete that profits from muscular strength and endurance, flexibility, a lean body, and high-level cardiorespiratory endurance. These ingredients of balanced fitness are needed by people from all walks of life, including college students. Expand your fitness program to include cross training activities. The time and energy you invest will give big pay offs. Look at the advantages:

1. Cross training builds overall fitness. This occurs because all five fitness components are emphasized. Cross training entices the exerciser to apply the overload principle in workouts, thus improving fitness gains in every component.

2. Cross training develops high levels of fitness. By participating in a variety of activities, new muscle fibers are recruited and neuromuscular pathways, formerly left untapped, are developed. Higher levels of cardiorespiratory endurance can result.[16]

3. Cross training reduces risk of overtraining and injury. By using a single type of activity to develop cardiorespiratory endurance, the same body parts are continually stressed. This is especially true in weight-bearing activities such as running. Repetitive impact injuries (i.e.,

shin splints) can result. Because the stress imposed by cross training is spread around the body to different muscle groups, a high volume of training can be performed without overtraining and injury.

4. Cross training develops muscle symmetry. Muscle symmetry involves the balance of both strength and flexibility in opposing muscle groups. Without the appropriate ratio, selected sites of muscles can become strong and their opposing muscles disproportionately weak. Well-balanced muscle pairs working in concert allow for more effective and efficient movement and eliminate some of the risk for injury.

5. Cross training reduces boredom and provides motivation. Cross training, with its variety of activities, stimulates interest in exercise, thereby improving adherence.

Table 2.7

Cross Training Activities for the Five Components of Fitness

Flexibility
Yoga, stretching, swimming, water exercise, or other activities that allow muscles to move through a full range of motion are excellent methods of developing flexibility.

Cardiorespiratory Endurance
Running, fitness walking, aerobic dance, bench and stair stepping, rope jumping, cross-country skiing, swimming, cycling, rowing, and water exercise (aqua-aerobics), etc. are recommended for developing cardiorespiratory endurance.

Muscle Strength
Weight machines, free weights, rubberbands, gymnastics, calisthenics (push-ups, abdominal curls, etc.) provide ways to enhance muscle strength.

Muscle Endurance
Lighter weights or resistance with increased repetitions of the exercises used to develop muscle strength are advised.

Body Composition
Minute for minute, activities that develop cardiorespiratory endurance expend the most calories. Muscular strength and endurance activities also help maintain the appropriate lean to fat ratio.

The Relationship between Activity and Health

The proof is in! We can no longer ignore the scientific evidence that documents how a sedentary lifestyle is killing us (see table 2.8). Stop for a moment to think about the impact exercise has on heart disease, cancer, and other causes of death. Americans worry about cholesterol in their diets and are giving up cigarettes, yet, continue to get more obese every year. Why do Americans ignore the reports on the relationship of exercise to health and weight control? The thought of not brushing our teeth everyday seems ridiculous to most of us. After all, our teeth have to last a lifetime. But exercise everyday? Even though mortality statistics overwhelmingly point to the health value of activity,[17] most people still do not include exercise in their daily schedule. Doesn't your heart have to last a lifetime, too? How sad it is that we pay more attention to our teeth than to our hearts.

Is it because we don't know what is involved in getting fit? Perhaps most people think that fitness takes too much time, energy, money, and that athletic ability is required. We all know the value of exercise. The problem is few make it a priority in their lives. Only about 10 percent of our population exercises intensely enough to protect their cardiorespiratory system.[18] These fitness enthusiasts practice the advice recommended by Dr. R. Paffenbarger and colleagues in their famous Harvard Alumni Study. The study reported that protection for the cardiorespiratory system through exercise was possible if the exerciser burned about 2,000 calories per week beyond what was required for normal energy needs. This can easily be accomplished by burning approximately 200–300 calories per day in exercise. Two-to-three miles of fitness walking/jogging, swimming 800–1,000 yards, bicycling about 5 miles, 30 minutes of aerobic dance/stairstepping/treadmill running, etc., all meet this caloric expenditure and provide protection for the cardiorespiratory system.

Table 2.8

Exercise and Health

Source: Institute for Aerobics Research, "Physical Fitness and All-Cause Mortality," Journal of the American Medical Association. *Nov. 3, 1989, Vol. 262, No. 17.*

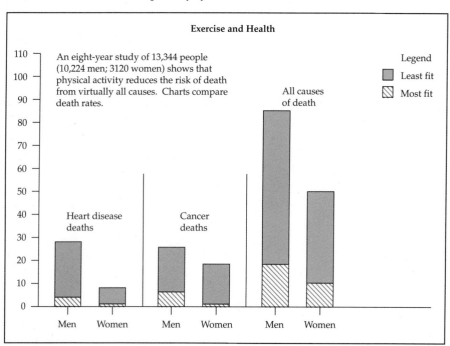

Exercise and Health

An eight-year study of 13,344 people (10,224 men; 3120 women) shows that physical activity reduces the risk of death from virtually all causes. Charts compare death rates.

Those who adhere to the FITT guidelines are not the segment of our population we need to reach, though. It is the remaining 90 percent—the sedentary segment. This group needs to realize that sedentary living affects mortality as much as high blood pressure, high cholesterol, and obesity.[19] We now know that exercise gives powerful health benefits and that inactivity is a major public health problem in the United States. People don't have to run marathons or swim the English Channel to reap the benefits of exercise. The real issue is getting people moving again; to convince sedentary Americans that exercise is a normal human need.

An important study conducted at the Institute for Aerobics Research in Dallas by Steven Blair, et al., provides evidence that physical fitness is associated with longevity (table 2.8). In this eight-year study, physical fitness was quantified using an exercise tolerance test on a treadmill. The subjects were categorized into five levels of physical fitness based on the treadmill test. As table 2.9 shows, the greatest reduction in risk of death occurs between the lowest level of fitness and the next lowest level. Therefore, a modest improvement in fitness among the most unfit can bring about substantial health benefits!

Table 2.9

Comparison of Fitness Levels and Risk of Death. Notice that the death rates for the least fit men (level 1) were 3.4 times higher than for the most fit men (level 5). Death rates for the least fit women (level 1) were 4.6 times higher than for the most fit women (level 5). The most dramatic drop in risk of death occurs between levels 1 and 2 (from 3.4 to 1.4 for men; from 4.6 to 2.4 for women).

Source: Steven Blair, et. al., "Physical Fitness and All-Cause Mortality: A Prospective Study of Healthy Men and Women," Journal of the American Medical Association. Nov. 3, 1989, Vol. 262, pp. 2395–2401.

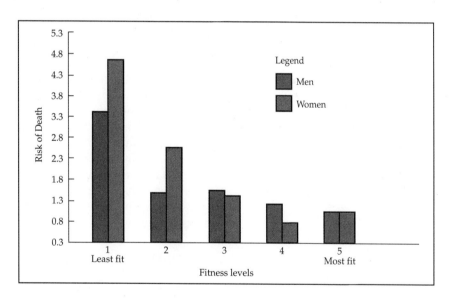

Even the recently published *Healthy People 2000* (see chapter 1) includes exercise objectives.[20] One of these objectives is "for 50 percent of all Americans to participate in fitness activities." This is important, but just as critical is the next objective, which is "for 60 percent of all Americans to participate in *moderate* physical activity." This is a significant objective—to get Americans involved in *moderate* activity. This alone would greatly improve mortality rates. Then, perhaps, these individuals will enjoy the new active lifestyle and begin to "see and feel" the benefits of exercise. Eventually, they may invest additional time and energy increasing the potential to acquire greater benefits from increased levels of activity.

What's involved in adopting a moderately active lifestyle?

First, realize physical activity does not have to be punishing to be beneficial. The emphasis should be on exercise of *moderate* intensity. Exercising for 30 minutes a day in the "fairly light" zone on the Borg RPE scale will produce measurable health gains. This would be equivalent to walking approximately 2 miles at a 15–20-minute-mile pace.[21] You don't have to be soaked with sweat for improvements in health to occur.

Second, exercise does not have to be all in one bout. We know that 20–30 minutes of vigorous exercise is recommended for high-level fitness (full cardiorespiratory benefit), but every bit of activity is beneficial to our health. Something is better than nothing. Incorporate bits of activity into every day whenever and wherever you can. The theme is to *pulse* activity into our daily lives. For example: ride your bike to mail a letter; play racquetball/walk/swim/run at noontime; take a walk after dinner; walk to the grocery when you need only a few items. *Look* for opportunities to add daily activity—get up earlier, utilize TV commercial time, or when working out a problem, when visiting a friend, etc.

Third, we should deemphasize the medical/scientific approach. Although medical screening and precise exercise prescription (exact THR) is recommended, it is more important to get moving. In the past, the scientific approach to exercise may have turned some people off to exercise. They may have had the impression that exercise was too complicated, took too much time, involved special equipment, and wasn't convenient. Our society is at a point where the best advice is "Just do it."

You are faced with a tremendous challenge. As our nation's future homemakers, parents, and leaders, the responsibility for the health and well-being of the next generation rests in your hands. Each one of you can make an enormous impact on the activity patterns of your own children, family, friends, and neighbors by setting a good example. So go to it . . . get up off the sofa, turn off the TV, put away the video games. Accept the challenge today to make exercise a daily habit, one as important as brushing your teeth.

Encourage your friends and neighbors to get out and work in the garden, walk around the block, mow the lawn, walk the dog, participate in recreational sports (bowling, tennis, golf, softball), and go dancing. Anyone can begin the journey toward wellness with a single step and begin reaping health benefits immediately.

Summary

The sedentary lifestyle of most Americans is seriously undermining the health and welfare of our nation. We are fast becoming over-fat and under-fit, resulting in reduced levels of well-being. From the information you have acquired in this chapter, you now have the necessary tools to confidently develop a personalized physical fitness program, based on sound scientific principles and utilizing your own age, resting heart rate, interests, and abilities. You also have gained a better understanding of the health benefits that can be achieved by incorporating moderate levels of physical activity into your daily life. By applying the FITT prescription factors, the concept of a three-segment workout, and finding ways to increase daily activity, you can be on your way to a lifetime of improved health, fitness, and wellness.

References

1. Stephens, L., D. R. Jacobs, Jr., and C. C. White. "A Descriptive Epidemiology of Leisure-Time Physical Activity." *Public Health Review 100* (March–April 1985): 147–58.

2. Bar-Or, O. "A Commentary to Children and Fitness: A Public Health Perspective." *Research Quarterly for Exercise and Sport.* 1987, Vol. 58.

3. Ignico, Arlene, "A Comparison of Fitness Levels of Children Enrolled in Daily and Weekly Physical Education Programs." *Journal of Human Movement Studies.* 1990, Vol. 18, pp. 129–39.

4. "The National Children and Youth Fitness Study II." *Journal of Health, Physical Education, Recreation and Dance* (November–December 1987): 50.

5. Bar-Or, O. "A Commentary to Children and Fitness: A Public Health Perspective."

6. Blair, S., Kohl, H., Paffenbarger, R., Clark, D., Cooper, K., Gibbons, L., "Physical Fitness and All-Cause Mortality: A Prospective Study of Healthy Men and Women." *JAMA.* Nov. 3, 1989, Vol. 66, No. 17.

7. "The Health Benefits of Exercise (Part I): A Round Table." *The Physician and Sports Medicine,* Vol. 15, No. 10, 1987: 131.

8. Hoeger, Werner. *Principles and Labs for Physical Fitness and Wellness.* Morton Publishing Co., Englewood, Colorado, 1988.

9. "1992 Health Guide, Fitness, No Pain and Lots of Gain." *U.S. News and World Report,* May 4, 1992.

10. "1992 Health Guide, Fitness, No Pain and Lots of Gain."

11. Karvonen, M., K. Kentala, and O. Mustala. "The Effects of Training on Heart Rate: A Longitudinal Study." *Annals of Medicine and Experimental Biology.* 35:307–15 (1957).

12. *Running and Fitness.* American Running and Fitness Association. Vol. 10, No. 6, June, 1992.

13. Borg, G. "Psychophysical Bases of Physical Exertion." *Medicine and Science in Sport and Exercise,* Vol. 14, 1982.

14. "Sticking to an Exercise Program" *American Journal of Health Promotion.* Vol. 4, No. 6, 1991.

15. "Sticking to an Exercise Program."

16. *Reebok Instructors News.* Edited by the Cooper Institute for Aerobics Research, Dallas, Texas, Vol. 5, No. 2, 1992.

17. Hahn, R., Teutch, R., Rothenberg, R., Marks, J. "Excess Deaths from Nine Chronic Diseases in the U.S., 1986." *JAMA,* Nov. 28, 1990, Vol. 264, No. 20.

18. "Physical Fitness and All-Cause Mortality: A Prospective Study of Healthy Men and Women."

19. "Excess Deaths from Nine Chronic Diseases in the U.S., 1986."

20. *Healthy People 2000: National Health Promotion and Disease Prevention Objectives.* U.S. Dept. of Health and Human Services, 1990.

21. *Reebok Instructors News.*

Suggested Readings

American College of Sports Medicine, 1992. *ACSM Fitness Book.* Champaign, IL: Human Kinetics Publishers.

Blair, S. N. 1991. *Living With Exercise.* Dallas, TX: American Health Publishing Company.

Brian, Sharkey, 1990. *Physiology of Fitness.* Champaign, IL: Human Kinetics Publishers.

Brooks, Christine, "Active Lifestyle Motivation," *Fitness Management* May, 1992.

Corbin, Charles and Lindsey, Ruth, 1991. *Concepts of Physical Fitness with Laboratories.* Dubuque, IA: Wm. C. Brown Communications.

Dawber, T. R. 1980. *The Framingham Study.* Cambridge, MA: Harvard University Press.

Deena, Balboa. 1990. *Walk for Life: The Lifetime Walking Program for a Healthy Body and Mind.* New York: Perigee Books.

Dishman, Rod. 1988. *Exercise Adherence.* Champaign, IL: Human Kinetics Publishers.

Dishman, Rod. "Exercise Adherence Research: Future Directions." *American Journal of Health Promotion.* Summer 1988, Vol. 3, No. 1, pp. 53–56.

Exercise, Fitness and Health. 1990. Hagberg, J. M. Champaign, IL: Human Kinetics.

Gavin, James. 1992. *The Exercise Habit.* Champaign, IL: Human Kinetics Publishers.

Golding, Lawrence and Myers, Clayton. 1989. *Y's Way to Physical Fitness.* The

Complete Guide to Fitness Testing and Instruction. Champaign, IL: Human Kinetics Publishers.

Guidelines for Graded Exercise Testing and Exercise Prescription. 1991. American College of Sportsmedicine, Philadelphia: Lea and Febiger.

Haywood, K. M. 1991. "The Role of Physical Education in the Development of Active Lifestyles" *Research Quarterly for Exercise and Sport,* 62, 151–156.

Howley, Edward, 1992. *Health Fitness Instructor's Handbook.* Champaign, IL: Human Kinetics Books.

Howley, Edward and Franks, Don. 1992. *Health Fitness Instructor's Handbook.* Champaign, IL: Human Kinetics Publishers.

International Federation of Sports Medicine. 1990. *"Physical Exercise: An Important Factor for Health"* The Physician and Sports Medicine, 18(3), 155–156.

Klug, Gary and Lettunich, Janice. 1992. *Exercise and Physical Fitness.* Guilford, CT: The Dushkin Publishing Group, Inc.

Mackinnon, Laurel. 1992. *Exercise and Immunology.* Champaign, IL: Human Kinetics Publishers, Inc.

Monahan, Terry. "Is Activity as Good as Exercise?" *The Physician and Sportsmedicine.* Vol. 15, No. 10 October 1987, pp. 181–86.

Paffenbarger, R. S., Jr., A. L. Wing, and R. T. Hyde. 1978. "Physical Activity as an Index of Heart Attack Risk in College Alumni."*American Journal of Epidemiology* 108 (September): 161–175.

Paffenbarger, R. S., Jr., R. T. Hyde, A. L. Wing, et al. "Physical Activity, All Cause Mortality, and Longevity of College Alumni," *New England Journal of Medicine* 314 (March 10, 1988): 605–13.

Roberts, Glyn. 1992. *Motivation In Sport and Exercise.* Champaign, IL: Human Kinetics Publishers.

Rowland, Thomas. 1990. *Exercise and Children's Health.* Champaign, IL: Human Kinetics Publishers.

Safran, M. R., W. E. Garrett, A. V. Seaber, et al. 1988. "The Role of Warm-up in Muscular Injury Prevention." *American Journal of Sportsmedicine* 16(2): 123–129.

Stretching Scientifically, Kurtz, Thomas. 1990. Island Pond, VT: Stadion Publishing.

Summary of Findings from National Children and Youth Fitness Study II. *Journal of Health, Physical Education, Recreation and Dance.* November/December 1988, pp. 49–96.

"The Health Benefits of Exercise (Part II)." A Round Table. *The Physician and Sportsmedicine.* Vol. 15, No. 11. November 1987, pp. 120–31.

Training for Sports and Fitness, 1991. Rushall, Brent Pyke, Frank, *Mac Millian of Australia* 107 Moray St., S. Melbourne 3205, Australia.

Van Camp. S. P. 1984. "The Fixx Tragedy: A Cardiologist's Perspective." *The Physician and Sportsmedicine* 12(9): 153–55.

3
Strength and Flexibility

Chapter Objectives

After reading this chapter, you will be able to:

1. Identify five out of ten benefits of strength training.
2. List two out of eight cautions/disadvantages for strength training.
3. Identify two differences between training programs for strength and programs for muscular endurance.
4. Describe three types of muscle contraction and give an example of each.
5. Define three principles of strength training.
6. Identify correct safety guidelines for weight training.
7. List four out of five different types of strength programs.
8. List and define two types of stretching.
9. Identify correct guidelines for flexibility development.
10. Define the chapter terms.

Terms

- Agonist
- Antagonist
- Circuit
- Concentric contraction
- Dynamic flexibility
- Eccentric contraction
- Isokinetic

- Isometric
- Isotonic
- Muscular power
- Plyometrics
- Progressive overload
- Proprioceptive neuromuscular facilitation (PNF)

- Repetition (rep)
- Repetition maximum (1 RM)
- Set
- Static flexibility
- Stretch reflex
- Valsalva maneuver

*A*t one time, physical fitness programs consisted almost entirely of strength and flexibility exercises. Then, in the 1970s aerobic activities rose to prominence. As a result, strength and flexibility exercises were swept into the role of supplemental activities added to the main workout if time permitted. As people flocked to gyms for aerobics, they were exposed to weight training and began to value the benefits of muscular fitness. Today, as the emphasis on balanced fitness grows, strength and flexibility assume new importance. They can enhance ability to perform daily tasks as well as athletic performance. Muscular strength and endurance make it easier to perform routine activities such as carrying groceries upstairs or moving the couch. Flexibility enables us to reach, bend, twist, and perform movements without excessive tightness or stiffness. Enhanced strength and flexibility allow you to perform vigorous activity with less risk of straining muscles or connective tissue, so they are important in the prevention and rehabilitation of injuries.

Muscular Fitness

Many people start a muscular fitness program in order to look better, to shape and tone muscles, or to increase lean muscle mass. At the same time they increase muscular strength and endurance. In this section, we will first examine benefits, muscle structure and function, general principles, safety, and specific exercise programs for muscular strength and endurance. Flexibility development will be covered in the second part of the chapter.

Strength Training: Benefits and Cautions

An advantage of aerobic activities is their cardiorespiratory benefits. Strength training can offer additional benefits to the participant:

Weight Control   The more muscle a person has, the higher the metabolism, and the more calories are burned, even at rest. This is one reason why men can consume more calories than women of equal size and not gain weight—the average male has roughly twice the muscle mass of the average female. Muscle is active, high-metabolic tissue, while fat is storage tissue. Weight training increases muscle mass, so weight control is easier. While women do not appear to gain as much muscle as men do from weight training, when differences in body size are taken into account, gains are comparable. Over a 4 to 6 month period, a man may gain 4 to 6 pounds of muscle, a woman 2 to 3 pounds. Muscle is denser than fat, and pound for pound takes up less space, so as muscle is gained, if fat is lost, the result is a loss of unwanted inches. While aerobic exercise and a nutritious low-fat diet are the quickest ways to reduce body fat, weight training does offer advantages in long-term weight control.

Weight Gain   For those who wish to gain weight, increasing lean muscle mass, not fat, is a desirable goal, and there is no better way than weight training. Rate and quantity of muscle tissue gains vary from person to person, however, because they are partially genetically determined. Those with a naturally tall, lean build tend to gain muscle slower than those with a stockier build, and men gain faster than women. A weight gain program is outlined in the weight training section for those who wish to increase lean weight.

Appearance   Developing a lean, well-toned body is the main reason many people exercise. If you feel that you need to lose weight, but your body fat percentage is in the average range, reevaluate. Weight loss alone does not give a firm, well-toned appearance to flabby thighs or abdominals. Weight training is the most effective way to shape and tone muscles, resulting in a trimmer appearance. Posture improves. Strengthening weak muscles and stretching tight, inflexible muscles helps develop good body alignment so that you move more fluidly, feel and look better.

Time Economy   Instead of doing 50 leg lifts without weights, you can cut your workout time by adding resistance. Lift a weight heavy enough to produce fatigue in 8–12 repetitions, and you will get more benefit in fewer lifts. For basic strength fitness, a balanced weight-training workout of 10–12 exercises takes approximately 30 minutes to complete. Despite what you may observe in the gym, more is not necessary. While a body builder, competitive weightlifter, or other strength-event athlete will work out much more than this, keep in mind that they have different goals. Health-related fitness levels can be developed and maintained in much less training time than needed for competition.

Energy   Performance and efficiency improve—more work can be done with less effort as muscular strength and endurance increase.

Injury Prevention   Aerobic exercises such as jogging and aerobic dance have the potential to cause injury through repetitive, forceful impact against unyielding surfaces. Strong, flexible muscles and connective tissue can better withstand the stress of many forceful landings during a workout. When ligaments, tendons, muscle, and bone are strengthened through muscular exercise, risk of injury is decreased. Many aerobic activities tend to develop strength in only a few groups of muscles, leaving others weak. For example, jogging strengthens quadriceps but leaves the hamstrings weak. Weak muscle groups are more susceptible to strains or pulls. A well-designed strength-training program develops balanced, proportional strength in both agonists (prime movers) and antagonists (opposing muscle groups). If injury does occur, it may be less severe and may heal more quickly if the muscle is well-conditioned. A carefully designed program can also rehabilitate injuries to regain normal (or better) strength levels. For more detailed information on injury prevention, see chapter 5.

Bone Strength   Resistance exercises decrease risk of osteoporosis. The pull of muscles on bone in weight-bearing exercise stimulates development of increased bone density and preserves existing bone. Lifting heavy weights, a few repetitions may be more important than lifting many repetitions of a light weight for increasing bone mass.

Flexibility   Moving weights through a full range of motion, from full extension to full contraction both stretches and strengthens muscles. This is an important training technique to master in order to maintain flexibility. Muscles become shortened if exercises are performed repeatedly through a partial range of motion.

Cholesterol   Although little significant change in max VO_2 occurs, studies have shown a significant reduction in total cholesterol and total cholesterol/HDL ratio after 3–4 months of weight training. This may lower cardiovascular disease risk.

Social Benefits   In addition to the physical benefits, lifting with a partner or friend offers social benefits. There are a lot more opportunities for conversation and interaction when working out together than sitting watching a movie.

Disadvantages and Cautions   Although strength training has many benefits, it does have disadvantages, and you need to be aware of some cautions. Strength training is not a complete exercise program since it does not develop cardiorespiratory endurance. As in any physical activity, injury is possible if you are careless or ignore safety procedures. You may need access to equipment. Also, you can expect some mild muscle soreness during the first week of your program.

Medical guidance should be sought for individuals with cardiovascular problems or high blood pressure due to the tendency of blood pressure to increase during strength training. Those who have a hernia, arthritis, or lower back problems should also seek medical clearance. Individuals with these health concerns may benefit from strength training but should be aware that they may need special exercise modifications.

Avoid use of hand and ankle weights when jogging, doing high-impact aerobic dance workouts, or other activities involving running and jumping. Ankle weights, particularly, distort proper form, increase stress to legs and feet, and increase risk of strains and sprains. While small increases in oxygen consumption and caloric expenditure do result from using light weights, the same effect can be produced with less risk by exercising longer or harder.

When used with controlled form and rhythm in a muscle toning or walking program, however, light weights are beneficial for increasing heart rate and upper body strength. All in all, strength training offers few drawbacks and major advantages for the time invested.

Muscle Function

Muscles are made of individual muscle fibers, bound together and sheathed in connective tissue. They end in a tendon that connects the muscle to a bone. An example is the Achilles tendon, which you can feel above your heel, connecting your calf to your foot. Muscle fibers can contract to shorten the muscle or relax and return to their resting length. They are also elastic. They can be stretched and will spring back to their resting length. Muscles cannot expand and push. Movement is produced as muscle contracts, shortens, and pulls on bones across a joint. As a muscle on one side of a bone contracts, a muscle on the other side must

Figure 3.1
Bicep curl demonstrating muscle function.

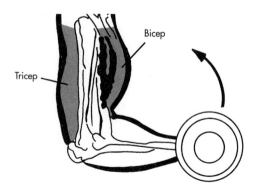

relax to allow movement to occur. The contracting muscle that initiates movement is called the **agonist.** The opposing muscle is called the **antagonist.** Performing a bicep curl, shown in fig. 3.1 for example, the agonist is the bicep, and the antagonist is the tricep. When performing a tricep extension, the roles reverse.

Determinants of Muscular Strength

Your potential for development of muscular strength is determined by the number and size of muscle fibers you possess and how well your muscular system can recruit them during muscular effort. The more muscle fibers you have, the larger they are, and the better your system is at activating them during muscular effort, the greater your strength. While the number of muscle fibers you possess is genetically determined, size and muscle fiber recruitment are a product of training.

Muscle Fiber Recruitment   When a muscle contracts, only the number of muscle fibers required for that momentary effort will shorten. Individual muscle fibers cannot contract partially. They either are working as hard as possible or not at all. This is called the "All-or-Nothing Principle." For example, when a bicep curl calls for a 50 percent effort, all fibers in the muscle do not contract at 50 percent effort; rather, only 50 percent of the muscle's fibers contract while the other 50 percent rest. After these first muscle fibers contract, fatigue slightly decreases their ability to apply force. On each subsequent contraction, more fibers must be recruited to continue to lift the same weight. After several muscle contractions, enough fibers are fatigued that the muscle temporarily can no longer generate the same effort. This is called temporary muscular failure. Muscle fibers increase strength only if they are stimulated by intensity of effort. If your goal is to develop maximal muscular strength, try to recruit, or activate, as many muscle fibers as possible by working a muscle to a state of temporary muscular failure. If you are working for health-related fitness levels, a less intense effort is adequate.

Muscle Hypertrophy   When muscles grow stronger, muscle fibers hypertrophy or increase in size. This occurs in both men and women and is proportional to muscle mass. Since the average man has about twice the muscle mass of the average woman, hypertrophy is more pronounced.

   Women are sometimes concerned that they will develop a massive, masculine musculature by weight training, and this myth is reinforced by televised images of women's bodybuilding competitions. Be assured that such significant muscle gains require years of strenuous daily effort. They don't occur by accident, nor with a 30-minute muscle toning workout three times a week.

Muscular Strength, Muscular Endurance, and Muscular Power

To increase muscular strength, endurance, or power, the key variables are resistance, repetitions, and speed. Strength is developed by contracting your muscles hard, at 80 percent to 95 percent or higher effort a few (3-6) times. Muscular endurance is enhanced by contracting repeatedly (i.e., 1-2 sets of 15–20 reps) with moderate (50%–60%) effort.

There is some crossover effect between muscular strength and muscular endurance. Development of muscular strength also produces some increase in muscular endurance; for example, if you can lift a 100-pound weight 5 times, you can probably lift a 5-pound weight 20 times. However, muscular endurance does not enhance strength. If you can lift a 5-pound weight 20 times, you may not be able to lift a 100-pound weight even once. If you want to develop both muscular strength and endurance, a muscular strength program can pay double benefits.

Muscular power, a function of strength and speed, is the ability to apply force rapidly. Power is increased by performing a muscle contraction quickly, as in plyometric exercises, discussed later in this chapter. While muscular power is not necessary for health-related physical fitness, it is an asset in many sports.

Types of Strength Training Programs

Three basic types of muscle contraction are isometric, isotonic, and isokinetic. Different strength programs have been developed for each type.

Isometric   *Iso* means equal or constant and *meter* refers to length. In **isometric** exercise, the muscle contracts but does not change length, and no movement occurs. If you pushed your palms together hard, your pectoral muscles would contract and try to shorten, but your arms would not move (fig. 3.2). An advantage of

Figure 3.2

Isometric Exercises (A) Pectorals (B) Upper back/triceps

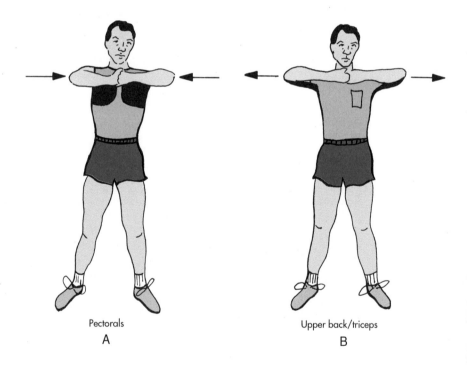

Pectorals
A

Upper back/triceps
B

Figure 3.2—*Continued*
(C) Inner thigh (D) Outer hip

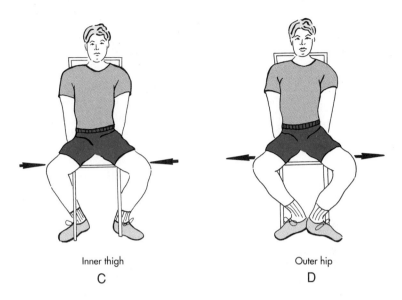

Inner thigh
C

Outer hip
D

isometric exercise is that it requires little or no equipment and can be done almost anywhere, for instance, while sitting at a desk. However, because resistance is applied at only one point in your range of motion, strength development is limited. Also, it is difficult to know how much force is being exerted, so strength gains are not as easy to observe as when equipment is being used. Three additional isometric exercises are illustrated in figure 3.2. Caution: For these and other strength exercises, breathe throughout the exercise. Do not hold your breath during exertion, as this can produce a potentially harmful elevation in blood pressure.

A. Pectorals. Press palms together at chest level for a count of five. Repeat 5 times.

B. Upper back/Triceps. Clasp hands together at chest level. Pull outward for a count of 5. Repeat 5 times.

C. Inner thigh. Sitting, place your knees outside the chair legs. Squeeze your thighs together for a count of 5. Repeat 5 times.

D. Outer hip. Sitting, place your feet inside the chair legs. Press out for a count of 5. Repeat 5 times.

Isotonic *Tonic* refers to tone or tension, so in **isotonic** exercise as the muscle contracts, tension, or force, is controlled throughout the motion. Isotonic contractions may be either concentric or eccentric. In a **concentric contraction,** a muscle shortens as it overcomes resistance. For example, a weight is lifted as the bicep contracts during the lifting phase of a bicep curl.

Eccentric contraction occurs when a muscle lengthens and contracts at the same time, gradually allowing a force to overcome muscular resistance; that is, the bicep contracts eccentrically during the lowering phase of a bicep curl. Eccentric contraction is an important component of strength development because it is half of the muscular effort.

Advantages of isotonic exercise are that it strengthens through a full range of motion, the load is measurable, and a variety of isotonic programs are available. Calisthenics, free weights, or machines such as Universal or Nautilus use isometric exercise.

Isokinetic   *Kinetic* means motion, and in **isokinetic** exercise, speed of movement is controlled. If you apply great force or a light force, the resistance is adjusted to maintain a constant rate of contraction. The advantage of isokinetic work is that the load is totally controlled by the efforts of the user. The disadvantage is that it requires special machinery, such as a Cybex or Orthotron, often used by athletic trainers for injury rehabilitation. You can get a sense of isokinetic movement by sweeping an arm through water. The harder you press, the more resistance you create.

Principles of Strength Training
Principles of strength development include progressive overload, specificity, and recovery.

Progressive Overload   **Progressive overload** is the most important principle of strength development. To stimulate a muscle to increase strength, it must gradually be overloaded, or forced to work at a higher than normal effort. Either the number of lifts performed, or amount of weight must gradually be increased. Increasing the number of repetitions increases muscular endurance. Increasing the weight lifted increases strength. General programs increase both until a desired maintenance goal is reached.

You must exercise three times per week to improve muscular fitness. To maintain strength, two intense workouts are adequate.

Specificity   The speed of contraction, range of motion, amount and type of resistance, and number and types of exercises are a few of the variables that determine results gained from strength training. If you desire a specific result, such as an increase in muscle mass, your program must be designed and executed to produce that result.

Recovery   Exercise provides a stimulus to the muscle to take in more protein and nutrients and undergo changes that increase its ability to forcefully contract. After a workout, you will be weaker, not stronger, due to fatigue. Improvement occurs during recovery, which gives the muscle fibers time to repair and grow. Strength workouts are best done every other day (48 hrs. rest) to allow recovery/improvement to occur.

Table 3.1

Safety Guidelines for Strength Training

> 1. Warm up before each workout, and stretch afterward.
> 2. Use good technique—keep your abdominals tight, back straight, hips tucked under, knees relaxed.
> 3. Work each exercise through a full range of motion from full extension without lockout to full contraction.
> 4. Perform each exercise smoothly, with control. Do not swing the limbs or use momentum. Faster is not better.
> 5. Before you lift, inhale, then exhale on the exertion. Do not hold your breath.

Guidelines for Strength Development

Optimal results can be obtained from any strength training program and risk of injury can be minimized if you follow the guidelines below and in table 3.1.

Sequence   Ideally, work large muscle groups first, ending with small muscle groups. It is difficult to adequately exercise large muscle groups if you have already fatigued the smaller supporting muscles. The suggested order of exercises is: hips/legs, torso, arms, abdominals (see sample weight training program).

Form   Never sacrifice form for weight. After progressive overload, correct exercise form is the most important (and most neglected) factor in maximizing strength gains and minimizing risk of injury. Improvement is more rapid if correct technique, not just quantity of weight, is emphasized. Always work through a complete range of motion for flexibility and maximum strength gains. Move from full extension without lockout to full flexion. Keep the back straight and abdominals tight to protect the lower back. In addition, when doing standing exercises, keep knees slightly bent and hips tucked under to support the back.

Avoid "cheating," a breakdown in exercise form that occurs when extra muscles are utilized to complete the exercise, decreasing the load to the prime mover. Cheating generally occurs when the load is too heavy or you are fatigued. Remember quality of work is more important than simply the amount of repetitions or weight lifted.

Muscle Balance   Since muscles work in pairs, it is important to strengthen muscles on both sides of a bone so that they pull evenly across joints and maintain body alignment. For example, if pectorals are stronger than upper back muscles, rounded shoulders result. When upper back muscles are strengthened, shoulders are naturally held erect. Tight lower back muscles opposed by weak, sagging abdominals pull the back into an exaggerated curve. This stresses lumbar vertebrae, increasing back fatigue and risk of lower back pain. Well-toned abdominals support the back, improve appearance, and prevent back problems. Strength programs must be planned to develop proportional strength in the following muscle pairs: biceps/triceps, pectorals/trapezius-rhomboids, abdominals/lower back, hamstrings/quadriceps, gastrocnemius/anterior tibialis, deltoids/latissimus dorsi (see figure 3.3).

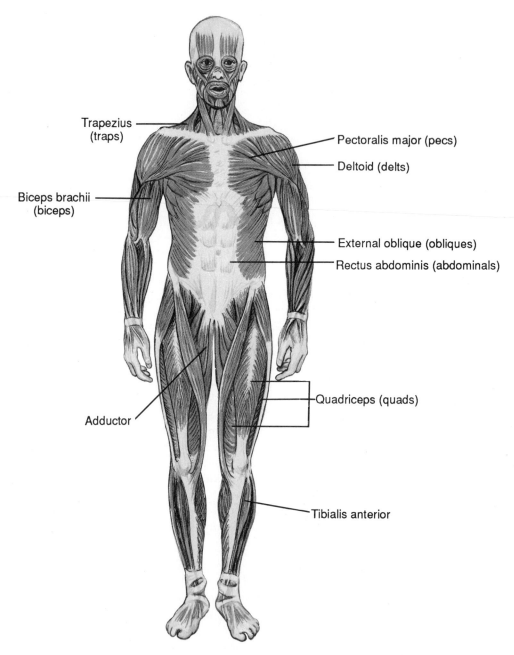

Figure 3.3A

Major muscles of the body (front).

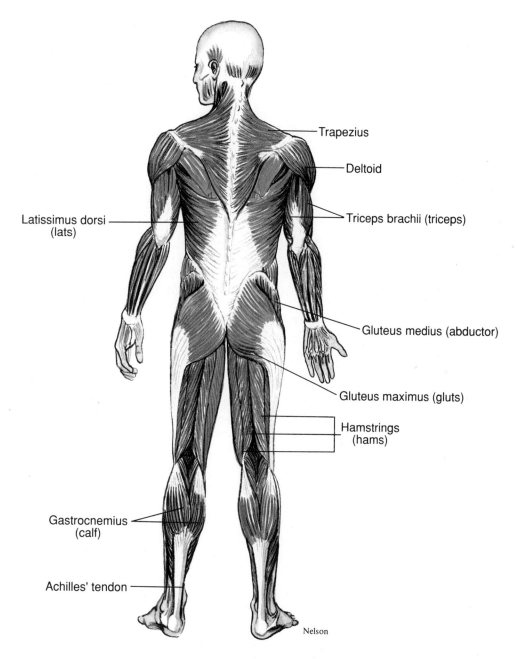

Figure 3.3B
Major muscles of the body (back).

Breathing   Exhale on the exertion, inhale on the release. Holding your breath while you strain against a closed epiglottis is called the **Valsalva maneuver** and can elevate blood pressure dangerously.

Speed of Movement   Exercising in a smooth, controlled manner maximizes strength gains and reduces injuries. Take two seconds to lift (concentric or shortening contraction), and two to four seconds to lower (eccentric or lengthening contraction). Control the movement, do not fling, swing, or kick. Jerky movements will cause excessive wear and tear on your joints. Also, when you use momentum to perform an exercise, you apply force and develop strength only through the first part of the movement. Lower a limb with the same control used to lift it. Do not drop weights with a crash. You are stronger lowering a weight than lifting.

Strength Training Programs

There are many different kinds of strength training programs. The type of program you select will depend on your goals and the type of equipment (if any) you plan to use. Regardless of the type of program you select, you can keep track of your progress with the Strength Training Log on page 421.

Weight Training

Weight training is a noncompetitive exercise program used to develop several health-related physical fitness components: muscular strength, muscular endurance, flexibility, and body composition. It differs significantly in its goals from competitive sports of weight lifting and bodybuilding. Male, female, young, old, athlete or fitness exerciser—all benefit from weight training. Beginners with low levels of muscular fitness benefit the most and will notice results more quickly than experienced lifters. Weight training can build strength levels so that recreational, competitive, or daily activities are accomplished more easily with less strain and fatigue.

What to Wear   Any comfortable workout gear will do. Shorts, T-shirt, and non-slip rubber-soled shoes are appropriate. A towel is useful for keeping sweat wiped off hands. Lifting gloves, which improve your grip, and a lifting belt to support the lower back and abdominals are not essential, though some lifters prefer to use them.

Equipment   For beginners, it really doesn't matter what type of equipment is used. A beginner will improve on almost any type of program as long as an adequate overload is provided. Two major types of equipment used in weight training are free weights and machines. Both have advantages and disadvantages.

Free weights are far less expensive than machines, so you can have your own set at home. Free weights cost about $100 on sale, double that if you add a padded bench and rack. Machines can cost upward of $500–$5,000. You have

Table 3.2
Safety Using Weights

1. Never attempt to lift more than you know you can handle. Work out—don't show off.
2. Always make sure that the weight pins, bars, or collars are secure.
3. Don't lift weights alone. Always work with someone else.
4. Keep sweat wiped off your hands; it makes weights slippery.
5. When using free weights, work with a trained spotter.

more variety of exercises on free weights than on machines because you have the freedom to lift in so many different positions. Lifting with proper technique is crucial. A wrong move can cause injury with any lifting, but particularly with free weights. To lift free weights safely, you must have a skilled spotting partner who can handle the weight in case you start to lose control. For strength development, free weights have an advantage over machines since they develop strength not only in the prime movers, but in muscles required to balance and control the weight. Follow the guidelines in table 3.2.

Machines such as Nautilus and Universal are easy to use and safer than free weights because they guide your movements and control the weights. An advantage of Nautilus equipment is that it prestretches the muscle and takes the joint through the full range of motion. Also, it provides variable resistance, adjusting the load to allow for strength variations throughout a lift. Universal gives the exerciser more control over range of motion and allows people to work more closely together. Because of their cost, it is best to start your program at a health club or Y. Proper lifting technique is easier to learn on machines, and you won't need a spotting partner. Loads can be changed quickly, so the workout may take less time than with free weights. For safety, convenience, and time, machines have the edge.

Program for General Conditioning A conditioning program should develop balanced strength. Many muscle strains occur because of weakness in the pulled muscle or its opposing muscle. A general strength program prevents strength imbalances. If you exercised only problem areas you would increase imbalances. The following exercises listed from large to small muscle groups may be done on Universal (see figure 3.4). Alternate free weight exercises are listed in parentheses. These may be done with a set of barbells or hand weights. If you plan to use Nautilus equipment, your first workouts should include instructions on how to adjust and efficiently use the equipment.

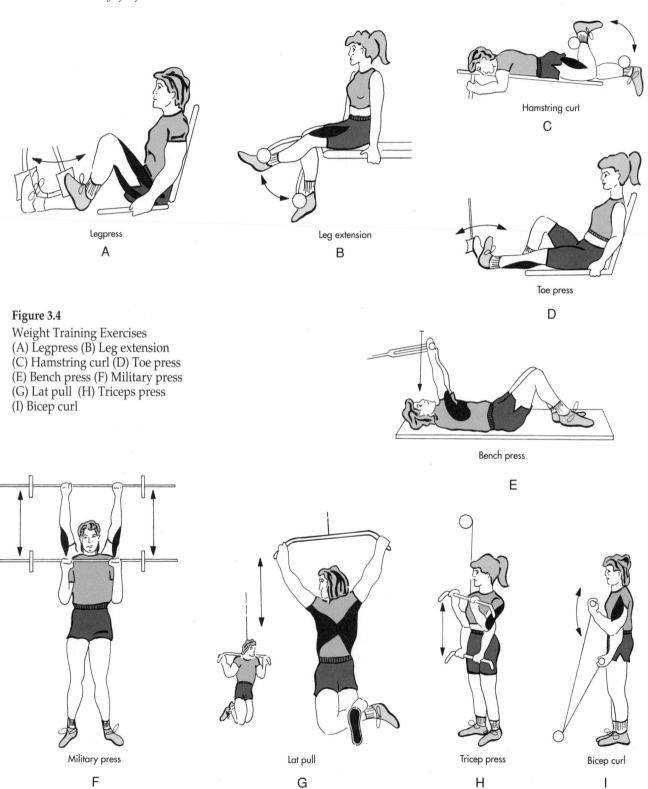

Figure 3.4
Weight Training Exercises
(A) Legpress (B) Leg extension
(C) Hamstring curl (D) Toe press
(E) Bench press (F) Military press
(G) Lat pull (H) Triceps press
(I) Bicep curl

Legpress
A

Leg extension
B

Hamstring curl
C

Toe press
D

Bench press
E

Military press
F

Lat pull
G

Tricep press
H

Bicep curl
I

Weight Training Exercises

A. Leg press (squats on free weights)
Prime movers: Quadriceps, hamstrings, and gluteus maximus

On leg press, sit on seat, adjust position to last slot or to a 90 degree knee angle. Place feet squarely on pedals, press out smoothly (do not lock knees), and return to starting position.

B. Leg extension (lunge on free weights)
Prime movers: Quadriceps

Sit on bench with both feet under the rollers. Toe in slightly. Do not lie back. Extend your legs, hold 1 second, and return to starting position.

C. Hamstring curl (squats)
Prime movers: Hamstrings and gluteus maximus

Lie face down on the bench, hook both heels under the rollers. Position your knees at the pivot point where the rollers attach to the bench. Pull up to 90 degrees, hold for one second, and return to starting position.

D. Toe press (calf raise with free weights)
Prime mover: Gastrocnemius

On leg press station, place feet squarely on pedals, press out to full leg extension without knee lockout. Press with toes from flat-footed position to foot extension, and return.

E. Bench press (same with free weights)
Prime movers: Pectorals and triceps

Lie on bench, head next to the machine. The grips should be lined up approximately with the shoulders. Place your feet flat on the bench with knees bent and back flat. Press to extension, and return.

F. Military press (same)
Prime movers: Deltoids and triceps

Sit on the stool or stand with abdominals tight, back flat, and knees slightly bent. With shoulders close to handles, extend upward with arms until they are straight but not locked, and return.

G. Lat pull (pullups or rowing with free weights)
Prime movers: Latissimus dorsi

Grip bar directly above shoulders or at handles. Pull down until you are kneeling or sitting. From this position, pull down chest or touch the back of shoulders, and return.

H. Tricep press (standing tricep press)
Prime movers: Triceps

Stand facing lat bar. With palms facing down, grasp the bar so that your hands are shoulder width apart. Keep elbows at waist. Press down to extension, and return.

I. Bicep curl (same)
Prime movers: Biceps

Stand facing the weights, hold bar with both hands, palms up. Flex arms until the bar meets your shoulders. Return to starting position. Keep back straight, abdominals firm.

How to Begin and Progress   A good general conditioning program would involve lifting 1–2 sets of 8–12 repetitions 3 times per week (for instance, M–W–F). A **repetition** (**rep**) is one lift; a **set** is a group of lifts.

The first week, a beginner should lift one set of 8–12 repetitions under the supervision of a trained professional. The first workouts should use light weights and concentrate on form, rhythm, and breathing. This will also minimize muscular soreness. The second week, an additional set can be added, and the third week, a starting load can be established.

Establishing Your Workload   To establish your workload, for each exercise find the maximum amount of weight you can lift once with good form (1 **repetition maximum** or **1 RM**). Take 75 percent of that weight, and that will be your workload. In the workout, lift to fatigue at each station. If you can do fewer than 6 repetitions, the weight is too heavy. If you can do 12 or more repetitions at that load, the weight is too light. Increase or decrease the load the next workout if necessary. At the correct workload, the last 2 repetitions of each exercise should be difficult for you to do, and you should reach fatigue between 8 and 12 repetitions.

Increasing Your Workload   When you can do 12 repetitions, increase the amount of weight. If you can do at least 6 repetitions at the new weight, stay with that weight until you can do 12 repetitions. If, when you increase the weight you cannot do at least 6 repetitions, drop back to your old weight and increase the number of repetitions each time until you can do 15. You should then be able to increase the weight and do at least 6 repetitions.

Variety   Variety can be incorporated by changing the workload, recovery period, number of sets, repetitions, rhythm, number or order of lifts. Here are a few examples of different programs:

1. General—2 sets of 8–2 reps at 70%–75% 1 RM. Rest 1–2 minutes between sets.

2. Strength—3 sets of 4–6 reps at 80%–90% 1 RM. Rest 2–4 minutes between sets.

3. Endurance—1–2 sets of 20 reps at 50%–60% 1 RM. Rest 30–60 seconds between sets.

4. Eccentric emphasis (negatives)— Lift 2 counts, lower 8. Some experts say that lowering the weight is more important to strength development than lifting it. This does tend to promote more muscle soreness. Strength increases occur with eccentric lifting alone.

5. Supersets—Work opposite muscle groups immediately (triceps/biceps, hams/quads)

6. Continuous set—Lift to muscular exhaustion at your regular weight, lower one plate and lift to exhaustion, continue to lower weight as you fatigue. This is a type of muscular endurance program. It is supposed to increase muscular definition, can be done with machines, but is difficult with free weights.

7. Pyramid—Lift 6 reps at 70% 1RM, 4 reps at 80% 1 RM, 2 reps at 90% 1 RM, 1 at 100% 1 RM. This program emphasizes strength.

8. Split routine—Work upper body one day and lower body the next day, or pushers (i.e., quads, triceps) one day, pullers (hams, biceps etc.) the next. You must work 6 days per week. This reduces total body fatigue but requires more time.

9. Aerobic circuit—Lighten weight to 40%–60% of 1 RM. Lift quickly 30 seconds (20 lifts), 30 seconds recovery while switching to the next station and setting the weight. Alternate a leg station with an arm station as you proceed through the circuit. As the goal is aerobic conditioning, you may also include a jump rope, bench step, jumping jack, or jogging in place station. Begin with 1 set of 10–12 exercises and work up to 3 sets, maintaining a target pulse. This is designed to strengthen the heart as well as develop muscular endurance. Be very careful to maintain good form—it is easy to get sloppy and hurt yourself in this workout because the lifting rhythm is so quick.

10. Weight gain program—A bulk-up of 3–5 sets of 5, gradually increasing to 10 repetitions at 70%–80% effort should be performed for several months to increase lean weight.

Common Discomforts   After lifting for a few weeks, you may notice a buildup of callus on your palms. If it bothers you, lifting gloves will offer some protection. If you experience nausea or lightheadedness, stop and figure out the cause. Did you allow enough time since your last meal? Are you exhaling on the effort? Are you trying to progress too quickly? If you experience pain, particularly joint pain, pay attention. It could be an early warning sign of injury. You may be lifting too heavy a weight or stressing your joints with poor form. Have a professional check your form periodically to make sure you are not falling into bad habits.

How to Shape and Tone without Weights

There are many different ways to develop muscular strength and endurance. While weight training is an excellent program, it is not always convenient. The programs described below can be done at home. The abdominal, hip and thigh, or upper body programs require no special equipment. Partner exercises add a social dimension to a workout. Elastic resistance produces results without bulky equipment. Finally, for those who enjoy a special challenge, add plyometrics to one or two workouts a week.

Abdominals, Hips, and Thighs   While weights add intensity to a workout, they are not always necessary when the goal is to shape and tone. Muscles develop firmness by working against a resistance, and that resistance can be your own body weight. This program emphasizes muscular endurance rather than strength by increasing repetitions. Abdominals, in particular, benefit from a muscular endurance routine because their function is one of endurance—sustained contraction. If you would like a total body program, combine this with the upper body routine that follows it.

These (fig. 3.5) exercises will not burn calories like aerobic work, so if you want to remove inches, diet and aerobic exercise are still important. Also, fat will not burn off just in the area exercised. While you can't spot reduce fat, say, in the thighs by doing leg lifts, you can spot tone flabby muscles. Be patient, and you may begin to see a difference in 8–12 weeks. You will want a mat or carpeted surface to work on. You do not need to count repetitions. Select one exercise for each body area, and perform it for one minute. Start with one set, and build up to two or three sets, three days a week. Variations are given to add variety to your program. If you wish to add intensity without purchasing weights, a sand-filled sock can be tied on as an ankle weight.

Figure 3.5

Abdominals, Hips and Thighs.(A) Abdominal curl "crunch"/Reverse abdominal curl (B) Oblique abdominal curl (C) Side leg lift (D) Inner thigh lift (E) Rear leg lift/Glute squeeze (F) Backward lunge/Wall sit

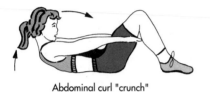

Abdominal curl "crunch"

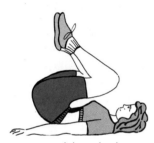

Reverse abdominal curl

A

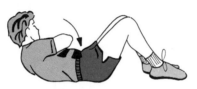

Abdominal curl "crunch"

B

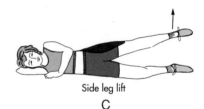

Side leg lift

C

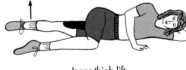

Inner thigh lift

D

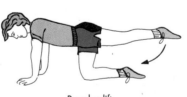

Rear leg lift

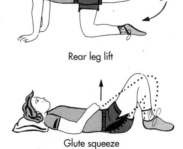

Glute squeeze

E

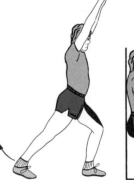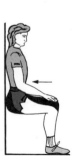

Backward lunge   Wall sit

F

Abdominals, Hips and Thighs

A. Rectus abdominis
  1. Abdominal curls
      Lie on back with knees bent, heels next to buttocks. Keep lower back on the ground, curl shoulders up 3 inches and return.

      Variations: Place one hand behind the shoulders to support the head, and reach the other hand through the knees. Do with feet raised or resting on a chair. Add resistance by moving hands from across chest to behind shoulders, or holding a 2 pound weight on each shoulder or behind the neck. Do not pull or jerk on the head.
  2. Reverse abdominal curls:
      From the starting position above, hold trunk steady and curl hips 1–2″ off the ground, then lower slowly.

B. Oblique abdominals
    Start in the same position as for abdominal curls, but add a twist bringing first right shoulder toward left knee, then left shoulder toward right knee. Variations: Cross right foot over left knee and twist right, then switch. Cross ankles, raise feet, and twist right, then left. Lay both knees to the left, curl toward the right hip, then switch. To increase resistance, hold a 2 pound weight on each shoulder.

C. Outer hip (hip abductors)
  1. Lying side leg lift
      Lying on one side, head resting on arm and lower leg bent for balance, slowly raise and lower top leg.

      Variations: This can be done standing. Keep foot level and leg lifting directly to the side, not toward the front.
  2. Kneeling side leg lift
      Take a hands and knees position with one leg extended to the side. Tighten abdominals, and round the back to protect it. You may also support weight on one forearm if desired. Tense the hip and raise and lower leg slowly no higher than 6 inches. Variations: Circle leg forward, reverse.

D. Inner thigh (thigh adductors)
  1. Inner thigh lift
      Lying on left side, raise and lower leg, keeping foot turned to the side (not upward). Repeat right. To increase resistance, press gently on left calf with right foot as you raise and lower leg, or add an ankle weight.
  2. Plié
      Standing with feet 3 feet apart and knees bent, place hands lightly on inner thighs. Press thighs against hands, pulling in hard for a count of 5. Repeat.

E. Gluteus
  1. Rear leg lift
      On hands and knees, hollow abdomen and round the back to protect it. Extend right leg to the rear. Tense gluteus. Raise and lower leg slowly 6–8″. Repeat left.
  2. Glute squeeze
      Lying on back with knees bent, squeeze gluteus hard, raising hips no more than 3 inches from floor. Do not arch back. Hold for a count of 5, relax, repeat.

F. Quadriceps, hamstrings
1. Backward lunge
    Keeping shoulders erect and weight centered over right foot, step back and touch lightly with the left foot, then return to starting position.

Repeat. Switch legs after 1 minute of repetitions.
2. Wall sit
    Hold a sitting position with your back against a wall for balance. Keep hips above knee level.

Upper Body Exercises Upper body exercises can improve appearance by straightening rounded shoulders, firming upper arm muscles, and toning pectorals that underlie and support the breasts. You do not need to count repetitions. Select one exercise for each body area and repeat for one minute. If you wish to increase resistance, bricks, books, or cans of food can serve as hand weights. Upper body exercises are illustrated in figure 3.6.

Figure 3.6
Upper Body Exercises (A) Push-ups
(B) Dips (C) Negative Pull-ups
(D) Shoulder shrug (E) Rhomboid row

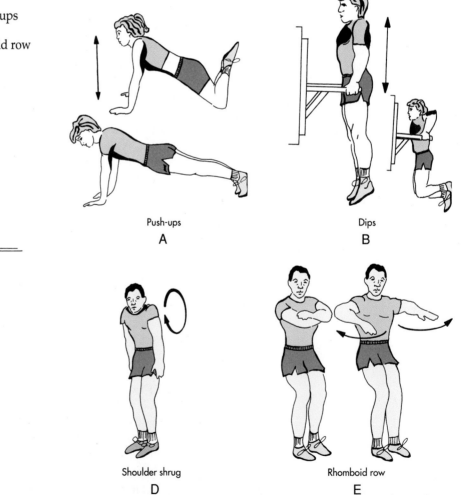

Push-ups
A

Dips
B

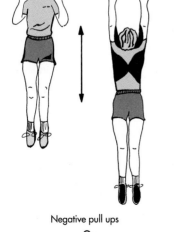

Negative pull ups
C

Shoulder shrug
D

Rhomboid row
E

Upper Body Exercises

A. Pushups (Pectorals/triceps)

These may be done standing, with hands against a wall and feet placed about 3 feet away from the wall (easiest), on the floor with knees bent (medium), or with weight supported on hands and feet (hardest). Keep abdominals firm and hips slightly flexed to support the back. Lower to right angles of the arms, then press back to arm extension. Variations: hands close emphasizes triceps. Hands wide increases pectoral strengthening.

B. Dips (Pectorals/triceps)

Dips are an alternative way to tone the same muscle groups as pushups. They may be done on a dip bar or using chairs. With weight evenly distributed between bars or two sturdy chairs, place a hand on each. Bend knees or extend legs so that weight is on arms, not feet. Bend arms to right angles, and return to extension.

C. Negative pullups (Latissimus dorsi/biceps)

Negative pullups offer the same benefits as full pullups for upper back and arms. Stand on a chair if necessary to grasp a pullup bar with arms flexed. S-L-O-W-L-Y lower yourself to a count of 5. As you gain strength over several weeks, try to start with a few full pullups and finish with negatives.

D. Shoulder shrugs (Trapezius)

Shoulder shrugs can tighten upper back muscles to reduce rounded shoulders. Combine this with pectoral stretches for best results. Rotate shoulders in full circles up-back-down, working to pull shoulder blades together. Variations: Add resistance by holding a weight in each hand.

E. Rhomboid row (Rhomboids)

Rhomboids are muscles that pull the shoulder blades back, down, and together. These also need to be strengthened to reduce rounded shoulders. With arms slightly below shoulder level, elbows bent, pull elbows fully back, squeezing shoulder blades together, and hold for a count of 5. Rest 2 counts. Repeat.

Elastic Resistance

Elastic resistance exercise was developed in the 1950s. It was originally used by physical therapists who gave patients surgical rubber tubing to add resistance to rehabilitative exercise programs. Elastic bands and tubing are lightweight, portable, and readily available at fitness centers and medical supply companies. They are inexpensive but do not last forever and need to be replaced as they wear out. Safety tips are listed in table 3.3. They come in different strengths, based on thickness of the elastic. Thin bands are best for beginners and upper body work. Thicker bands are useful for lower body work. Two thin bands can be used in place of one thick band. All principles of form, rhythm, and breathing apply here as for any strength training program. Elastic resistance exercises are illustrated in figure 3.7.

Table 3.3

Safety Tips for Elastic Resistance Exercise

1. Check the band for tears before every workout. Do not use it if it shows cracks or tears because it may break.
2. Point the band away from your face.
3. Sweat makes the band slippery—keep sweat wiped off.
4. Keep the wrist in line with the forearm—flexion against resistance stresses the carpel joints of the wrist.
5. Stretch the band slowly and release slowly, leaving light tension in the band. Do not let the band go slack.
6. Wearing socks can prevent the band biting into the ankles in the leg exercises.
7. Begin with 30 seconds of repetitions, and work up to 1 minute for each. Completing 2 sets is a good goal.

Figure 3.7

Elastic Resistance Exercises (A) Leg extension (quadriceps) (B) Hamstring curl (hamstrings) (C) Side leg lift (thigh abductors) (D) Inner thigh lift (thigh adductors) (E) Chest crossover (pectorals) (F) Deltoid raise (deltoids) (G) Left pull down (lats) (H) Rhomboid row (rhomboids) (I) Bicep curl (biceps)

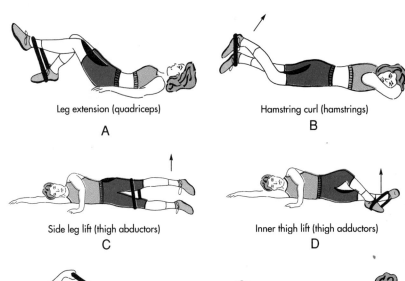

Leg extension (quadriceps)

A

Hamstring curl (hamstrings)

B

Side leg lift (thigh abductors)

C

Inner thigh lift (thigh adductors)

D

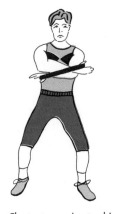

Chest crossover (pectorals)

E

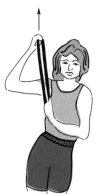

Deltoid raise (deltoids)

F

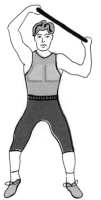

Lat pull down

G

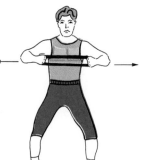

Rhomboid row (rhomboids)

H

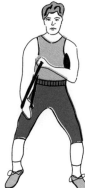

Bicep curl (biceps)

I

Elastic Resistance Exercises

A. Leg extension (Quadriceps)
Step on one end of the band with the right foot and hook the other end around the left foot. Lie back, knees bent and feet on floor. Keeping knees and thighs together, straighten knee, lifting the left foot as high as possible. Release and repeat. Change legs.

B. Hamstring curl (Hamstrings and gluteus)
Place the band around right ankle and arch of the left foot. Lie face down with arms under the chin or hands under hips. Bending knee, slowly lift left foot. Release slowly, maintaining some tension in the band. Repeat. Change legs.

C. Side leg lift (Hip abductors)
Place the band one inch above both knees. Lying on right side, torso supported by arms, slightly bend lower leg. Keep hips facing forward and lift left leg. Lower, keeping tension on the band, and repeat. Change sides.

D. Inner thigh lift (Thigh adductors)
Place band around right arch and left leg. Lie on left side, with trunk supported by arms. Lift left leg slowly, hold briefly, lower slowly, repeat. Switch legs.

E. Chest crossover (Pectorals)
Standing with back straight and abdominals tight, hold band in both hands, cross forearms in front, palms facing down, and press across chest. Keep arms slightly below shoulder level.

F. Deltoid raise (Deltoid and triceps)
Standing with good posture, hold one end of band under armpit and press other arm directly upward.

G. Lat pull (Latissimus dorsi)
Hold band overhead, elbow extended but not locked. Pull down behind head to shoulder level with other hand. Be careful not to get hair caught.

H. Rhomboid row (Rhomboids)
Hold band in front of body. Pull elbows back, pulling shoulder blades together. Release with control and repeat.

I. Bicep curl (Biceps)
Hold band in both hands, placing left hand on hip, palm down, and turning right hand palm up. Keeping elbow at your side, curl right arm to shoulder and slowly release.

Plyometrics

Plyometrics became popular in the 1960s when athletes in the Soviet Union and Eastern Block countries began using bounding and jumping drills to increase explosive power. They use the stretch reflex to convert the rapid stretching of a muscle into a forceful contraction.

For the experienced strength trainer, plyometrics can offer variety and additional challenge. Plyometrics are not for everyone, however. This is an intense high-impact activity that can injure joints not prepared for repetitive landings at 3–6 times body weight. A thorough warm-up beforehand is imperative. The safest application for plyometrics is as part of a water exercise program. Jumping, skipping, and bounding exercises can be done in waist-to-chest deep water safely with minimal impact stress.

Plyometrics should comprise no more than 10 percent to 15 percent of a program and should be done no more than twice a week. The landing surface should be resilient—mats, wood floor, grass, not concrete. It is best to do these at the beginning of a workout, before fatigue affects coordination. Do not do these if you are overweight, have leg or back problems, or are not in good fitness. The stress on muscles and joints is very high. With these precautions in mind, you might wish to work 1–2 of the exercises below into a circuit training program to increase lower body strength and power. A **circuit** is a group of exercises, each performed a certain number of reps or amount of time, generally at different exercise stations. Once all exercises have been completed, the circuit may be repeated. The plyometric exercises shown in figure 3.8 progress from elementary to advanced.

Figure 3.8
Plyometrics (A) Lunge walk
(B) Lunge jump

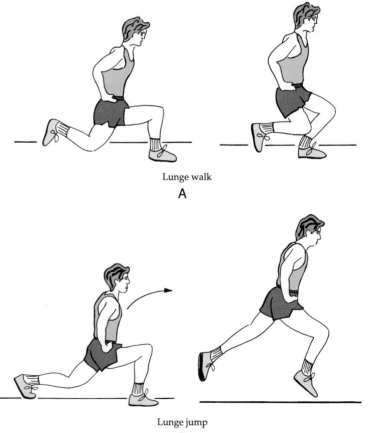

Lunge walk

A

Lunge jump

B

Figure 3.8 (Continued)
(C) Bounding run
(D) Bounding skip (E) Tuck
jump (F) Vertical squat jump
(G) Long jump

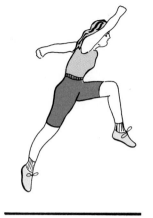
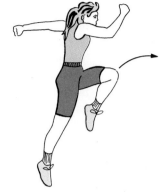
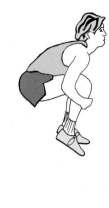

Bounding run
C

Bounding skip
D

Tuck jump
E

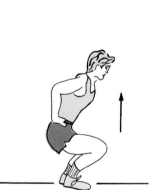
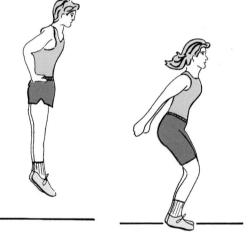

Vertical squat jump
F

Long jump
G

Plyometrics

A. Lunge walk
Step into a forward lunge, with
trunk erect and front leg forming
a 90 degree angle. Continue for
10 feet to 30 feet.

B. Lunge jump
Start in a lunge, dip slightly, and
explode upward, switching legs
to land with the other leg
forward. Continue for 10–30 feet.
To increase difficulty, keep
hands on hips.

C. Bounding run

Leap into the air, leading with the right leg and left arm. Land on the right leg and immediately drive the left leg and right arm into the air. There should be maximum hang time. Height, not forward momentum, is the object.

D. Bounding skip

Skip into the air, driving right knee and left arm high. Take off and land on the same leg, then switch. Again, aim for air time.

E. Tuck jump

From a standing position, bend at the knees and waist as you swing your arms behind you. Swinging the arms forward, jump vertically and grasp knees briefly with both hands. Land in place.

F. Vertical squat jump

With hands on hips, squat, explode up, and land, flexing knees.

G. Long jump

Using arms to add momentum and balance, perform a series of standing long jumps over a 10- to 30-foot distance.

Box Plyometrics

Box routines are excellent for building explosive leaping power. If you do not have a sturdy box, a bench or stair could be used.

Using an 8 inch–18 inch box or set of boxes placed 2 feet to 3 feet apart

1. Jump with two feet on, off, on, off.
2. Jump with left foot on, off, on, off. Repeat with the right.
3. Jump, two feet, over, over, over.
4. Step off a box forward/backward and rebound as high as possible.

Stair drills

Keep a hand on a rail for balance and use sets of 10 to 15 steps. *Walk down.*

1. With feet together, jump up one step at a time.
2. Jump up using only the left foot. Repeat with the right.
3. Jump, two feet, touching every other step.
4. Jump, one foot, touching every other step.
5. Sprint as quickly up stairs as possible, hitting every step.
6. Sprint, hitting every other step.

Partner Strength Exercises

Exercising with a partner can be both challenging and enjoyable. Partner communication and sensitivity to your levels of strength and fatigue are important. The partner must vary resistance for different muscle groups and increase resistance during the eccentric part of each contraction. While many of these exercises can be done without equipment, to add variety, you may wish to try them using a towel to pull on (bicep curls) or a broomstick (overhead press). This is a balanced program of 4 lower body and 5 upper body exercises. Do not count repetitions. Perform each exercise for a minute and work up to 2–3 sets (see figure 3.9).

Figure 3.9

Partner Strength Exercises (A) Leg extension (B) Hamstring curl (C) Inner/outer thigh press (D) Foot flexion (E) Overhead press (F) Lat pull (G) Elbow press forward (H) Elbow press backward (I) Bicep curl

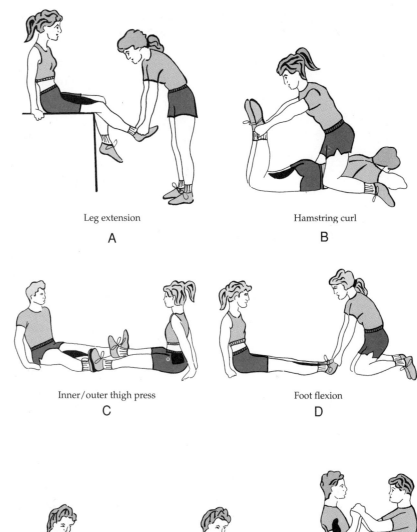

Leg extension

A

Hamstring curl

B

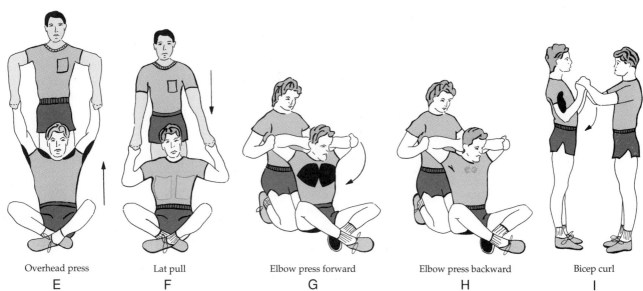

Inner/outer thigh press

C

Foot flexion

D

Overhead press

E

Lat pull

F

Elbow press forward

G

Elbow press backward

H

Bicep curl

I

Partner Strength Exercises

A. Leg extension (Quadriceps)
Sit on a bench or chair. Move one leg from flexion to full extension and back as partner resists by pressing on the front of the lower leg.

B. Hamstring curl (Hamstrings, gluteus)
Lie face down while partner straddles your thighs and places a hand on each ankle. Bend your knees and curl your calves toward your buttocks as your partner resists. Continue the resistance as you return to the starting position.

C. Inner/outer thigh press (Thigh adductors and abductors)
Partners sit, facing each other, legs forward, hands behind hips for balance. One partner places both feet inside the other's feet and presses outward as the other partner resists by pressing inward. Switch positions after 6–8 repetitions.

D. Foot flexion (Anterior tibialis)
Sit with legs extended. Partner kneels and presses down on top of both feet as you flex them, then return to extension.

E. Overhead press (Deltoids, triceps)
Sit with hands at shoulder level, palms up. As partner resists, press up toward the ceiling, then return to the starting position.

F. Lat pull (Latissimus dorsi)
Sit and reach high overhead to grasp partner's hands. As partner resists, pull down to shoulder level and slowly return to the starting position.

G. Elbow press forward (Pectorals)
Sit with elbows out and hands touching shoulders. As partner resists at the elbows, pull them in toward your midline and return to the starting position.

H. Elbow press backward (Rhomboids)
Sit with elbows out or with arms crossed. Partner sits behind, pressing on your elbows as you press back, pulling shoulder blades together. As partner continues resistance, return to starting position.

I. Bicep curl (Biceps)
Stand, palms facing upward. Partner resists on your palms as you curl your arm from extension to flexion and back. This may also be done holding a towel in one hand in front of body. Partner sits or kneels facing you, resisting on the other end of the towel as you curl your arm.

Flexibility

The ability to move your joints through their full range is an asset that can be maintained throughout life. As children, we are naturally flexible, but as we age, flexibility tends to decrease. Disuse, injury, excessive body fat, and muscle imbalances are common factors in this loss of range of motion. Youthful flexibility can be maintained by incorporating stretching into your regular workouts.

The flexibility exercises in this section are grouped as follows: a basic fitness flexibility program with exercises for joggers, walkers, aerobic dancers, cyclists, swimmers, and water exercisers; and examples of PNF partner-assisted stretches.

Flexibility Development: Benefits and Cautions

There are five main benefits to be gained from flexibility development:

- It decreases risk of injury. When tight muscles restrict the natural range of motion of a joint. The slightest unusual twist can cause a strain or pull, such as a strained hamstring. Inflexibility also is a precipitating factor in overuse injuries such as tendinitis, because inelastic muscles transfer excessive stress to even less pliable connective tissue.
- It decreases aches and pains. Tight, inflexible muscles pull unevenly across joints, causing skeletal misalignment, poor posture, unnecessary fatigue, and muscle and joint pain. Stretching can alleviate these problems.
- It increases ability to move freely and easily and to perform activities such as bending down to tie your shoes, scratching your back, or turning to look back as you are driving.
- It enhances athletic performance. In racquetball, golf, tennis, volleyball, or swimming, greater range of motion and ability to apply force through that range of motion can give a winning edge.
- It feels good to stretch. Stretching reduces muscular tension, promoting relaxation.

Cautions If carelessly done, stretching can cause injury. You must be careful not to overstretch, particularly when muscles are cold and tight. Stretching is not a competitive activity, so don't try to imitate the most flexible person in your class. Injured areas should be stretched with great care and not into pain, which risks reinjury. If you feel pain during stretching, particularly joint pain, stop!

Types of Flexibility

There are two basic types of flexibility: static and dynamic. **Static flexibility** refers to the range of motion you can achieve through a slow controlled stretch. **Dynamic flexibility** is the range of motion achieved by quickly moving a limb to its limits.

Static stretching techniques are those in which you slowly stretch a muscle to the point of tension and hold, such as holding a sitting hamstring stretch. The stretching force is provided by gravity or the force of one limb pulling on another. When a muscle is stretched and held at a constant length, after a period of time there is a slow loss of tension and gradual muscle lengthening.

Dynamic stretching programs employ swinging or ballistic moves, such as a high forward kick. Ballistic exercises may be useful in preparation for athletic activities requiring such moves, but they do carry increased risk that a muscle or joint could be overstretched, resulting in muscle or tendon tears and joint injury. Also, ballistic exercises initiate the **stretch reflex,** a natural response that causes the stretched muscle to contract. This contraction is designed to protect the muscle from being overstretched, but it also limits flexibility gains. While both types of stretching can increase flexibility, static stretching is preferred in health-related fitness programs because it is highly effective and carries little risk of muscle or joint strain.

Principles of Flexibility Training

Both types of flexibility are specific to the joint; that is, flexibility in one leg does not guarantee identical flexibility in the other leg, and flexibility in the shoulders does not ensure flexibility in the lower back.

An individual's flexibility range for any particular joint is not only specific but also partially genetically determined. You may have observed that some people seem to be naturally more flexible than others, even "double jointed" (they aren't really). Flexibility is determined by joint structure and elasticity of muscle and connective tissue. While you may not be able to change your genetics, you can improve your degree of flexibility within your genetically determined range of motion. A person who has never been able to touch his toes may, for example, be able to get inches closer with practice but may never be able to wrap his palms around his feet without bending the knees.

Flexibility gains are proportional to the overload applied; to the frequency, intensity, and time (duration) of stretching. Frequency: stretch at least 3–4 days a week, daily if possible. Greater flexibility is produced by more frequent stretching. Intensity: Low-intensity stretching is best. Progress at your own speed. Stretching is not competitive. Flexibility changes from day to day, and some days you might not be able to stretch as far as you did the day before. Stretch just slightly beyond the normal range of motion, to the point of tension and hold. Do not force a stretch. Time: many programs recommend a 10- to 30-second stretch, though holding up to 60 seconds in a cool down stretch can increase flexibility retention. The optimal number of repetitions has not been determined, but one 10- to 30-second sustained stretch for each muscle group should be considered a minimum, repeating once or twice if time permits.

While less flexible individuals may envy those who can do splits with ease, keep in mind that with flexibility, more is better only up to a point. There is concern (though no hard evidence) that excessive flexibility, unless accompanied by muscular strength, may increase joint laxity and susceptibility to injury.[1] For this reason, it is wise to combine stretching with muscle strengthening for optimal fitness benefits.

Guidelines for Flexibility Development

Everyone can benefit from flexibility. To maximize results from the time invested, implement the following guidelines into your next stretching session:

- Warm up before stretching. An increase in muscle temperature produced by fast walking, slow jogging, jumping jacks, or other large muscle exercise will make stretching safer and more productive. You are sufficiently warmed up when you begin to sweat.

- After warm-up, stretching is often used as preparation for activity. While some feel that stretching during warm-up decreases risk of injury in the activity that follows, there is no evidence that this is true. Warm-up stretching is different from a planned program of stretching for general flexibility. Warm-up stretching can be limited to what is essential, being careful not to overstretch. Stretch muscle groups used in the activity, hold at the point of tension for 5 to 10 seconds, and do not push for flexibility increases. Any gains will be minimal due to the tightening effect of the workout that follows.[2]

- Stretching for flexibility is most effective during a cool-down. Muscles are warmest and most elastic at this point. Stretching is easier. More permanent changes in muscle lengthening occur with low-force, long-duration stretching if muscles are allowed to cool in a stretched position. Cooling muscles before releasing tension apparently causes muscle collagen (connective tissue), like stretched taffy, to stabilize toward its new stretched length.[3]

- Stop at the point of tension, not pain. Stretching to the point of pain, or until muscles quiver, can risk overstretching injury.

- Don't bounce. A sustained stretch is more effective.

- Since flexibility is specific to a joint, a well-planned program for general flexibility will contain 8–12 stretches, one for each major muscle group. Warm-up or cool-down stretching may contain fewer exercises because they are activity specific and have different goals. Pay particular attention to body areas that are least flexible, and stretch them more often.

- Strive for muscle balance. When stretching muscles on one side of a joint, stretch those on the other side as well; for example, if you stretch hamstrings, stretch quadriceps too.

Flexibility Exercises for Basic Fitness

As part of a warm-up or cool-down, exercises 1–6 are important for runners, walkers, and aerobic dancers. Cyclists, swimmers, and water exercisers should add upper body stretches 7–10. If time is limited, save stretching for the cool down. For basic fitness flexibility, perform the full program of exercises in figure 3.10. Hold each 10 to 30 seconds, and repeat once or twice.

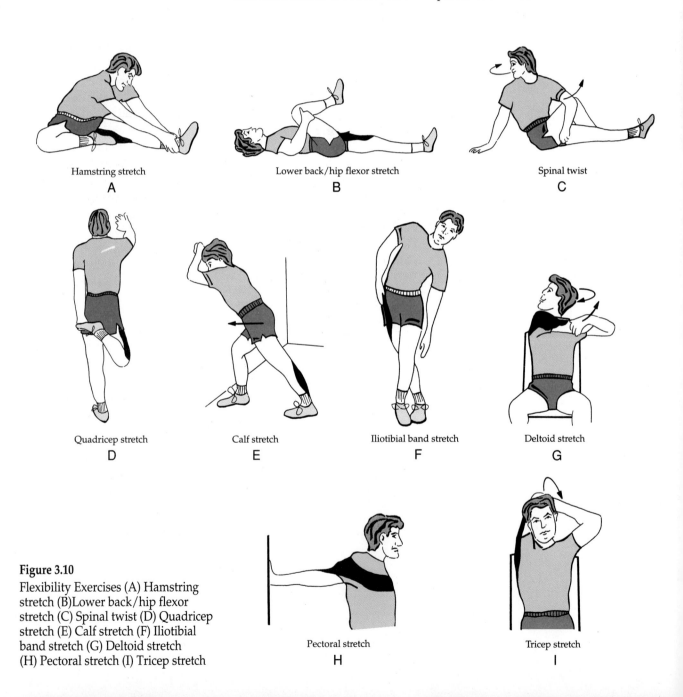

Figure 3.10
Flexibility Exercises (A) Hamstring stretch (B) Lower back/hip flexor stretch (C) Spinal twist (D) Quadricep stretch (E) Calf stretch (F) Iliotibial band stretch (G) Deltoid stretch (H) Pectoral stretch (I) Tricep stretch

Flexibility Exercises

A. Hamstring stretch
Keeping shoulders erect, press abdomen forward. Hold. Repeat with other leg.

B. Lower back/hip flexor stretch
With hands behind thigh, press thigh toward chest. Keep extended leg straight. Repeat left.

C. Spinal twist (Lower back and hip abductors)
Sit with right leg extended, step left leg over right, and turn upper body toward the left. Repeat on the other side.

D. Quadricep stretch
With left hand, pull right heel toward buttocks. Keep shoulders up, abdominals tight, and hips tucked under to prevent back hyperextension. Omit if you have knee problems.

E. Calf stretch
Standing in a forward lunge position, toes pointing forward, press heel toward floor. Repeat with other leg.

F. Iliotibial band stretch
Cross left foot over right, press hips to the left. Repeat to the other side.

G. Deltoid stretch
Cross right arm in front of body, pull it in toward midline with left hand.

H. Pectoral stretch
Place right hand on wall, elbow extended but not locked. Twist shoulders left. Repeat with left arm.

I. Tricep stretch
Pull left elbow behind head. Repeat right.

PNF Partner-Assisted Stretches

A type of static stretching called **proprioceptive neuromuscular facilitation** or **PNF,** a partner-assisted stretch often used by athletic trainers, is one of the most effective methods known for increasing flexibility. To perform a PNF stretch, you first perform a static stretch, then contract the muscle to produce fatigue, then relax while a partner stretches your limb.

It is important to be sensitive to your partner's needs and flexibility levels. Be sure to communicate when more/less resistance or pressure is needed throughout each exercise. Work with the same partner throughout the series. Switching partners can lead to injury because of unfamiliarity with the flexibility limits of the person being stretched. Some examples of PNF stretches are illustrated in fig. 3.11. Consult suggested readings for more ideas.

Figure 3.11
PNF Partner-Assisted Stretches
(A) Hamstring stretch (B) Inner thigh
stretch (C) Gluteal/lower back stretch
(D) Pectoral stretch

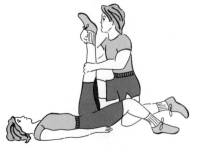

Hamstring stretch

A

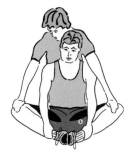

Inner thigh stretch

B

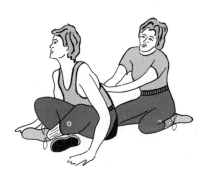

Gluteal/lower back stretch

C

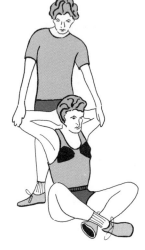

Pectoral stretch

D

PNF Partner-Assisted Stretches

A. Hamstring stretch
Lie on your back and lift one leg
into the air. Partner supports
ankle and knee in a static stretch.
Next, keeping knee extended but
not locked, push against your
partner as he resists. Then relax,
as partner eases leg into a new
stretch.

B. Inner thigh stretch
Sit with knees out and bottoms of
feet together. Press down on
knees in a static stretch. Next,
partner kneels behind and resists
on knees as you press them
upward. Finally, relax as partner
gently presses them toward the
floor in a stretch.

C. Gluteal and lower back stretch
Sit cross-legged and stretch
forward. Partner kneels behind
you with hands on your upper
back. Next, resist back against
partner. Then, stretch forward as
partner assists.

D. Pectoral stretch
Sit cross-legged with your fingers
interlaced behind your head and
back supported by your partner's
thigh. Partner gently pulls your
elbows back for 10 seconds, then
resists as you attempt to pull
them forward. Next, relax as
partner gently stretches them
back.

Summary

Muscular strength, muscular endurance, and flexibility exercises are a vital supplement to a regular program of aerobic exercise. They can enhance appearance by improving the shape, firmness, and tone of muscles. Enhanced posture, decreased risk of lower back pain, greater ease of movement, and more energy are benefits. While injury is possible in any exercise program if safety guidelines are ignored, sensible strengthening and stretching programs generally decrease risk of injury for those who participate in health-related fitness programs or athletics.

References

1. Alter, Michael J. *Science of Stretching* Human Kinetics Books, Champaign, IL, 1988.

2. Alter.

3. Alter.

Suggested Readings

Alter, Michael J., 1990. *Sport Stretch.* Champaign, IL: Leisure Press..

Berger, Richard A., 1991. *Introduction to Weight Training, 2nd ed..* NY, NY: Prentice-Hall.

Chu, Donald A., 1992. *Jumping into Plyometrics.* Champaign, IL: Leisure Press.

Hesson, James, 1991. *Weight Training for Life, 2nd ed.* Englewood, CO: Morton Publishing.

Institute for Aerobics Research Staff, 1990. *The Strength Connection: How to Build Strength and Improve the Quality of Your Life.* Dallas, TX: Institute for Aerobics Research.

Kalvin-Stiefel, Judy, 1992. *Defining Woman: Natural Body Workout for Body and Mind.* Peelsicin, NY: Bywood Publications.

Lycholat, Tony, 1991. *The Complete Book of Stretching.* Crowood, UK: Trafalgar Publishing.

Miele, Mark, 1992. *The Dumbbell Book: Fitness without a Gym.* West Palm Beach, FL: Sand Dollar Publishing.

Moran, Gary and George McGlynn, 1990. *Dynamics of Strength Training.* Dubuque, IA: Wm. C. Brown Publishers.

Robinson, Jerry, 1993. *The Weightless Workout.* Los Angeles, CA: Health for Life.

Seidler, et al., 1991. *Weight Training and Fitness for Health and Performance.* Dubuque, Ia: Kendall-Hunt.

Spring, H., 1990. *Stretching and Strengthening Exercises.* New York: Thieme Medical Publishers.

Tobias, Maxine. 1993. *New Stretching Book.* New York: David McKay Co, Inc.

Wescott, Wayne, 1991. *Strength Fitness: Physiological Principles and Training Techniques, 3rd ed.* Dubuque IA: Brown and Benchmark Publishers.

4
Fitness Assessment

Terms

- Exercise tolerance test
- Fat-free tissue
- Lean body mass
- Skinfold calipers
- Subcutaneous fat

*P*hysical fitness tests are often divided into two categories: health-related and skill-related. Skill-related tests, such as a vertical jump or shuttle run, are performance-based and are related to athletic ability. Health-related tests are related to functional well-being in the areas of cardiorespiratory endurance, muscular strength and endurance, flexibility, and body composition. These areas of physiological functioning can be improved or maintained through regular exercise and offer protection from the negative effects of a sedentary lifestyle.

Do you know how fit you are? We all seem to have a natural curiosity about how we compare to others. The main purpose of fitness testing is to help you identify your current fitness levels in several health-related categories. Such an evaluation should tell you whether your current lifestyle is effective in developing and maintaining a level of fitness conducive to optimal wellness. Your results can be used as a basis for setting personal fitness goals, for developing an appropriate individualized exercise prescription, and finally, for measuring the effectiveness of your fitness program in reaching your goals. This chapter gives norms that enable you to compare your fitness levels with other college-age students. *Norms are for people under 30 years of age* and reflect achievements of people who have completed a fitness course.[1] If you are over 30, you may wish to consult the suggested readings at the end of this chapter for resources containing norms appropriate for your age group. When evaluating your fitness and setting goals, keep in mind that scoring in the "poor" category does not reflect negatively on you as a person. While "superior" is an attainable goal for some, relatively few people achieve this level in one or more areas of fitness. Bodies are different. Physical capacity to achieve any particular level of fitness is partially genetically determined. You may find that you gain strength easily but must constantly work on flexibility, or vice versa. Health-related fitness benefits can be experienced at the "average" fitness level. Also keep in mind that all tests are subject to some measurement variability. Use these norms as guidelines. Finally, testing should not dominate your program but help you measure its effectiveness. You may wish to measure at the beginning of your program, and remeasure eight weeks into the program to see how you are progressing.

A Personal Fitness Profile is located in the student activities section at the back of the book. When completed, it will indicate areas of fitness you can maintain and areas needing improvement. It will help you decide where to begin in your fitness program.

Guidelines for Medical Clearance

According to American College of Sports Medicine guidelines[2], it is generally safe to begin a vigorous exercise program if you are under 40 years of age for men, under 50 for women, are healthy, and have had a satisfactory medical checkup in the past two years. Also, if you have been exercising regularly, it is probably safe to continue progressing gradually from your current activity level. Prior to participation, you should complete the Health/Exercise Assessment Form found in the student activities section to identify any potential health concerns.

If you are over the age guidelines, or if, regardless of age, you have had health concerns noted on the Health/Exercise Assessment Form, it is important to check with your personal physician before taking a cardiorespiratory fitness test or participating in vigorous exercise. The Exercise Clearance Form in the student activities section is designed to assist your instructor in individualizing your fitness program according to your physician's recommendations. You may need to have a medical checkup and diagnostic exercise test. If you smoke cigarettes, have been sedentary over the past several months, have diabetes, are 20 or more pounds overweight, or have family members who have positive risk factors for heart disease, it is particularly important that you see your physician. Also, check with your physician if you are unsure or have concerns about your health.

Cardiorespiratory Endurance

A high level of cardiorespiratory fitness permits a person to do more work with less fatigue as compared to a person with a low cardiorespiratory fitness. Increased cardiorespiratory fitness can enhance quality of life by increasing the rate of energy production during physical activity. Low levels of cardiorespiratory fitness may result in a limited lifestyle due to low energy reserves, quick exhaustion with moderate exertion, and resulting inability to participate in vigorous, oxygen-demanding activities. High-level wellness is inextricably tied to a physically active lifestyle. If you want to be an active participant in life—not just a spectator—cardiorespiratory fitness is essential. The ability of your heart and lungs to supply oxygen during activity is one of the best indicators of overall physical fitness. There are several ways to measure your body's ability to use oxygen. The most accurate method is an **exercise tolerance test** on a treadmill or on a bicycle ergometer in a laboratory (fig. 4.1). In an exercise tolerance test, a person exercises strenuously while heart rate and oxygen consumption are measured. This, however, is complex, expensive, time consuming, and requires elaborate equipment and trained personnel. It is impractical for testing large numbers of people.

Figure 4.1
Treadmill exercise tolerance test

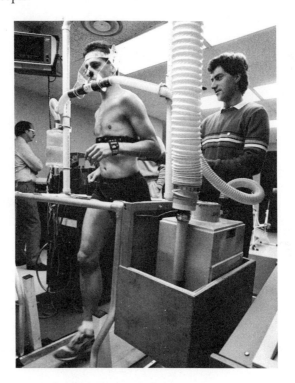

Cardiorespiratory fitness can also be measured in field tests conducted out of the laboratory setting. What they lose in accuracy, they make up in the practicality for self-testing or testing many people at the same time. Field tests of cardiorespiratory endurance are generally based on physiological performance (distance or time tests) or a parameter such as pulse rate (step test).

A field test used to estimate oxygen consumption is to measure the time it takes you to jog 1.5 miles. Studies have shown that time on the 1.5-mile run correlates well with maximal oxygen uptake. The faster you cover the distance, the more efficient your heart and lungs are at their job of supplying oxygenated blood and nutrients to the working muscles and in carrying away waste products. Field tests make it easy for you to measure your own fitness and to detect progress as you train. You should only take the 1.5-Mile Run Test if you are conditioned

Cardiorespiratory potential varies among individuals.

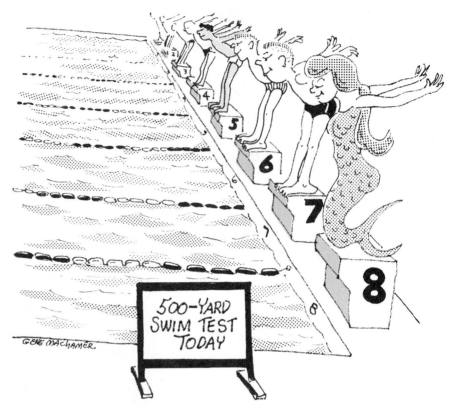

for it. Other field tests that measure cardiorespiratory endurance include the 1-Mile Walk Test, the 5-Mile Bicycling Test, the 500-Yard Swim Test, the 500-Yard Water Run Test, and the Step Test. You can choose the test most appropriate for your chosen physical conditioning activity.

General Instructions

For any of the cardiorespiratory endurance tests you will need comfortable clothes appropriate for the activity and a stopwatch or a watch with a second hand. If possible, avoid taking the test under conditions of extreme heat or cold, particularly if you are not accustomed to exercising under those conditions. Do not eat a heavy meal or smoke for up to three hours prior to the test. Rest from vigorous exercise at least one day prior to taking the test. Warm up and stretch before taking the test, then cool down and restretch afterward. If at any point during the test you begin to feel ill, dizzy, faint, or extremely short of breath, stop! Your body is telling you that you are not yet ready for this level of exertion. Do not be ashamed of stopping before completing the test, especially if you are unfit. Test performance may be limited by local muscular endurance or by aerobic capacity. You may record the amount of time in the test you were able to complete and work toward a fitness level that will enable you to complete the test.

1.5-Mile Run Test

The 1.5-Mile Run Test requires six laps around a standard quarter-mile track, or it can be done on a measured section of road. You should consider taking this test only if you have been exercising previously. The 1-Mile Walk Test may be more appropriate for you if you are over 35 years of age, 20 or more pounds overweight, or have been out of shape for quite some time, but are otherwise in good health.

Goal: To run 1.5 miles as quickly as you can.

Directions:

1. Locate a standard quarter-mile track, or measure a section of road that has few stoplights.
2. Have a stopwatch or a watch with a second hand.
3. Warm up before taking the test.
4. This is a test of your maximum capacity, so do the best you can. Push yourself to cover the distance as fast as possible without overdoing. Try to maintain a continuous, even pace. Run as long as you can, then walk when necessary. If you are running with a group, it is helpful if runners are given the right-of-way on the inner lanes and if people will move to the outer lanes when they need to walk.
5. When you complete the 1.5-mile distance, record your time and cool down with walking and stretching.
6. Check table 4.1 for your fitness level.

Table 4.1

1.5-Mile Run Norms

	Men	Women
Excellent	<8:26	<10:52
Good	8:26–10:21	10:52–13:40
Average	10:22–12:17	13:41–16:28
Poor	12:18–14:14	16:29–19:16
Very Poor	>14:14	>19:16

1-Mile Walk Test

For those starting a walking program, or for whom the 1.5-Mile Run Test may be too vigorous, the 1-Mile Walk Test is an option. You will need a one-mile measured course (four laps of a quarter-mile track), your walking shoes, and a watch with a second hand.

Goal: To walk one mile as quickly as you can.
Directions:

1. Warm up and stretch before beginning.
2. Walk one mile as quickly as you can.
3. Record your time to the nearest second.
4. Cool down and stretch.
5. Locate your fitness level in table 4.2.

Table 4.2
1-Mile Walk Norms

	Men	Women
Excellent	<11:07	<12:02
Good	11:07–12:31	12:02–13:05
Average	12:32–13:56	13:06–14:10
Poor	13:57–15:20	14:11–15:14
Very Poor	>15:20	>15:14

5-Mile Bicycling Test

If your main fitness activity is bicycling, you can test your cardiorespiratory fitness with a timed 5-mile bicycle ride. This test can be done on a bike track or on a measured section of road with few stoplights or stop signs.

Goal: To bicycle five miles as quickly as possible.
Directions:

1. Warm up by riding for a few minutes and stretching.
2. Cycle the five miles as quickly as you can. If you are doing this on the road, be careful to obey all traffic rules.
3. Try to pace evenly. Time the ride with a stopwatch or a watch with a second hand. Record the time.
4. Cool down and stretch.
5. Check your results with table 4.3.

Table 4.3
5-Mile Bicycling Norms

	Men		Women	
	Track	**Road**	**Track**	**Road**
Excellent	<12:13	<14:00	<13:18	<15:30
Good	12:13–13:16	14:01–15:20	13:18–14:28	15:31–16:50
Average	13:17–14:20	15:21–17:00	14:29–15:38	16:51–18:30
Poor	14:21–15:24	17:01–18:30	15:39–16:49	18:31–20:00
Very Poor	>15:24	>18:30	>16:49	>20:00

500-Yard Swim Test

If your fitness program primarily involves swimming, you will find a swimming endurance test useful. A regulation 25-yard pool is recommended, and you will need a friend to time you. You may swim any stroke, although best results will be obtained with the front crawl.

Goal: To swim 500 yards as quickly as you can.

Directions:

1. Warm up.
2. Have a friend time you and count lengths. In a 25-yard pool, 500 yards is 20 lengths.
3. Record your time, cool down, and stretch.
4. Check table 4.4 for your fitness level.

Table 4.4

500-Yard Swim Norms

	Men	**Women**
Excellent	<6:12	<7:05
Good	6:12–7:44	7:05–8:49
Average	7:45–9:19	8:50–10:34
Poor	9:20–10:52	10:35–12:19
Very Poor	>10:52	>12:19

500-Yard Water Run Test

The 500-Yard Water Run Test (fig. 4.2) was designed for those involved in an aerobic water exercise program in which swimming skills are not required. It can be done lengthwise in a pool of constant depth or widthwise across the shallow end of a pool of variable depth. It helps to work in pairs, with one partner on deck counting completed laps for the other. For most accurate results, runners should carve their own paths through the water and avoid drafting in the wake of another runner. Runners should use their arms to pull as they run but must maintain a vertical body position. No swimming is allowed.

Goal: To run 500 yards in the water as quickly as possible.

Directions:

1. Measure pool width and calculate the number of lengths required to cover 500 yards.
2. Have a partner on deck count laps and keep the time.
3. Warm up with a couple minutes of easy jogging in the water.
4. To give runners of different heights a similar level of water resistance in a variable depth pool, select a starting point along the pool wall where the water level is at a midpoint between the runner's navel and nipple. Shorter runners will start in

Figure 4.2
The 500-Yard Water Run is a valid field test for nonswimmers. (Note: the water level should be midpoint between navel and nipple.)

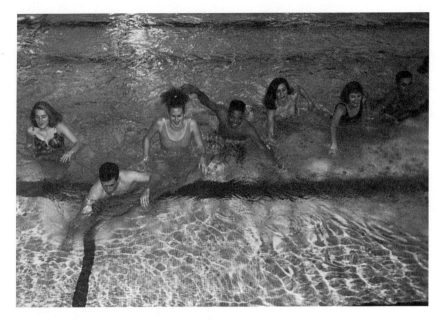

shallower water, taller runners in deeper water.

5. Take a position in the water, note your starting time, and run the necessary number of widths.

Record your time to the nearest second.

6. Cool down and stretch.

7. Check table 4.5 for your fitness level.

Table 4.5
500-Yard Water Run Norms

	Men	Women
Excellent	<6:48	<7:57
Good	6:48–7:26	7:57–8:37
Average	7:27–8:05	8:38–9:18
Poor	8:06–8:44	9:19–9:59
Very Poor	>8:44	>9:59

3-Minute Step Test

There are a variety of step tests useful for testing cardiorespiratory fitness indoors. They involve stepping on and off a bench for a 3- to 5-minute period and measuring the heart rate recovery. The step test is based on the fact that the heart rate of a person who is physically fit is lower at any work load and recovers faster than the heart rate of a person who is unfit. Although it is not the best measure of cardiorespiratory fitness, it is a quick and simple way to evaluate the heart's response to exercise. It is easy to administer to an individual or to large groups, requires no special skill to perform, and requires little equipment (see fig. 4.3).

Figure 4.3
Step test

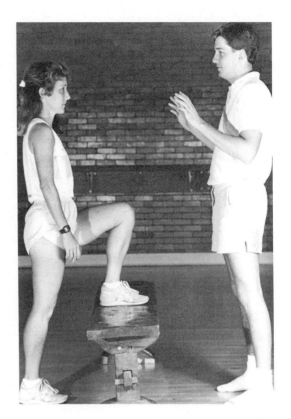

Goal: To step on and off a bench for three minutes.
Directions:

1. Locate a 15-inch bench or a 16-inch rollout bleacher step.
2. Warm up.
3. Work with a partner. While one partner is stepping on and off the bench, the other partner (tester) stands in front of the person being tested, to stop the partner from falling, should he stumble.
4. You will need to step up and down at 96 counts per minute. A metronome or recorded music at a tempo of 96 beats per minute will help you keep cadence, or your instructor will call the cadence, "Up-up-down-down." At the signal "Begin," step up with your right foot, left foot, then down right, left, and continue for three minutes. Straighten your knees as you step up on the bench. To prevent leg soreness, you may want to switch lead legs about halfway through the test.
5. Stop at the end of three minutes and sit down. Five seconds after completing the test, the tester counts the partner's pulse for 15 seconds. The tester can check the partner's carotid pulse by lightly pressing against the neck under the jawbone. The partner being tested can double-check his or her own pulse at the radial artery, located on the thumb

side of the wrist. The partners' pulse counts should not vary more than one or two beats if they count accurately.

6. Record the pulse.
7. Cool down and stretch.

8. Compare your pulse with norms given in table 4.6 to assess your cardiorespiratory fitness. If you are unable to keep the cadence for the full three minutes, consider yourself to have very poor cardiorespiratory endurance.

Table 4.6
3-Minute Step Test Norms

	Men	Women
Excellent	<31	<37
Good	31–37	37–41
Average	38–41	42–44
Poor	42–45	45–49
Very Poor	>45	>49

Muscular Strength and Endurance

Muscular strength and endurance are assets in the ability to perform daily activities—lifting, carrying, pushing, pulling—without strain or undue fatigue. Strength and endurance of the abdominal muscles are particularly important for good posture and lower back health. Muscular fitness activities add shape and firmness to muscles, resulting in a trim, well-toned appearance.

Muscular strength and muscular endurance tests have been used as a measure of physical fitness for years. Physical conditioning activities require and can develop both components. Strength is best developed by weight training and is often measured by one maximal lift with weights (see chapter 3). Muscular endurance can be measured without special equipment, using tests provided here. Abdominal curls are perhaps the best way to assess the endurance of the abdominal muscles. The traditional bent-knee sit-up test requires use of the thighs and hip flexors as well as abdominals and may put the back at risk. Abdominal curls isolate and test only abdominal muscles, decreasing risk to the lower back. Directions and norms for abdominal curls are given. To test the muscular endurance of the arms and upper body muscles, norms are also given for push-ups.

Abdominal Curls

Goal: To complete as many abdominal curls as possible in one minute.
Directions:

1. Tape a strip on the floor three inches wide and lie on the floor with fingertips at the edge of the strip. Bend your knees and bring your heels as close as possible toward your hips.

2. Curl forward until your fingertips have moved forward three inches, then curl back until your shoulder blades touch the floor. Your shoulders should lift from the floor with each curl, but the lower back should stay on the ground. If you are working with a partner, your partner should not hold your feet down, nor should your feet lift off the ground, or you are curling too high (fig. 4.4).

3. Complete as many curls as possible in one minute; then check the results in table 4.7.

Table 4.7

1-Minute Abdominal Curl Norms

	Men	Women
Excellent	>95	>88
Good	82–95	76–88
Average	68–81	63–75
Poor	54–67	49–62
Very Poor	<54	<49

Figure 4.4

Abdominal curls (fingertips move forward 3 inches)

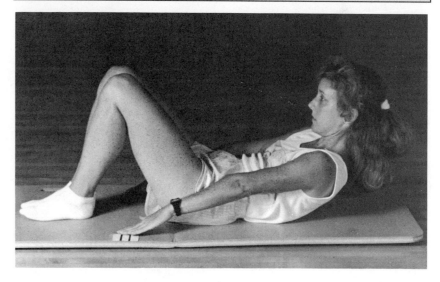

Push-Ups

Goal: To complete as many push-ups as possible in one minute.
Directions:

1. Start in an "up" position with your weight on your toes (men) or knees (women) and hands (figs. 4.5 and 4.6).

2. Lower yourself until your elbows form a right angle and your upper arm is parallel to the floor.

3. Complete as many full push-ups as you can in one minute. Be sure to keep your abdominals tight, hips slightly piked, and your back straight to protect your lower back. Record, and check your score in table 4.8.

Table 4.8
1-Minute Push-Up Norms*

	Standard Position	Modified Position
Excellent	>64	>54
Good	51–64	44–54
Average	37–50	32–43
Poor	23–36	20–31
Very Poor	<23	<20

*Norms are based on men using the standard position and women using the modified position.

Figure 4.5
Push-up—standard position
(Note the 90° elbow angle)

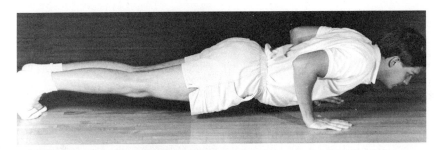

Figure 4.6
Push-up—modified position

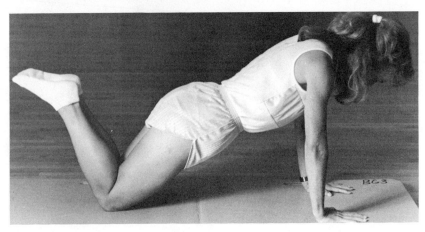

Flexibility

Flexibility is a valuable asset in daily activities or in any type of vigorous exercise program. The ability to move joints through a full range of motion without stiffness or tightness makes exercise more comfortable and decreases risk of injuries. The tests included in this section will indicate whether you have a normal range of motion in the lower back and other important areas.

Quick Checks for Flexibility

The following quick checks for flexibility are easy ways of measuring flexibility of major muscle groups often shortened and tightened in daily activities. Each quick check is also a stretch, so if your range of motion is limited or if you feel excessive tightness in a joint or muscle group, use the same position to improve flexibility in that area (see chapter 3 for basic fitness flexibility guidelines).

Figure 4.7

Lower back flexibility test

Muscle: Erector Spinae (lower back)

Test: Lying on your back, pull both thighs to chest.

Passing: Thighs should touch chest.

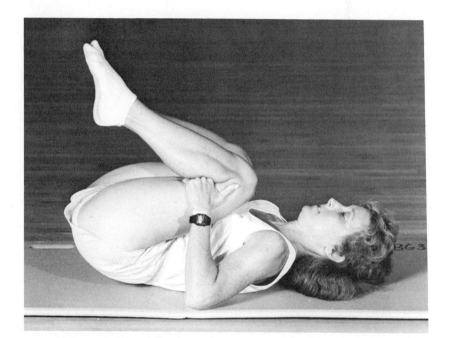

Figure 4.8

Hip flexor flexibility test

Muscle: Iliopsoas (hip flexor)

Test: Lying on your back, pull one knee to chest, keeping the other leg fully extended on the floor.

Passing: Calf of the extended leg must remain on the floor; the knee must not bend.

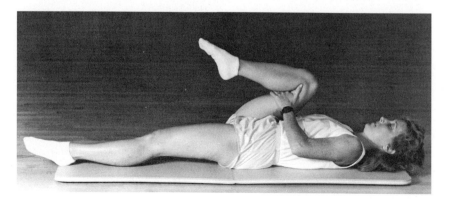

Figure 4.9

Quadricep flexibility test. Caution: Avoid if you have or experience knee problems.

Muscle: Quadriceps (front of thigh)

Test: Lying face down with knees together, pull heel toward buttocks.

Passing: Heel should comfortably touch buttocks.

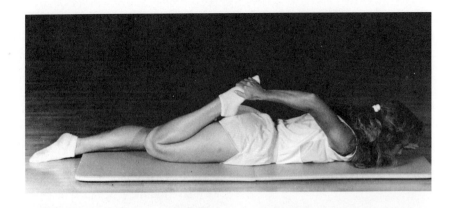

Figure 4.10

Hamstring flexibility test

Muscle: Hamstrings (back of thigh)

Test: Lying on your back, lift one leg, keeping other leg flat on the floor without bending either knee.

Passing: The raised leg must reach vertical (90 degrees).

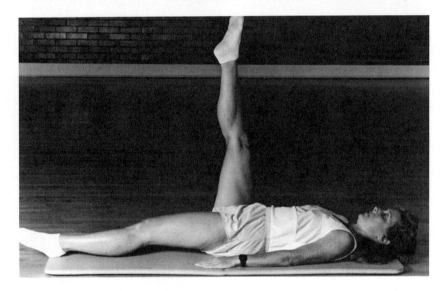

Figure 4.11

Calf flexibility test

Muscle: Gastrocnemius (calf)

Test: Standing without shoes, raise one forefoot off the floor, keeping the knees relaxed and the heels down.

Passing: The ball of the foot should clear the floor by a height equal to the width of two fingers.

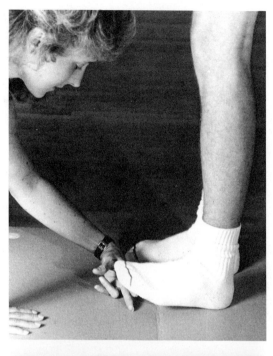

Figure 4.12

Shoulder girdle flexibility test

Muscle: Shoulder girdle

Test: Try to touch fingertips behind your back both ways.

Passing: Fingertips touch.

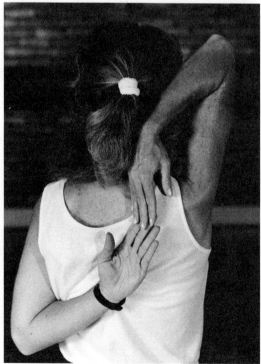

Sit and Reach

The sit and reach test, which measures hamstring flexibility, can be done with a flex box. If you do not have a flex box, the test can be performed with a ruler on a bench or on the ground with feet flexed (fig. 4.13). Norms are given using the soles of the feet as the zero inches mark.

Goal: To measure flexibility of the hamstrings.

Directions:

1. Warm up.
2. Sit with feet flat against the flex box about five inches apart and legs straight.
3. Place hands together. Without bending the knees, reach as far forward as possible, extending fingertips along the box. Hold the position three seconds.
4. Find your flexibility in table 4.9.

Table 4.9
Sit and Reach Norms (inches)

	Men	Women
Excellent	>7.0	>8.5
Good	4.0–7.0	6.5–8.5
Average	1.0–3.9	4.0–6.4
Poor	–2.0–0.9	1.0–3.9
Very Poor	<–2.0	<1.0

Figure 4.13
Sit and reach test

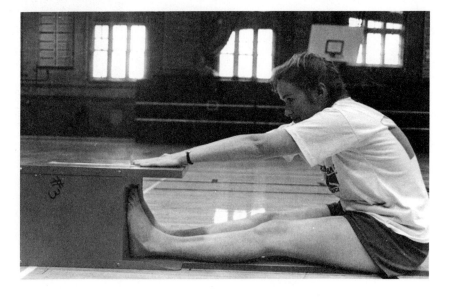

Sit and Reach Wall Test

The sit and reach wall test is a self-check for flexibility and can quickly be performed by a large number of people. All you need is a wall! (see fig. 4.14.)

Goal: To measure flexibility of the hamstrings.

Directions:

1. Warm up by walking and static stretching.
2. Remove shoes, sit facing a wall, feet flat against the wall and knees straight.
3. Reach forward as far as possible to touch fingertips, knuckles, or palms to wall, and hold position for 3 seconds (fig. 4.14).
4. Check your flexibility evaluations in table 4.10.

Table 4.10
Sit and Reach Wall Test Scores

Result	Flexibility
▪ Cannot touch wall	▪ Poor
▪ Fingertips touch wall	▪ Average
▪ Knuckles touch wall	▪ Good
▪ Palms touch wall	▪ Excellent

Figure 4.14
Sit and reach wall test

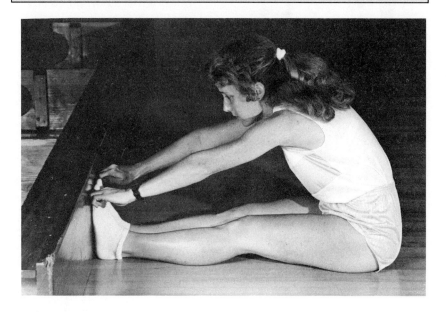

Body Girth Measures

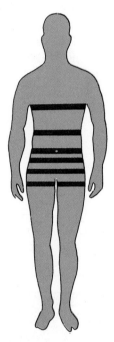

Figure 4.15
Body girth measurement sites

One reason many people begin a fitness program is because they are concerned about their physical appearance. Basic body build is an inherited characteristic, and only about 5 percent of the population can aspire to the current cultural "ideal," of model-like proportions. Take a look at your parents and grandparents to get an idea of your genetic endowment and what is realistic for you. While your basic structure cannot be altered, nevertheless, as fitness improves, fat may be lost from deposit areas and muscles become firmer, enhancing body contours. You may notice a loss of unwanted inches from the waist, hips, or thighs, or a desirable reshaping of body contours before noticing any weight change. Body girth measures will help you set goals to work for a trim, healthy body shape.

Goal: To measure body girths.

Directions:

Recruit a partner to measure you. You will need a measuring tape. For each measurement, pull the tape snugly, but do not indent the flesh. Take the measurements at the following sites (fig. 4.15):

- Chest—across the nipple line at the midpoint of a normal breath
- Abdominal 1—across the floating ribs, halfway between the chest and waist, at the midpoint of a normal breath
- Waist—the narrowest point, across the navel
- Abdominal 2—across the iliac crest (hip bones), midway between waist and hips
- Hips—feet together, across the pubic bone in front and widest part in back
- Thigh—right side, widest part, one inch below the crotch
- Calf—widest part
- Wrist—narrow part, above the bone, palm up

Body Composition

A certain amount of body fat is essential to good health. Fat acts as an insulator, conserving body heat. It pads bones and cushions internal organs, and it stores and supplies energy for later use.

In a diet-obsessed society in which both obesity and eating disorders abound, few people realize that excessive leanness can be as unhealthy as excessive fatness. Note that for young adults, an average range of body fat for women is 21 percent to 24 percent and for men, 14 percent to 17 percent (table 4.11). Each of us has inherited a certain body build and fat distribution; it is natural for some bodies to carry more fat than others.

While weight scales can tell you how much you weigh, they cannot tell you how much of your body is composed of fat or lean tissue. A sedentary individual may maintain a normal weight for height but increase fat and lose **lean body mass** (muscle tissue) over time. A body builder may be "overweight" according to height-weight charts, but this is due to development of muscle and bone rather than fat. Being overweight due to having a substantial amount of lean muscle tissue is not the same as being overweight due to excess fat tissue. A person who has a muscular build may think she is too heavy when the weight is mainly lean tissue. She could jeopardize her health trying to lose weight unnecessarily. On the other hand, a sedentary person who is satisfied with her weight may be shocked to discover her body fat percentage is over 30 percent, high enough to pose a health risk. In the early stages of a fitness program, excess fat will often be lost and lean muscle weight will increase as fitness improves. Even if no significant weight change occurs, the exerciser is leaner and appears trimmer because a pound of muscle is denser than a pound of fat.

Body fat is most accurately measured by underwater weighing in a laboratory. Because fat is more buoyant than muscle tissue, underwater weighing can estimate body composition within plus or minus 2 percent to 3 percent. However, this requires elaborate equipment, trained personnel, and considerable time to test each individual. Other laboratory tests of body composition currently being researched include bioelectrical impedance, near-infrared spectrophotometry, ultrasound, and photon absorptiometry.

Bioelectrical impedance is based on the fact that an electrical current travels through **fat-free tissue** (all parts of the body except fat) with its high water and electrolyte content more readily than through fat. This is not harmful, since the current is too mild to be felt. Results vary with differences in hydration, placement of electrodes, skin temperature, and type of machine used. The validity of this technique has not been determined, and studies have found both over- and underestimation of body fat when compared to other criterion measures.[3, 4, 5]

Infrared technology has been traditionally used to determine the moisture, protein, and fat composition of food. When used to measure body composition, it tends to underestimate body fat, though some feel it is more accurate than other methods for very lean or obese individuals.[6]

Ultrasound devices measure the variation in diffusion rates of ultrasound waves through fat and lean tissue. Accuracy varies with the pressure exerted on the skin, body fluid balance, and the number of sites measured.

Photon absorptiometry is based on the variations in the rate of photon emissions from bone, lean, and fat tissue after the body is exposed to low-dose radiation. It is not commonly used due to its limited availability, expense, complexity, and concern over radiation exposure.[7, 8]

A practical technique for measuring body composition involves the use of **skinfold calipers.** A caliper is a device that compresses the skin at a pressure determined by a spring. Skinfold measurements can be used to assess your proportion of fat to lean tissue because about 50 percent of your **fat** is **subcutaneous**—located directly under the skin. The amount of subcutaneous fat you have correlates highly with total body fat. An experienced measurer can assess body fat with skinfold calipers to within a range of plus or minus 2 percent to 5 percent. Two or more body sites may be measured, and accuracy increases with the number of sites sampled. Accuracy diminishes at the ends of the scale—for the very obese and the very lean, but for the average individual, skinfolds are quite reliable.

Self tests of body composition, though considerably less accurate than skinfold calipers, involve body girth measures of body fat and the pinch test. Keep in mind that greater fitness is not guaranteed by low body fat, and that a healthy fat percentage for you is an individual matter.

Body Composition Assessment Using Skinfold Calipers[9]

Goal: To accurately measure subcutaneous body fat.

Directions: Have a person trained in the use of skinfold calipers perform the following steps.

1. Measure skinfolds on the right side of the body using a skinfold caliper.
2. Grasp a fold of skin between thumb and forefinger, pulling it away from the underlying muscle.
3. Apply the calipers about one-quarter inch below the fingers holding the skinfold (fig. 4.16).
4. Tricep and thigh measurements are taken on a vertical skinfold. Subscapular and suprailiac measures are taken on a slight lateral slant along the natural fold of the skin.
5. Measure twice. Take readings to the nearest half millimeter. If the readings do not match, take a third measurement and average the closest two measurements.
6. Skinfold sites for women are:
   a. Tricep. Measure a vertical skinfold on the back of the arm midway between the shoulder and the elbow (fig. 4.17).
   b. Suprailiac. Measure a slightly lateral fold at the middle of the side of the body just above the hip bone (iliac crest) (fig. 4.18).
7. Skinfold sites for men are:
   a. Thigh. Measure a vertical fold on the front of the thigh midway between the inguinal fold (where the hip joint bends in front) and the top of the patella (knee cap) (fig. 4.19).
   b. Subscapular. Measure a diagonal fold just under the right shoulder blade (scapula) (fig. 4.20).
8. Mark your two skinfold measurements on the Percent of Body Fat Chart (fig. 4.21) and connect the marks with a straight line. Read your percent fat on the center scale.

Figure 4.16
Skinfold measuring technique

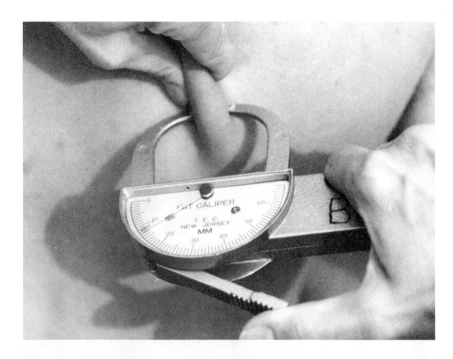

Figure 4.17
Tricep

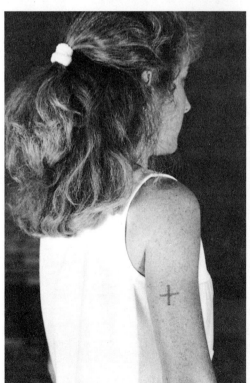

Figure 4.18
Suprailiac

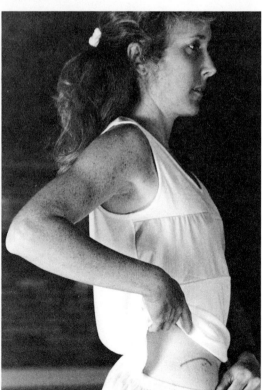

Figure 4.19
Thigh

Figure 4.20
Subscapular

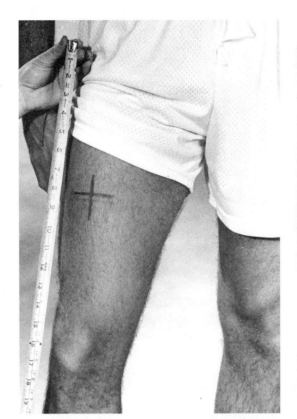

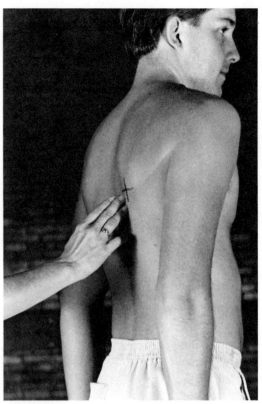

How to Determine Desirable Weight

Once you have measured your body fat percentage, it is useful to determine your desirable weight based on your present fat-free mass. For young adults, a reasonable body fat level in the trim range for women is 17 percent to 20 percent fat, and for men it is 10 percent to 13 percent fat (table 4.11). The following steps use an example of a female with 26 percent body fat and weighing 140 pounds to illustrate how to determine desirable weight at 18 percent body fat.

Goal: To calculate desirable weight at 18 percent fat for women and 12 percent fat for men.

Directions:

Body fat percentage 26 %.

Weight = 140 lbs.

1. Body fat percentage .26 × body weight 140 lbs = fat 36.4 lbs.
2. Body weight 140 – fat lbs. 36.4 = fat-free mass 103.6 lbs.
3. For women, desired weight at 18% fat = fat-free mass 103.6 lbs. ÷ .82 = 126 lbs.

For men, desired weight at 12% fat = fat free mass _____ lbs. ÷ .88 = _____ lbs.

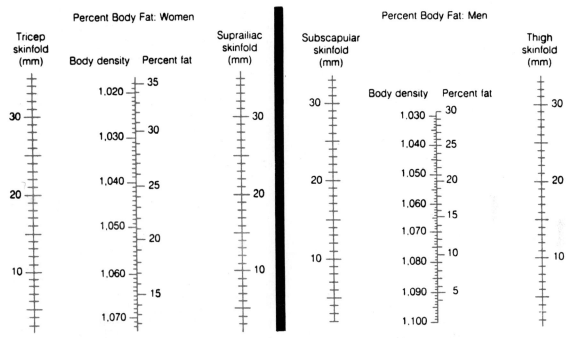

Figure 4.21

Percent body fat nomogram.

Source: Sloan, A. W. and Weir, J. "Nomograms for Prediction of Body Density and Total Body Fat from Skinfold Measurements" Journal of Applied Physiology 28 (1970): 221–222. Reprinted by permission of the American Physiological Society.

Table 4.11

Body Fat Norms

	Men	Women
Very Low Fat	<10	<17
Low Fat (Trim)	10–13	17–20
Average	14–17	21–24
Above Average (Fat)	18–20	25–27
High Fat	21–25	28–30
Obese	>25	>30

Based on the Sloan formulas for young adult men and women.

Body Girth Measures of Body Fat

Body girth measures of fatness are considerably less accurate than other measures of body fat such as skinfolds. However, their advantage is that they do not require special equipment nor training, and they can be done with a measuring tape at home.

Directions:

1. Men should measure waist girth at the navel and women should measure hips at the widest point. Pull the tape so it is snug but does not indent the skin (fig. 4.15, Body Girth Measurement Sites).

2. Remove shoes. Men measure their weight without clothing. Women measure their height.

3. Mark the measurements on the appropriate circumference chart and connect them with a straight line (fig. 4.22).

Figure 4.22
Circumference charts. Nomograms developed by Jack Wilmore, University of Texas. Used by permission.

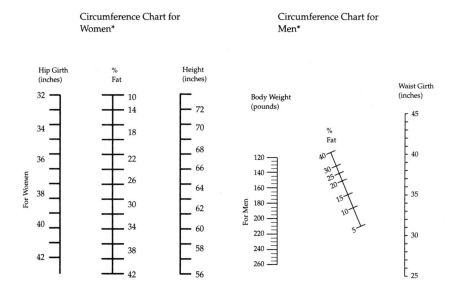

Waist-to-Hip Ratio

Recent investigations have begun pointing to the location of excess fat as a risk factor for heart disease and certain cancers. Fat distributed in the abdominal area is linked to increased health risks; hip/thigh fat is not as risky. As a result, the waist-to-hip ratio has become a common assessment used for health risk identification. To compute this ratio, divide the wait measurement by the hip measurement.

Examples: $\dfrac{29 \text{ in. (waist)}}{38 \text{ in. (hip)}} = .76 \qquad \dfrac{42 \text{ in. (waist)}}{36 \text{ in. (hip)}} = 1.17$

(See chapter 10 for more information on waist-to-hip ratio as a health risk factor.)

Pinch Test

Another simple measure of body fatness is the pinch test. Grasp a skinfold at the midpoint of your side, just above your hip bone (iliac crest). More than a one-inch skinfold thickness may indicate excessive body fat.

Summary

Assessment is an important tool to use in developing any dimension of wellness. It helps you to understand your own strengths and weaknesses, and to decide whether your current levels of cardiorespiratory endurance, muscular endurance, flexibility, and body fat are conducive to optimal wellness. With this knowledge, you can set reasonable fitness goals, establish a starting point for a fitness program, and develop a plan of action. Specific workout programs for different aerobic activities can be found in the appendix. A health/exercise assessment form and a personal fitness profile form are also available in the appendix.

As you progress in your fitness program, it may be useful to retest occasionally. While testing should not dominate your program, it will allow you to monitor your progress, and can give additional motivation to continue regular exercise.

References

1. Keener, E., Powers, D., Robbins, G., and Rushton, J. Undergraduate Student Physical Fitness Assessment, Ball State University, Muncie, IN, Spring 1989.

2. The American College of Sports Medicine, *Guidelines for Exercise Testing and Prescription, 4th ed.*, Philadelphia: Lea & Febiger, 1991.

3. Chumlea, W. C. and Baumgartner, R. N. "Bioelectrical Impedance Methods for the Estimation of Body Composition." *Canadian Journal of Sport Sciences* 15 (September 1990): 172–179.

4. Kaminsky, L. A. and Whaley, M. H., "Variability in Predicting Body Composition Using Bioelectrical Impedance and Skinfold Measurements." *Medicine and Science in Sports and Exercise* 21 (April 1989): S74.

5. Lukaski, H. C., et. al. "Body Composition Assessment of Athletes Using Bioelectrical Impedance Measurements." *Journal of Sports Medicine and Physical Fitness* 30 (December 1990): 434–440.

6. Israel, R. G., et. al. "Validity of a Near-Infrared Spectrophotometry Device for Estimating Human Body Composition." *Research Quarterly for Exercise and Sport* 60 (1989): 379–383.

7. Galea, V., et. al. "Body Composition by Photon Absorptiometry." *Canadian Journal of Sport Science* 15 (June 1990): 143–148.

8. Shephard, R. J. "Human Body Composition." *Canadian Journal of Sport Science* 15 (June 1990): 88.

9. Lohman, Timothy G. *New Dimensions in Body Composition.* Champaign, IL: Human Kinetics, 1992.

10. Sloan, A. W. and Weir, J. "Nomograms for Prediction of Body Density and Total Body Fat from Skinfold Measurements." *Journal of Applied Physiology* 28 (1970): 221–222.

Suggested Readings

American Alliance for Health, Physical Education, Recreation and Dance. 1988. *Physical Best: The American Alliance Physical Fitness Education and Assessment Program.* Reston, VA.

American College of Sports Medicine. 1991. *Guidelines for Exercise Testing and Prescription.* Lea & Febiger, Philadelphia, PA, 1991.

Barrow, Harold M. et. al., 1989. *Practical Measurement in Physical Education and Sport, 4th ed.* Malvern, PA: Lea and Febiger.

Baumgartner, Ted. A. and Jackson, Andrew S., 1991. *Measurement for Evaluation in Physical Education and Exercise Science, 4th ed.* Dubuque, IA: Brown and Benchmark

Corbin, C. B., and R. Lindsey. 1991. *Concepts of Physical Fitness with Laboratories.* Dubuque, IA: Wm. C. Brown Publishers.

Francis, Peter and Lorna. "Flexibility Screening." *Dance-Exercise Today.* (September 1987).

Hastad, Douglas N., and Alan C. Lacy. 1989. *Measurement and Evaluation in Contemporary Physical Education.* Scottsdale, AZ: Gorsuch Scarisbrick Publishers.

Heyward, V. H. 1991. *Advanced Fitness Assessment and Exercise Prescription,* 2nd ed. Champaign, IL: Human Kinetics Publishers.

Kravitz, Len and Vivian Heyward. "Getting a Grip on Body Composition." *IDEA Today* (April 1992): 34–39.

Lohman, Timothy G., et. al. 1991. *Anthropometric Standardization Reference Manual.* Champaign, IL: Human Kinetics.

Lohman, Timothy G. 1992. *New Dimensions in Body Composition.* Champaign, IL: Human Kinetics.

Safrit, Margaret J. 1986. *Introduction to Measurement in Physical Education and Exercise Science.* St. Louis, MO: Times Mirror/Mosby College Publishing.

5

Common Injuries and Care of the Lower Back

Chapter Objectives

After reading this chapter, you will be able to:

1. Identify four main reasons why injuries occur.
2. Explain how muscle weakness and inflexibility contribute to injuries.
3. Identify four common muscle imbalances.
4. List and explain the general recommended treatment for common injuries (i.e., R.I.C.E.).
5. Describe the basic causes and treatment of blisters, chafing, muscle soreness, side stitch, muscle cramp, muscle strain, tendinitis, plantar fasciitis, heel spur syndrome, shin splints, stress fracture, chondromalacia, and ankle sprain.
6. Identify the four symptoms of injury that indicate the need for medical attention.
7. Identify the two most important keys to preventing lower back pain.
8. List and describe six of the eight exercises recommended to reduce the risk of lower back pain.

Terms

- Blister
- Chondromalacia
- Cramp
- Heel spur
- Intervertebral disc
- Ischemia
- Ligament

- Orthotics
- Overpronation
- Overuse
- Plantar fasciitis
- Pronation
- R.I.C.E.
- Shin splint

- Side stitch
- Sprain
- Strain
- Stress fracture
- Supination
- Tendinitis
- Tendon

Y ou walk into your first jogging class, eager to improve your fitness. You have not exercised regularly and you hope this class will help you get into shape. Your instructor begins with a warm-up and an easy jog around campus. After your run you feel great and invigorated. The next morning you wake up and your whole body aches. You don't remember having been run over by a truck. You think "Where are the paramedics? What should I do now? Withdraw from class? Stay in bed? Buy stock in Ben-Gay? When will I be able to move again?"

Participation in fitness activities offers many benefits. These benefits far exceed the risk of injury. When you exercise, you intentionally use certain muscles to increase their strength and endurance. As your body adapts to these efforts, you may experience minor aches and soreness. Physical activity also carries some risk of overuse or injury. Fortunately, many of these discomforts are minor, and you will be able to continue or quickly resume your workouts. This chapter discusses how to prevent injuries, in addition to recognizing their signs, symptoms, and recommended treatments. It also includes how to maintain a healthy back, since back pain is a common problem. Finally factors that affect the musculature of the spine and how to avoid lower back injury are covered.

Injury Prevention

Prevention is the key to reducing the frequency of injuries. Understanding the cause of injury allows you to stop minor problems before they turn you into the "walking wounded." Prevention is far more conducive to wellness than any patch and repair job. There are four main reasons why injuries occur:[1]

1. Overuse—Doing too much too soon or too often, causing a breakdown at the weakest point—ankle, Achilles tendon, shin, knee, or back.

2. Footwear—Wearing improper or wornout shoes.

3. Weakness and inflexibility— Muscles so weak or tight that the slightest unusual twist strains them.

4. Mechanical problems—Caused by the way the foot hits the ground, or using poor form while exercising.

An individually adjusted workload, well-made and well-kept shoes, supplemental toning and stretching exercises, and mechanical improvements will prevent the majority of injuries.

Overuse

In order to improve or maintain fitness, you must overload, or push, beyond normal demands. Overload is necessary and good up to a point, but you must be able to recover between workouts. The goal is to exercise so that you improve, but not so much that you cause **overuse,** excessive overload leading to injury or illness (fig. 5.1). Overuse problems commonly occur at the beginning of a new exercise program and account for the majority of injuries. The first four months of a new program are the most critical. The body and muscles must be given time to gradually adapt to the new demands.

Figure 5.1

Overload is good up to a point, overuse can cause injury.

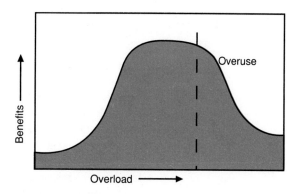

Set realistic goals early in a fitness program. Your instructor will help you determine an appropriate entry level conditioning program and progression. Gradually increase your exercise intensity and duration to attain your personal goals. For example, if you have never participated in aerobics, your first goal may be to perform 10 minutes of continuous aerobic exercise, although other members of the class may work out 25 or 30 minutes. Try not to compete or compare with your friends who may be able to exercise for a longer duration or at higher intensity. You will be able to catch up in time, but if you attempt to keep up with them before your body is ready, you risk the potential of an overuse problem.

A good rule of thumb to follow is to increase the duration of the workout no more than 10 percent weekly. A beginner should not jump from a 20-minute workout up to 40 minutes. This principle holds true in aerobics, lap swimming, water exercise, bicycling, fitness walking, and jogging. Studies show an increasing injury rate with increasing weekly jogging distance beyond 20 miles per week.[2] Many fitness buffs and athletes have a feeling of invulnerability. They think their bodies can adapt to increased exercise workloads without any problem. Realize that more is not always better. By allowing your body to gradually adjust to new exercise demands, you will greatly reduce the risk of suffering an overuse injury.

Consider alternating an impact activity with a low or nonimpact activity. This allows the muscles a period of rest and recovery and switches the demands to a new muscle group. It is repetitive stress on the body that causes problems. Some people enjoy alternating activities because it adds variety and develops total body fitness better than any single activity. For example, water exercise or bicycling is a good supplement to an impact exercise such as jogging.

It is crucial that you listen to your body during and after exercise. After a great workout, if you feel a little soreness, it should gradually decrease over the next couple of hours. However, if you develop excessive soreness or pain, cut back in your next workout, try a different activity, or take a day off. The importance of rest is often overlooked. It is when you are in a state of fatigue that you are most susceptible to developing a problem.

If you are getting the right amount of exercise, you should look good, feel good, and be alert and productive. Too much exercise, like too little, can be unhealthy. After a workout, you should get enough rest to be fully recovered by the next workout. Rest is probably the most neglected aspect of fitness. Your body does not improve during the exercise itself, but during recovery. Exercise provides the overload that stimulates that improvement. During the rest period between workouts, the body makes adaptations to the demands made upon it. When the recovery is adequate, you will begin the next workout feeling strong and energetic. If you feel tired and washed out, rest will do you more good than exercise. Also keep in mind that exercise isn't the only source of overstress. Other aspects of daily life, such as poor nutrition, emotional tension, job, social, or family problems, and lack of sleep can contribute to chronic fatigue.

The concept of "no pain, no gain" is outdated. Pain is the body's natural way of informing you that something is wrong. Pain may be localized in a specific spot or generalized over a broad area. However, pain is a subjective response, and each individual will tolerate it differently. Do not try to exercise through pain of injury. Almost every study shows that previous injury is a risk factor for future injuries.[3] Therefore, it is important to allow for complete healing and to correct mechanical problems before resuming activity.

Footwear

While many injuries are due to overuse, this is only part of the problem. Wearing improper or wornout shoes places added stress on your hips, knees, ankles, and feet—the sites of up to 90 percent of all sports injuries.[4] The feet are the most abused and neglected part of the body. Good footwear is the best investment you can make in an exercise program. Each time your foot hits the ground when jogging, the force of impact is approximately three times your body weight. Your

Improper footwear increases risk of injury.

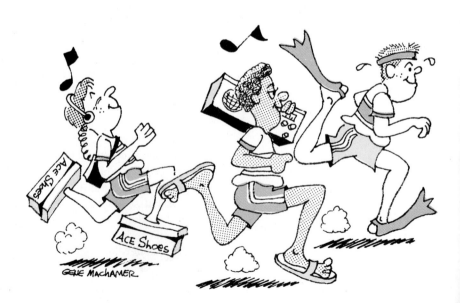

feet, ankles, shins, knees, hips, and lower back must absorb a tremendous amount of stress. If the stress is too great, breakdown occurs at the weakest link in the chain. A well-fitted pair of shoes is the first line of defense against impact injuries. Shoes should provide good shock absorption, support, and stability, yet maintain a reasonable degree of flexibility.[5] Your foot will naturally roll inward when you jog; therefore, the heel counter must be firm to prevent excessive heel movement. The bottom of the shoe must have good traction to prevent slipping. Shoes are manufactured to be used for a certain number of miles, and they can lose their cushioning ability even if the uppers still look good. Each step compresses the sole, causing it to flatten and gradually lose shock absorbability. Exercise shoes typically lose about one-third of their ability to absorb shock after 500 miles of use.[6] The upper part of the shoe stretches and weakens, decreasing lateral support. This happens so gradually you may not notice it until you try on a new pair of shoes. With less cushioning and support, there is a greater chance of injury. If you wear the shoes 5 to 10 hours a week during exercise (walking, jogging, aerobics, etc.), you should probably replace them every 6 months to retain adequate cushioning. Runners would be well advised to keep a log of their mileage as a reminder of when to buy new shoes.

Weakness and Inflexibility

Sit down with your feet extended in front. Slowly reach toward your toes. Can you touch them without bending your knees? Many exercisers who neglect flexibility exercises cannot pass this test for minimal flexibility. Their legs are too tight, and this increases susceptibility to muscle and tendon injuries that might not occur if they maintained flexibility. Aerobic activities are great for the cardiorespiratory system, but they alone do not develop balanced fitness. They tend to shorten and tighten muscles that are used repetitively, leaving opposing, relatively unused muscles weak. This can lead to muscle imbalance. If some muscles are too tight, joint movement is restricted. Table 5.1 lists some common muscle

Table 5.1
Common Muscle Imbalances

The rule of thumb to avoid injuries is to *stretch* the muscles that are tight and *strengthen* the opposing muscles that are weak.

Strong	Weak
gastrocnemius (calf)	tibialis anterior (shin)
quadriceps (front of thigh)	hamstrings (back of thigh)
erector spinae (lower back)	abdominals (stomach)
pectorals (chest)	rhomboids (upper back)

imbalances. The solution to this problem is to stretch the tight muscles and strengthen the weak ones. Flexibility is one of the most important factors in injury prevention. Incorporate a basic stretching routine into each workout, preferably during the cool-down. (See chapter 3 for recommended strength and flexibility exercises.) Stretch gently, placing only slight tension on the muscles. Hard stretching or bouncy movements may activate the stretch reflex. This causes the muscle to involuntarily contract and shorten—exactly the opposite of what you're trying to do—to protect itself from injury. Concentrate on event-specific exercises. For example, if you are a swimmer, you will want to spend additional time stretching the shoulders and arms. If jogging or aerobics is your activity, concentrate on stretching the hamstrings, quadriceps, lower back, and calf. Abdominal curls are an important supplement to any fitness workout. Strong abdominals and a flexible lower back are critical in preventing lower back problems.

Mechanics

Structural weaknesses, mainly affecting the legs, knees, ankles, and feet, are often revealed when a beginner starts a new exercise program, or when overuse occurs. Biomechanical difficulties often arise in the feet. The foot is a marvelous structure of 26 bones, with almost double that number of ligaments and muscles. It strikes the ground about 80 to 90 times a minute during exercise. When a weak foot pounds the ground several thousand times a day, the potential for injury is great. It is natural for your foot to **pronate** slightly—that is, the foot rolls inward slightly after the outer edge of the heel strikes the ground. Since all bodies are not created equal, different foot types, gait styles, and body mechanics vary in susceptibility to injury. For example, flat feet may cause **overpronation**—too much inward rotation (see fig. 5.2). This could cause tendinitis, plantar fasciitis, or knee strain. Overpronation can be detected by excessive shoe wear on the inside of the forefoot. **Supination,** on the other hand, is the rolling outward of the foot upon contact. People with high arches tend to supinate. When the foot hits the ground, it does not roll inward enough to absorb the shock of impact, increasing the risk of shin splints, stress fractures, and medial knee and hip problems. Supination causes excessive wear on the outside of the shoe sole.

Moderate pronation problems can be corrected by wise shoe selection. Most exercise shoes are designed to limit overpronation, not eliminate all inward rotation. Observing the wear pattern on your shoes can help you select a shoe designed for your specific mechanics. Many employees in sports shoe stores are trained to help you select a proper shoe. If discomfort persists, you may want to consult a physician or podiatrist, who will check your foot mechanics. They may prescribe **orthotics,** shoe inserts molded to your foot, to correct abnormalities. These allow the foot to operate mechanically efficient. They are highly effective for alleviating excessive ankle pronation/supination.

Figure 5.2

Supination and overpronation

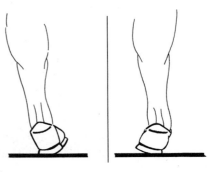

Left foot: supination   Left foot: over pronation

Regardless of body type, it is important to pay attention to form when participating in any aerobic activity. Participants in aerobic dance, water exercise, bicycling, step aerobics, and even those using stair climbing and rowing machines need to understand the proper mechanics of each activity. In this way, many injuries and discomforts can be avoided. You will find technique and safety tips for a variety of aerobic activities in the appendix. You may also want to refer to the "contraindicated exercises" listed in chapter 8.

The body is a marvelous mechanism. Considering its complexity, it is a wonder it doesn't break down more often. Exercise is vital to maintain wellness. Illness and injury are less common in those who maintain peak performance through regular exercise than in those who exercise sporadically. Even when injuries do occur, few are debilitating. Many simply cause some inconvenience. The recommended treatment for many injuries, whether mild or severe, is rest, ice, compression, and elevation **(R.I.C.E.).**

R.I.C.E.

Acute injuries to muscles, joints, and tendons are often accompanied by swelling. Rapid recovery requires keeping the swelling to a minimum. The aim of treatment is to assist the healing process.

R = Rest

The classic remedy of old-time coaches was "run it off." On the contrary, the injured area should be rested for 24 hours to 72 hours, depending on the severity of the injury.[7] Using crutches, rather than bearing weight, is one example of a

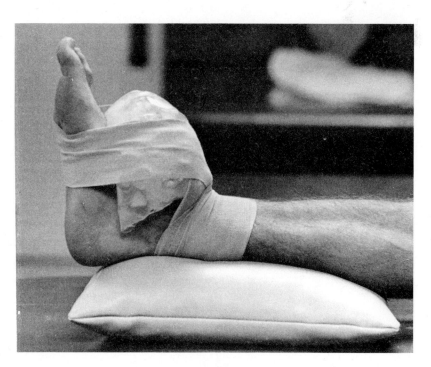

R.I.C.E.

way to "rest" an injured ankle or leg. A minor complaint can become a major problem if you keep aggravating the situation. Healing progresses more rapidly when stress to the area is reduced. Frequently, people will start back into full activity before they are ready and reinjure the area. Once you return to your usual workout routine, reduce your duration, frequency, and/or intensity by 25 percent.[8] Do not resume your normal workout level until you are free of pain both during and after exercise.

I = Ice

Apply ice to the injured part immediately. You can freeze a paper cup filled with water, peel some of the paper away, and rub it on the area (i.e., shin splints), or surround it with 2 to 3 plastic bags of ice (i.e., sprained ankle). Crushed ice or ice cubes from the freezer work best. Commercial cold packs may not stay cold long enough to reduce swelling. Apply the ice for at least 20 minutes (but be careful not to freeze the skin with excessive icing). The ice may make the injured part ache for the first 5 minutes to 10 minutes. Keep it on! After 10 minutes the part will become numb. This will give immediate pain relief by decreasing blood flow to the superficial tissues. It also reduces swelling, inflammation, and tissue damage. In deeper blood vessels, circulation increases, bringing blood, nutrients, and healing cells to the injured area. Ice the injured area every 3 to 4 waking hours for the first 48 hours to 72 hours.

If you feel mild discomfort when exercising and suspect an overuse injury, such as tendinitis, you should apply ice to the tender areas right after you work out, and reapply it several times a day for the next 48 hours.

C = Compression

When not icing the injury, wrap the part with an elastic wrap to prevent fluid buildup in the injured area. Wrap it snugly, but not tightly enough to interfere with circulation. If the part starts throbbing, the wrap may be on too tight. Remove the wrap and reapply more loosely. Do not sleep with the wrap on.

E = Elevation

Raise the injured area above the level of the heart. This will reduce the swelling by combatting the effect of gravity pulling blood and fluids down to the injured area. Most people with an injured ankle or knee will place it on a pillow for elevation when going to sleep. However, you may move during the night and lose the elevation. Instead, place 3 or 4 books under your mattress to raise it approximately 6 inches to 8 inches.

Heat and Pain Relievers

Many people mistakenly apply heat to an acute injury. Heat actually stimulates blood flow and increases inflammation. You should stick with ice for at least the first 48 hours to 72 hours after an injury, and only then, *after swelling has subsided*, try heat. At that point, heat may speed the healing and help relieve pain, relax muscles, and reduce stiffness. Either dry heat (heating pad or lamp) or moist heat (a hot bath, whirlpool, hot-water bottle, damp heat pack) will do. Apply the heat for 20 minutes to 30 minutes, two or three times a day. You can also use it for 5 minutes to 10 minutes before exercising to reduce stiffness.

Over-the-counter liniments and balms are popular methods for producing a warm feeling in muscles. The effect of these much-advertised products is only superficial—the active ingredients stimulate sensory nerve endings in the skin to produce a sensation of heat. This does little or nothing to promote healing and may actually mask the pain.

Aspirin or ibuprofen (such as Motrin or Advil) can reduce the pain and inflammation of minor sprains, strains, and tendinitis. In this case, acetaminophen (such as Tylenol) is less helpful because it has no anti-inflammatory effect. Your doctor should be consulted before using any drugs.

Common Injuries

In pursuit of wellness, you may occasionally push yourself beyond the current capabilities of your structure. Finding your peak and keeping it is a challenge and a process of learning about your body's own unique strengths and weaknesses. If, in your zeal to experience peak performance, you develop an athletic ailment, it will generally be minor and you will be able to resume activity within a few days. Here we will discuss the potential causes, symptoms, and treatments for the most common injuries.

Blisters

Blisters are a common problem, especially for beginning exercisers. They are, essentially, burns caused by the friction of the foot rubbing against the shoe. They are usually only a problem if they become infected or if they cause you to limp. The most common areas for blisters are the bottom of the foot, the side of the big and little toes, and the back of the heel. A blister is a hot, red, and inflamed area, occasionally containing water or blood. Blisters can be prevented by eliminating the friction that causes them. Wear 100 percent acrylic (orlon) socks. Acrylic is best at dissipating moisture and preventing blisters from forming. Cotton socks produce twice as many blisters that are three times as large, and even worse is a cotton-acrylic blend.[9] Never wear new shoes for a workout without first breaking them in by walking around in them at home for a few days. Should a blister be opened? Some say no, let the fluid reabsorb into the system since an open blister invites infection. Others say to pop the blister if it is painful and causes you to limp. The best treatment is to apply a donut pad and lubricant to the blister to reduce friction and pressure. Some runners wear their socks inside out to avoid the abrasion of the rough interior seam. It may also help to wear two socks on the affected foot—a thin nylon sock inside an acrylic sock. If the blister is lanced, keep the area clean to prevent infection. Consult your physician if you think it may be infected.

Chafing

When skin rubs against skin or against clothing, it becomes irritated and can crack and bleed. The most common problem areas are between the thighs, under the armpits, and the nipples (runner's nipples). While chafing can happen to anyone, frequency increases with body fat percentage. To prevent chafing, select clothing of smooth, nonabrasive material with few or well-covered seams. Avoid clothing that is tight or bunches under the arms or between the legs. Treat chafing by applying petroleum jelly to the affected area. Wearing tights or knee-length exercise shorts can protect chafed thighs. Nipple chafing can be decreased by going shirtless in warm weather or by applying petroleum jelly and band-aids to the nipples. Women should select a good exercise bra that has no seams across the nipple area.

Muscle Soreness

This may be fairly mild and usually is just a reminder that you had a good workout. Other than following a sensible progression, there is no real prevention for muscle soreness. It indicates that some muscles that were out of shape have been stimulated to tone up, usually occurring at the beginning of any new exercise program. For example, a person who has not recently lifted weights will develop muscle soreness following the first workout. Duration of activity and eccentric (lengthening) contractions are highly correlated to muscle soreness. For example, running downhill repeatedly will produce more quadricep soreness than an equal amount of flat or uphill running. Muscle soreness is thought to be caused by microscopic tears or spasms of the connective tissue. There is no long-term damage from this. Muscle soreness may develop immediately or over a 24- to 36-hour period following unaccustomed exercise and will usually disappear within 1 to 3 days. There is no real pain, but rather a mild achiness when moving the major muscle groups used in the activity. After several sessions of the same activity, soreness will diminish or disappear entirely. There is little or nothing that can be done for mild muscle soreness. While stretching is beneficial for flexibility it has little effect on reducing soreness.[10]

Side Stitch

A **side stitch** may result from participating in vigorous activity before the body has had sufficient warm-up. It may be related to a lack of conditioning, weak abdominals, shallow breathing, consuming a meal before exercise, dehydration, excessive exercise intensity, or **ischemia** (inadequate oxygen) to the diaphragm or intercostal muscles between the ribs. A side stitch is basically a diaphragm spasm. It can be treated by stopping activity and stretching or holding the side. After cessation of the activity for a few minutes, the pain and spasm should subside. Taking a deep breath may also break the spasm. Once the pain has dissipated, activity may resume.

Muscle Cramp

A **cramp** is a sharp, involuntary muscle contraction. It may occur during exercise or at rest. The calf is the most common area for a muscle cramp to occur, but cramps may occur anywhere in the body. Muscle cramps may be caused by fatigue. This is a protective mechanism, your body telling you to quit or you will do yourself damage. They may also be related to a strength imbalance, an electrolyte imbalance, or dehydration. Occasionally, low levels of circulating calcium and potassium in the blood can contribute to cramps. Frequently, a muscle cramp will occur in the summer when the weather is hot and humid. Nighttime calf cramps can happen in bed when you suddenly stretch your toes downward, causing the calf muscle to contract. Cramps can be treated with fluid intake and gradually stretching the muscle. A calf cramp may be treated by flexing the foot to a 90 degree angle. Occasionally, gentle massage may help.

Muscle cramps may be prevented by taking precautions when exercising in the heat. Wear light, loose clothing; drink water freely; gradually acclimatize yourself to the heat; and exercise during the cooler hours of the day. Extra salt is not needed. A regular program of stretching may also help prevent muscle cramps.

Muscle Strain

A muscle **strain** is a tear or rip in a muscle or tendon and is sometimes referred to as a pull. There are many different causes, but it most often happens from a violent contraction of the muscle. A strain may be caused by fatigue, overexertion, muscle imbalance or weakness, or electrolyte or water imbalance.

A strain may range from mild (more painful than just soreness) to a complete rupture of the muscle. Muscles most likely to be affected are the gastrocnemius, hamstrings, quadriceps, hip flexors, groin, and the rotator cuff muscles of the shoulder. Generally, symptoms include sharp pain, weakness with possible loss of function, spasm or extreme tightness, and tenderness to the touch. R.I.C.E. is used to treat muscle strain. Reduce or eliminate activity until the injury starts to heal. The severity of the injury and which muscle is injured will affect the recovery time. The hamstrings usually take the longest to heal and rehabilitate, while the quadriceps and hip flexors heal more quickly. If the strain is severe, it will heal with a significant amount of scar tissue. Scar tissue is not elastic like muscle, so stretching and strengthening exercises are important to return to normal function. To prevent strains, complete a full-body warm-up before working out, take care not to overdo, and work toward balancing the strength and flexibility in opposing muscles.

Tendinitis

Anytime you see *-itis*, think inflammation. **Tendinitis** is the inflammation of a tendon from repetitive stress. **Tendons** are the fibrous cords that connect muscles to bones. The most commonly known is the Achilles tendon, which can be felt at the back of the ankle. Tendons are vulnerable to inflammation because the force of muscle contractions is transmitted through them. When inflamed, the tendon may become hot, red, and swollen in moderate to severe cases. There will be pain on movement and activity. Normal daily activities, such as opening a door or walking up the stairs, can be painful. The most common areas to suffer tendinitis are the Achilles tendon, knee, shoulder, and elbow ("tennis elbow"). Tendinitis often affects participants in swimming, tennis, baseball, and volleyball. Achilles tendon problems, common to runners, fitness walkers, and aerobic dancers, are almost always due to tight calf muscles. When the foot flexes to push off, the powerful Achilles pulls the heel up. If the calf is too tight, it yanks the heel up prematurely, stressing the Achilles tendon. Rest from the activity that caused the injury and stretching to alleviate excessive tightness are recommended. It may take 2 to 3 weeks to completely heal and rehabilitate. Continuing activity will only delay healing. Meanwhile, you may include alternate activities to maintain fitness. A regular program incorporating stretching and strengthening can help prevent tendinitis.

Plantar Fasciitis

The plantar fascia is a long thick band of connective tissue on the undersurface of the foot that attaches the base of the calcaneus (heel bone) to the base of the toes. An inflammation of the plantar fascia, **(plantar fasciitis)** is usually felt as heel or arch pain before, during, or after activity. Injury to the fascia may result from excessive impact, worn shoes, or poor foot mechanics. Anatomical problems frequently cause plantar fasciitis—high arches, tight Achilles tendon, flat feet, excessive pronation. Also, with age and repeated weightbearing stress, the fat pad under the heel becomes flattened and less shock-absorbent. Rest, ice, and elimination of causal factors are the recommended treatments. Orthotics will reduce symptoms in 95 percent of cases of plantar fasciitis.[11]

Heel Spur Syndrome

A **heel spur** is a bony growth found on the underside of the calcaneus, behind the insertion of the plantar fascia. A heel spur is caused by chronic irritation of the plantar fascia at its insertion. Not all heel spurs cause pain. Heel spur syndrome is generally attributable to heel trauma from overuse, excessive impact, or a continuous pull on the plantar fascia, which strains the arch. It is most painful when a person first steps down on the foot in the morning, but pain may continue throughout the day. Treatment involves rest, anti-inflammatory medication, and insertion of a heel pad in the shoe to alleviate inflammation of the plantar fascia.[12]

Shin Splints

A **shin splint** refers to any pain in the front of the lower leg (shin). Early signs are acute burning pain or irritation in the lower third of the anterior tibialis. This may progress to slight swelling, redness, warmth, and inflammation. A variety of causes contribute to shin splints. They often come early in an exercise program and are particularly common in those who are out of shape, overweight, wide-hipped, knock-kneed, or duck-footed. Working out on very hard or very soft surfaces can bring them on, even if a person is well-conditioned. Switching from a hard to a soft surface or vice versa, excessive mileage, improper footwear, poor foot mechanics, running on a road slope, and running the same direction all the time on an indoor track may cause them. Women, particularly those who wear high heels, are affected nearly three times more often than men.[13]

Shin splints may be a sign of a long arch problem in the foot. As the long arch begins to sag, it stretches lower leg muscles and causes pain. Another cause is a muscle imbalance between the strong calf muscle and the weak anterior tibialis, which may lead to inflammation of the membrane between the tibia and the fibula. This imbalance can be corrected by flexion exercises to strengthen the anterior tibialis and by stretching the calf. These should be done each workout. If mechanical problems are not corrected, shin splints tend to recur.

To treat shin splints, rub ice on the affected area for 20 minutes 3–4 times a day. Occasionally, aspirin therapy may be indicated for a few days to reduce inflammation. If the pain is persistent, reduce your activity level and consult a physician to eliminate the possibility of a stress fracture.

Stress Fracture

A **stress fracture** is a microscopic break in a bone caused by overuse. Unlike a broken bone, which occurs with a distinct traumatic event, a stress fracture is the result of cumulative overload that occurs over many days or weeks. Doing too much too soon (overuse) is the major cause. Bone is living tissue that adjusts to exercise force demands placed on it. As force is applied, bone will remodel itself to better handle the force. If too much force is applied, the bone may fracture before it can successfully remodel. Running extreme mileage, impact aerobics, wearing wornout shoes, exercising on hard surfaces such as asphalt or concrete, and poor foot mechanics may cause a stress fracture. While it can occur anywhere in the lower legs and feet, it is most common at the end of the tibia near the ankle. Because they have smaller, lighter bones, women are more susceptible to stress fractures than men. A stress fracture may be debilitating if not treated correctly. Frequently, a stress fracture may be confused with a case of severe shin splints. Stress fractures are difficult to detect clinically. Frequently they will not show up on X-ray until 3–4 weeks after the onset of symptoms. A bone scan can detect a stress fracture much earlier in the injury because it reveals the active bone formation that occurs while the fracture is healing.[14] The pain of a stress fracture will not go away with conventional treatments (ice, ultrasound) or medication. Only rest will decrease the pain.

Stages in the progression of a stress fracture include (1) pain during activity that subsides after the completion of exercise; (2) pain during activity that continues during the rest of the day into the evening; and (3) continuous pain throughout the day and night.

The best treatment for a stress fracture is rest from the activity that caused it. This does not mean elimination of exercise altogether. Riding a bicycle or swimming are good alternatives during the healing phase. Depending on the severity of the stress fracture, activity may be resumed within 2 weeks to 6 weeks after diagnosis. "Running through the injury" is not recommended. This may lead to a nonunion fracture of the bone and a 6-week to 8-week recovery period in a cast.

Chondromalacia

Chondromalacia, knee cap pain, is a condition in which the cartilage on the underside of the patella is being irritated and worn away. Symptoms include pain when walking up and down stairs, pain when sitting with knees flexed, grating or roughness felt behind the kneecaps, the knee "locking up" or "giving away," and joint swelling, commonly called "water on the knee." It can be caused by excessive mileage, always running the same direction on the track, bouncing, and rapid ballistic movements such as those done in aerobics. One common cause is structural. Wide hips tend to make the quadriceps pull the kneecap out against the femur, producing inflammation. Loose kneecaps or a quadriceps muscle not strong enough to keep the patella in its groove also may lead to chondromalacia. The knee will not get better if you continue your activity during the injury. Rest and ice are the conventional treatments for this injury. To prevent recurrence, the knee must be rehabilitated. To stabilize the knee and to assist in correcting the tracking mechanism of the patella, strengthen the quadriceps with leg extension exercises. Stretching should increase hamstring and iliotibial band flexibility. In severe cases, surgery may be indicated.

Ankle Sprain

A **sprain** is an injury to a **ligament,** the fibrous connective tissue that binds bones together to form a joint. A sprain is most often a result of a sudden force, typically a twisting motion that surrounding muscles are not strong enough to control. Both ankles and knees are vulnerable to sprains. An ankle sprain will typically exhibit signs of swelling and tenderness on the outside of the ankle. The amount of swelling depends upon the severity of the injury. In severe cases, discoloration or bruising will develop. Range of motion in the ankle may be decreased by swelling and pain. R.I.C.E. for the first 72 hours is the best treatment for sprains. It is extremely important to control the amount of swelling in the joint in order to return to activity quickly. Strong, flexible muscles help protect against sprains. For example, to prevent ankle sprain, strengthen ankles with flexion, inversion, and eversion exercises. High-top shoes or a commercial ankle wrap may also be worn to provide additional support to the joint.

When to Seek Medical Help

You should seek medical assistance for an injury if you experience any of the following symptoms.

1. The body part is not in its natural anatomical position.

2. The injury is extremely painful or the pain has not decreased in intensity over the course of several days.

3. You heard a "pop" or a "snap" when the injury occurred.

4. You are unable to bear complete weight on the part or there is some loss of strength.

Once injured, who should you see? Your family doctor will be able to treat common sprains and strains. However, there are other sports injury specialists who can help. Table 5.2 describes some of these specialists.

Table 5.2
Injury Specialists

> **Orthopedists**—are M.D.s with specialized surgical training. They treat injuries to any part of the musculoskeletal system. Many specialize in athletic injuries.
>
> **Podiatrists**—are D.P.M.s (doctors of podiatric medicine). They treat foot-related problems that are common to fitness-related injuries. Though not M.D.s, they receive special training and are state licensed. They can prescribe medications, design orthotics, and perform some surgeries.
>
> **Physical Therapists**—are licensed by the state to administer rehabilitative techniques—from massage to strength and flexibility exercises. Most states require a doctor's referral to visit a registered physical therapist.
>
> **Sports Medicine Clinics**—Because sports medicine is a rapidly growing field, many communities and medical centers have specialized sports medicine clinics. Many clinics have "walk-in" hours and are likely to include some of the specialists mentioned above as part of their staff.
>
> **Athletic Trainers**—Many colleges, universities, and sports medicine clinics have athletic trainers who have extensive knowledge and experience in dealing with injuries. They are highly trained and must pass rigorous written and practical examinations to become certified.

Communicating with a doctor is an important step in assuming an active role in your health care. Be sure to tell the physician everything that happened leading to the injury: what you felt, signs and symptoms, and any additional information to aid in diagnosing the injury. Do not feel rushed or intimidated by confusing terminology and tests. You are the consumer and are paying for the doctor's time and services. To get your money's worth, follow these suggestions when planning to see a physician.

1. Write down a list of complaints and questions you have, such as, "I twisted my ankle last week, and it hasn't gotten any better," or "The swelling is still in my knee after applying ice and taking the medication you prescribed." Do not leave the office until you have asked all of your questions and feel completely satisfied with the responses.

2. Understand the terminology the doctor uses. If you are confused, ask him to use common, everyday terms. For example, the physician may say, "You have a second-degree anterior talofibular sprain." You would better understand it if he said, "You moderately injured a ligament on the outside of the ankle."

3. Understand the reason for the treatment. Don't be satisfied with the response, "You must rest the part for two weeks and then see

When in doubt, see a physician.

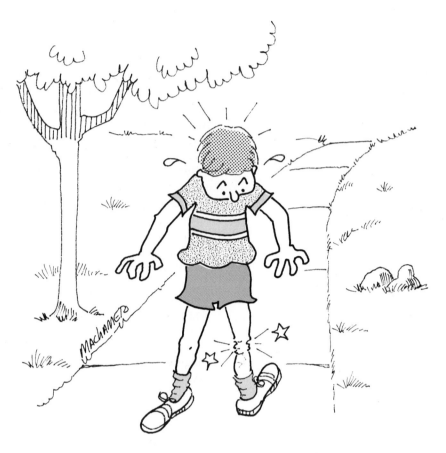

me again." Frequently, rehabilitation can be started much sooner. If not, find out which alternate activities can be done while recovering from the injury.

4. Ask about the medication prescribed. What will it do and how will it help in the recovery process? Question the physician about the side effects. Will it make me drowsy? Nauseated? Are there any special instructions I should follow?

5. Inquire of any diagnostic test that may be performed. What will it show? Where do I have to go for it? Is there any pain associated with the test?

6. If the doctor says, "You need surgery," have him explain the procedure in detail. What are the risks and benefits? How long until I can resume normal activity? What happens if I choose not to have surgery? Ask questions until you are totally satisfied with the decision.

Remember, you are the consumer. Do not rely on the nurse, receptionist, or friends to explain your injury and treatment. Make sure you completely understand everything you must do to speed your recovery.

Getting Back into Action

To resume activity, you will need to regain normal range of motion and strength in the injured body part. Move the part as early as possible to regain flexibility. When moving, avoid creating excessive discomfort. Moving the part will increase circulation and reduce the amount of swelling. Work all the motions of a joint to gain freedom of movement. For example, in an ankle injury, move the ankle up and down, in and out, 10–20 times, 3–4 times a day. Gradually increase the repetitions. If after moving the part you feel pain, apply ice and reduce the amount of repetitions in the next session. You may be doing too much too soon.

After obtaining full range of motion, begin to build strength. Gradually increase the strength of a part to equal that of the uninjured side. You can use partner resistance, free weights, rubber tubing, and universal or nautilus equipment. Work under the supervision of a qualified physical therapist or other professional, especially in the early stages of rehabilitation, since this is when you are most susceptible to reinjury.

Gradually work your way back to your former activity level. You will not be able to start where you stopped. Frequently, exercisers will try to begin working out at their previous level after injury. They will generally reinjure themselves since the weakened area is unable to withstand the stress.

Exercise and Disease Resistance

During exercise, 75 percent to 85 percent of the energy produced is released in the form of heat, producing an increase in body temperature.[15] Much of this heat is dissipated at the skin, but still, body temperature is elevated during exercise. This regular increase in body temperature, it is speculated, is inhospitable to some viruses and might decrease incidence of viral infections in exercisers, as compared to nonexercisers. Moderate exercise also has been found to boost the immune system.[16] However, overtraining, leading to exhaustion, might weaken the system and increase susceptibility to colds and minor infections. Few people exercise so strenuously that they need to worry about any possible adverse effects on immunity. The problem for most Americans is too little exercise, rather than too much!

Should you exercise when ill? If you just have a minor head cold and otherwise feel fine, it is probably all right to work out. Avoid exercise to the point of exhaustion. Avoid exercise if you have the flu, have a fever, feel achy, tired, or congested. Exercise does not cure illness! The old adage "you can sweat out a cold" with exercise is untrue. When you do recover from illness, do not start exercising at the same level as before. Give yourself a few days to build back to normal levels.

Care of the Lower Back

Lower back pain accounts for more lost time from work and more visits to physicians than any other medical problem.[17] An estimated 85 percent of Americans suffer lower back pain at some time in their lives.[18] Fortunately, over three-quarters of all back pain can be prevented with exercise, good posture, and good lifting mechanics.

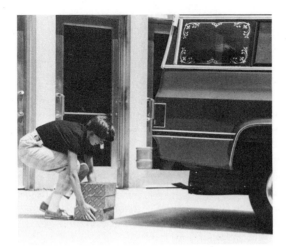

(a) Correct lifting technique.

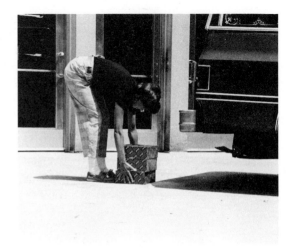

(b) Incorrect lifting technique.

Ways to Avoid Lower Back Pain

Why does back pain occur? How can risk of back injury be reduced? During the high school and college years, our bodies are relatively flexible. As we age, muscles begin to shorten and tighten, decreasing flexibility, especially in the back. With few exceptions, back problems can be resolved with improved fitness, living and work habits, and posture.

The most important keys to preventing lower back pain are to maintain strong abdominal muscles and back flexibility. Studies show that people who are physically fit have almost 10 times less back pain.[19] Many of those who suffer back pain are overweight, with weak, sagging abdominals. This puts the back into an overarched position, placing additional stress on the spinal column. Maintaining normal weight and keeping abdominal muscles strong and tight reduces strain on the spine. Strong abdominals keep the pelvis and spinal column stabilized in a normal position. At the same time, it is important to keep the opposing back muscles flexible.

The one-third of your life you spend sleeping should help, not harm, your back. This makes it very important to select a firm, but not extremely hard, mattress. Sleeping on a mattress that is too hard will leave the back unsupported. Sleeping on a sagging mattress places the back in an unbalanced position. Water beds, properly adjusted, may provide satisfactory back support as an alternative to a traditional mattress.

The fetal position is the best sleeping position for maintaining a healthy back. Lying on your side, pull your knees up to your chest. This will round the lower back and alleviate back stress. If you must sleep on your back, place a pillow or similar object under the knees to flatten the curve of the lower back. Sleeping on your stomach increases the arch of the back, shortening the back muscles. By placing a small pillow, or even your arm, under your pelvic bone (abdomen) may help straighten your spine enough to sleep without strain.

To decrease back stress when getting out of bed, roll to one side and sit up sideways, using your arms to help. This will eliminate using all of your back and abdominal muscles to get out of bed. This tip is especially helpful if you currently have a back problem.

Good lifting mechanics can reduce the risk of lower back injury. When lifting a heavy weight, bend your knees and use the large muscles of the buttocks and legs. Combining lifting with a twisting force is one of the most common causes of back injury. Instead, lift the object and pivot with your feet rather than your waist.

Keep your body close to the object. Standing far away from the object will place undue stress on the lower back. Lift with your back straight rather than bending at the waist. When carrying heavy objects such as books, backpacks, and groceries, try to distribute the load equally and close to the body. Finally, obtain help when lifting heavy objects.

Workplace Considerations

Many Americans will spend the majority of their work time behind a desk or in a car. Sedentary jobs and lifestyle make us vulnerable to back pain. How can you maintain a healthy back if your job entails a lot of sitting? Sit close to your work

Habitually carrying a heavy backpack on one side may cause back discomfort.

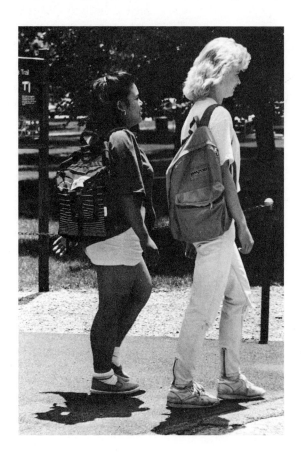

and keep your hips and knees at a 90 degree angle. This will straighten the lower back and prevent slouching. When you sit in a chair, place both feet on the floor. If the chair is too low, it will increase your back curvature excessively. Use a chair that supports your back in its normal slightly arched position. You can place a small pillow or towel against your lower back to maintain that position. Wearing high-heeled shoes is deadly for the lower back. This shortens the Achilles tendon and hamstrings, throws the back into an overarched position, and at the same time overstretches the abdominals. Wear low-heeled shoes to maintain back health.

Maintain good posture while driving, especially when driving long distances. Sitting for extended periods of time in an automobile is a frequent source of complaint of back pain sufferers. To maintain normal spinal curvature, place a small pillow between your lower back and the seat. Sit close enough to reach the accelerator and steering wheel without slumping.

If your job requires long periods of standing, you can minimize stress on the back by putting one foot on a low stool. Frequently shift your weight from one leg to another.

Finally, when driving or working in one position for an extended period of time, get up, stretch, and walk for several minutes. You will feel better, and your back will benefit from the change.

Lower Back Injuries

The lower back is made up of many tiny ligaments that hold the vertebrae together from the skull to the tailbone. A sudden severe twisting force can injure these ligaments. There are also several groups of muscles, called the erector spinae muscle group, which parallel the spinal column. These muscles may be injured by lifting a heavy weight, through excessive bending, or by sleeping on a sagging mattress.

If you suffer back pain, what symptoms indicate that you should see a physician? Numbness or tingling in the legs, buttocks, or back may indicate an impingement of a spinal nerve of an **intervertebral disc** injury. The intervertebral disc is a cushion that separates the bony vertebrae. Discs are filled with fluid and are flexible through early adulthood, but thin and lose their resiliency as we age. A ruptured intervertebral disc will compress the nerve, causing pain down the buttocks and legs. Consult a physician who specializes in back pain for these injuries.

Exercises for the Lower Back

There are several exercises you can do to maintain a healthy back. We recommend the exercise routine in figure 5.3. Practice this series daily for best results. These exercises should not cause any pain, numbness, or tingling in the back and legs. If they do, discontinue them and consult your specialist.

Figure 5.3

Exercises for the lower back.

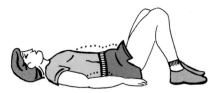

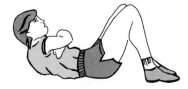

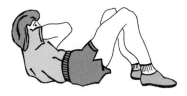

1. Lie on back, knees bent. Press smallof back firmly down to floor by tightening the abdominal muscles. Hold for a count of 5.

2. Do a pelvic tilt and, while holding this position, curl head and shoulders up until shoulder blades have been lifted from the floor. Hold briefly. Lower slowly.

3. Do a pelvic tilt and, while holding this position, curl head and shoulders up, twisting right shoulder toward left knee. Hold briefly. Lower slowly. Repeat other side.

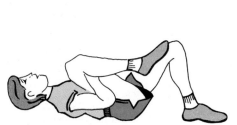

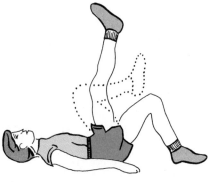

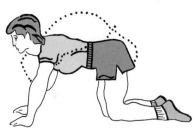

4. a. Lie on back. Pull one knee toward chest. Hold for a count of 5. Repeat other leg.
   b. Double knee pull. Pull both knees to chest; hold for a count of 5.

5. Lie on back. Bring knee toward chest and extend leg toward ceiling. Flex foot. (You may grasp the back of your thigh with your hands.) Hold 20 seconds. Repeat with other leg.

6. Start on all fours. Round the back upward like a cat. Tighten your abdominals. Hold for 5 seconds. Relax and return to starting position. Do not let back sag.

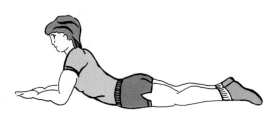

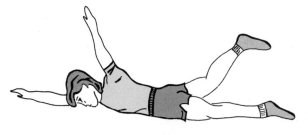

7. Lie on your stomach with forearms flat on the ground. Tighten abdominals. Lift upper body using back muscles. Do not press with arms. Hold for a count of 5.

8. Lie on your stomach with arms extended in front. Raise one arm overhead toward ceiling while simultaneously lifting the opposite leg. Hold for a count of 5. Repeat with the other arm and leg.

Summary

Much soreness and injury can be prevented. Stretching, strengthening, proper warm-up, sensible progressions, and avoiding overuse are the keys. It is better to block injuries at their source than to pay doctors' fees to treat breakdowns. The pursuit of excellence involves learning to balance your own individual strengths and weaknesses, and cooperating with your body instead of assaulting it.

You can prevent lower back problems with proper care and treatment. Maintain leg and back flexibility, strengthen abdominals, utilize correct lifting mechanics, and reduce sources of lower back stress. This is all within your control.

References

1. "Exercise Without Injury." *University of California, Berkeley Wellness Letter* 6 (March 1990): 4–5.

2. Macera, Caroline A. "Lower Extremity Injuries in Runners: Advances in Prediction." *Sports Medicine* 13 (January 1992): 50–57.

3. Macera. "Lower Extremity Injuries in Runners."

4. "Exercise Without Injury."

5. Cook, Stephen D., Mark R. Brinker, and Mahlon Poche. "Running Shoes: Their Relationship to Running Injuries." *Sports Medicine* 10 (July 1990): 1–8.

6. "Fascinating Facts." *University of California, Berkeley Wellness Letter* 8 (January 1992): 1.

7. "Relief: Exercise Injuries, Part II." *University of California, Berkeley Wellness Letter* 6 (May 1990): 4–5.

8. "Relief: Exercise Injuries, Part II."

9. Delhagen, Kate. "Health Watch." *Runner's World* 24 (July 1989): 21.

10. Buroker, Katherine C., and James A. Schwane. "Does Postexercise Static Stretching Alleviate Delayed Muscle Soreness?" *The Physician and Sportsmedicine* 17 (June 1989): 65–83.

11. Warren, Barbara L. "Plantar Fasciitis in Runners: Treatment and Prevention." *Sports Medicine* 10 (November 1990): 338–45.

12. Seder, Joseph I. "How I Managed Heel Spur Syndrome." *The Physician and Sportsmedicine* 15 (February 1987): 83–84.

13. Ellis, Joe. "Shin Splints: Too Much, Too Soon." *Runner's World* 21 (March 1986): 50–53, 86.

14. Matin, Philip, G. Lang, and R. Carretta. "Bone Scanning for Detection of Exercise-Induced Musculoskeletal Injury." *The Physician and Sportsmedicine* 17 (September 1989): 124–35.

15. Costill, David L. *Inside Running: Basics of Sports Physiology.* Dubuque, IA: Brown and Benchmark Publishers, 1986.

16. "Does Exercise Boost Immunity?" *University of California, Berkeley Wellness Letter* 8 (March 1992): 6.

17. Collins, John, and Barbara Agenbroad. *What You Can Do For Your Back.* Washington, DC: Department of Veterans Affairs, Fall 1991.

18. Harvey, Jack, and Suzanne Tanner. "Low Back Pain in Young Athletes." *Sports Medicine* 12 (December 1991): 394–406.

19. Collins, and Agenbroad. *What You Can Do For Your Back.*

Suggested Readings

Clayton, Lawrence, and Betty Sharon Smith. 1992. *Coping with Sports Injuries.* New York: Rosen Publishing Group.

Cook, Stephen D., Mark Brinker, and Mahlon Poche. "Running Shoes: Their Relationship to Running Injuries." *Sports Medicine* 10 (July 1990): 1–8.

Ellis, Joe. "The Match Game: Finding the Right Shoe for Your Biomechanics and Running Gait." *Runner's World* 20 (October 1985): 66–70.

Francis, Peter, and Lorna Francis. 1988. *If It Hurts, Don't Do It.* Rocklin, CA: Prima Publishing.

Guten, Gary N., M.D. 1991. *Play Healthy, Stay Healthy.* Champaign, IL: Human Kinetics Publishers.

"Improving Your Posture." *University of California, Berkeley Wellness Letter* 8 (March 1992): 4–5.

Macera, Caroline A. "Lower Extremity Injuries in Runners: Advances in Prediction." *Sports Medicine* 13 (January 1992): 50–57.

McKeag, Douglas B., and Cathleen Dolan. "Overuse Symptoms of the Lower Extremity." *The Physician and Sportsmedicine* 17 (July 1989): 108–23.

Ritter, Merrill A., M.D., and Marjorie J. Albohm. 1987. *Your Injury: A Common Sense Guide To Sports Injuries.* Dubuque, IA: Brown and Benchmark Publishers.

Root, Leon, M.D. 1990. *No More Aching Back.* New York, NY: Villard Books.

Swezey, Robert L., M.D., and Annette M. Swezey. 1990. *Good News for Bad Backs.* New York, NY: Knightsbridge Publishing Co.

White, Augustus A. III, M.D. 1990. *Your Aching Back.* New York, NY: Simon and Schuster Inc.

YMCA of the USA. 1991. *Y's Way To a Healthy Back.* Champaign, IL: Human Kinetics Publishers.

6

Heart Health

Chapter Objectives

After reading this chapter, you will be able to:

1. Identify the percentage of deaths in the United States attributable to heart disease.
2. Identify the four primary heart disease risk factors.
3. Identify the eight secondary heart disease risk factors.
4. Identify the controllable and uncontrollable risk factors for coronary heart disease (CHD).
5. Define arteriosclerosis, atherosclerosis, angina pectoris, myocardial infarction, and stroke.
6. Identify the symptoms of a heart attack.
7. Identify the role of cholesterol and saturated fats in the development of atherosclerosis.
8. Explain the roles of HDL and LDL in heart health.
9. Explain why smoking cigarettes increases heart disease risk.
10. Identify normal blood pressure range and the blood pressure reading that indicates hypertension.
11. Identify the cholesterol reading that indicates high blood cholesterol.
12. Recognize the personality traits of Type A behavior that increase heart disease risk.
13. Recognize five of eight heart disease risk factors that are positively affected by exercise.
14. Identify the two trends that will impact on cardiovascular disease in the future.

Terms

- Angina pectoris
- Arteriosclerosis
- Atherosclerosis
- Cardiovascular disease
- Cholesterol
- Collateral circulation
- Diabetes mellitus
- Diastolic blood pressure
- High-density lipoprotein (HDL)
- Hypertension
- LDL cholesterol receptors
- Low-density lipoprotein (LDL)
- Myocardial infarction
- Plaque
- Primary risk factor
- Risk factor
- Secondary hypertension
- Secondary risk factor
- Stroke
- Systolic blood pressure
- Triglycerides
- Type A, B, C personality patterns

Impact of Cardiovascular

The number one killer in America is not cancer, accidents, or AIDS. It is heart disease (fig. 6.1). Make no mistake, cancer and other diseases are a real threat, however, cardiovascular diseases kill more than twice as many victims as all other leading causes of death. The tragedy is compounded because cardiovascular diseases are often inaccurately perceived as diseases of the elderly. On the contrary, based on data from the Framingham Heart Study, (chapter 1) approximately 45 percent of all heart attack victims are under the age of 65, and 5 percent are under the age of 40.[1] These diseases demand attention because they are killing too many Americans who are in the prime of their lives. Don't become complacent! The way you are living your life now determines your future heart health. Many coronary heart disease deaths are preventable. You can reduce your chances of developing coronary heart disease by assessing your current level of risk and by learning ways to reduce those identified risk factors. Education and behavior change are the keys.

Cardiovascular disease (CVD) accounts for nearly half of all deaths in the United States according to the American Heart Association (AHA) statistics.[2] In other words, one out of two Americans who die each year do so from CVD. **Cardiovascular disease** (from "cardio" meaning heart and "vascular" meaning blood vessels) is a condition in which either blood flow through the heart and

Figure 6.1

Leading causes of death by sex.

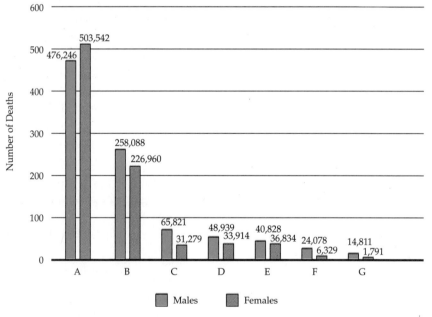

A Cardiovascular Disease and Stroke
B Cancer
C Accidents
D Chronic Obstructive Pulmonary Disease
E Pneumonia and Influenza
F Suicide
G AIDS

More Americans die each year from heart disease than the equivalent number killed in 10 Vietnam Wars.

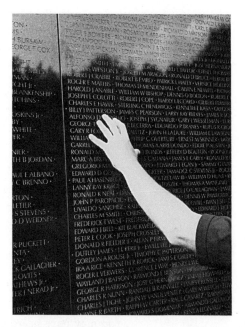

body is impeded, or the electrical impulse of the heart muscle is interrupted. Common forms of CVD include heart attack, stroke, high blood pressure, angina pectoris, irregular heartbeat, congestive heart failure, rheumatic heart disease, and congenital heart disease. More than one in four Americans suffer from these related disorders. Studies show that the incidence of death from heart disease is much greater for the least educated than for the most educated.[3]

Of all CVD deaths, 54.6 percent were from heart attack, making this disease the most prevalent form and the leading cause of death in America today. The cost of CVD in 1989 was estimated by the AHA at $108.9 billion. This figure includes the cost of physician and nursing services, hospital and nursing home services, the cost of medications, and lost productivity resulting from disability. While costs for treatment of CVD are spiraling upward, the death rate for these diseases appears to be declining. Advances in medical treatment, education, and healthy lifestyle changes can be credited for the declining death rate. However, don't become too complacent about these facts. We still have a long way to go. Cardiovascular disease is a killer; someone still dies every 34 seconds.[4]

Coronary Heart Disease

The heart is a muscle that works all the time. It never stops beating. Each day the average heart beats 100,000 times and pumps about 2,000 gallons of blood. Besides providing oxygen and other nutrients to all tissues of the body, the heart must supply itself with oxygen. It has a separate circulatory system, which nourishes only the heart muscle. This system has two coronary arteries, each about the size of a pencil, that subdivide and encircle the entire heart muscle (fig. 6.2).

Figure 6.2
Coronary artery system.

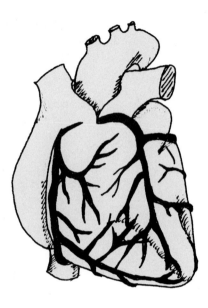

You may have heard of someone who has "hardening of the arteries." This is actually **arteriosclerosis,** which is a general term for the thickening and hardening of arteries. Some hardening of arteries normally occurs as we age. Coronary heart disease is most commonly the result of atherosclerosis. **Atherosclerosis** is a type of arteriosclerosis. It is a progressive condition in which deposits of cholesterol and other lipids, along with cellular waste products accumulate on the inner walls of coronary arteries. This buildup is called **plaque.** As the condition progresses, the inner walls of blood vessels become more and more inelastic and clogged and may become totally hardened and blocked. Sometimes a blood clot forms on the plaque buildup and blocks the entire artery. A heart attack or stroke may result.

There are a variety of causes of atherosclerosis, many of which are related to unhealthy lifestyle choices. One theory attributes atherosclerosis to minor injuries of the inner wall of coronary arteries, which create a roughened region where debris and materials in the blood can attach. Thus begins the atherosclerotic buildup. What injures the lining of our coronary arteries? High blood cholesterol levels, excessive dietary cholesterol and saturated fat, high blood pressure, your reaction to perceived emotional stress, and nicotine are often responsible. All are influenced by lifestyle. Besides causing damage to the smooth lining of our blood vessels, lifestyle factors also contribute to excess plaque in the bloodstream. Atherosclerosis does not suddenly develop at age 65. It is a long, progressive process beginning in childhood.

Angina Pectoris

Atherosclerosis may lead to **angina pectoris,** or chest pain. This pain occurs when a coronary artery becomes partially blocked, causing an oxygen debt in the heart muscle. Often, angina pectoris is brought on by sudden exertion or vigorous exercise when the blood flow to the heart is insufficient to meet its oxygen demands. The Framingham Heart Study estimated that 2.5 million people suffer from angina pectoris with 350,000 new cases occurring each year.[5]

Myocardial Infarction

Myocardial infarction, or heart attack, results when one or more of the coronary arteries is partially blocked by atherosclerosis and a blood clot (thrombus) plugs the remaining opening. The portion of heart muscle beyond the blockage is deprived of oxygen, resulting in injury or death of that portion of the heart muscle. If a damaged area is large enough or in a vital area of the heart, the individual will die. However, many people do survive a heart attack and are capable of living productive lives (table 6.1).

Table 6.1

Warning Signs of a Heart Attack

- Uncomfortable pressure, fullness, squeezing or pain in the center of the chest lasting two minutes or longer.
- Pain spreading to shoulders, neck, jaw, arms, or back.
- Severe pain, lightheadedness, fainting, sweating, nausea, and/or shortness of breath.

Not all of these warning signs occur in every heart attack. If some of these symptoms do occur, don't wait. Get help immediately!

Source: 1992 Heart Facts. American Heart Association.

A number of studies have shown that in some damaged hearts new blood vessels develop to nourish the area that is being starved of oxygen and other nutrients. This is called **collateral circulation.** Everyone has collateral blood vessels, which are microscopic and closed under normal conditions. However, in some people with coronary heart disease, these seem to enlarge and form a detour around the blockage to provide alternate routes for the blood. Exercise appears to be one practical way to increase myocardial oxygen demand, which in turn may stimulate the development of collateral vessels. In some cases, coronary angiography (x-ray) has revealed increased collaterization after exercise training.[6]

Stroke

A **stroke** occurs when blood flow to the brain is blocked. The brain needs a continuous supply of oxygen-rich blood to function. When a blood clot interrupts the flow of oxygen, the brain does not receive the nourishment it needs, and brain cells die. Atherosclerosis is a leading cause of stroke, which is the third largest cause of death behind heart attack and cancer. While declining, the death rate for strokes is still high, however[7] (see fig. 6.3). A stroke can result in death, paralysis of one side of the body, loss of ability to speak or to understand the speech of others, loss of memory, and behavioral change. Because brain cells

Figure 6.3

Death rate for stroke.

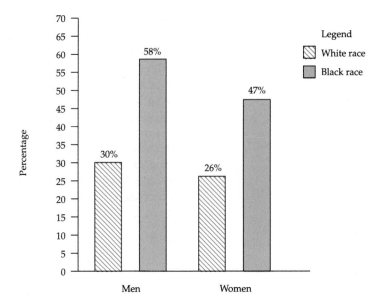

can't heal, modification of risk factors is very important in the prevention of this disease that affects 500,000 Americans every year.[8] Your risk of stroke increases with these factors:

- Hypertension—If you have high blood pressure, you are two to four times more likely to have a stroke than someone with normal blood pressure.

- Heart Disease—Sometimes blood clots forming in the heart can move up to the brain and block blood flow.

- Gender—About 19 percent more men than women have strokes.

- Diabetes—Those with diabetes have almost double the risk of stroke.

- Age—Eighty percent of stroke victims are 65 or older.

- Race—Black Americans have nearly twice as many fatal strokes as whites. Hypertension and sickle cell anemia are the suspected causes.

- Lifestyle—Factors that increase risk of stroke and can be controlled: high-fat, high cholesterol diet; *alcohol or cocaine abuse*; smoking; and sedentary lifestyle.

Risk Factors

Risk factors are the conditions, situations, and behaviors that increase the likelihood that an undesirable outcome (injury, illness, or death) will occur. The risk is generally established by multiple scientific studies. A risk factor does not cause the undesirable outcome 100 percent of the time, but of those people who engage in the behavior (or experience the condition), a certain number of them will experience the undesired outcome. The stronger the risk factors link with a negative outcome, the more likely it is that an individual will experience the undesired result.

The riskiness of various behaviors is determined in part through epidemiological research, which involves studying large populations in order to investigate the causes and control of diseases. The famous Framingham Study is an example of this type of research. Research studies on animals and humans, in which conditions are carefully set up to test a hypotheses, are often needed to confirm relationships among behaviors, conditions, illness, and death. Over time, clearer and clearer pictures emerge about the degree of danger or risk in a particular situation until health experts can say, "If you do this, chances are good that this will occur." An example of this is the link between smoking, cholesterol, hypertension, and heart attack seen in figure 6.4.

CHD researchers have identified several risk factors that may lead to the development of atherosclerosis. The more risk factors you possess, the greater your chances are of developing coronary heart disease. While no one can accurately

Figure 6.4

Danger of heart attack within 8 years by risk factors present.

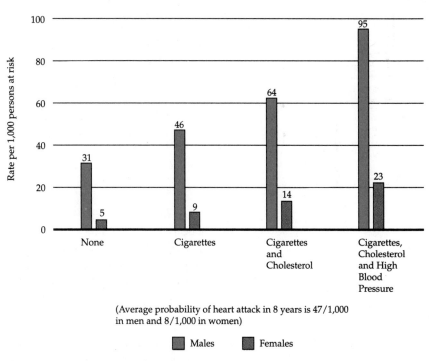

(Average probability of heart attack in 8 years is 47/1,000 in men and 8/1,000 in women)

■ Males   ■ Females

This chart shows how a combination of three major risk factors can increase the likelihood of heart attack. For purposes of illustration, this chart uses an abnormal blood pressure level of 150 systolic and a cholesterol level of 260 in a 55-year-old male and female.

*Risk ratios for men in the Framingham Heart Study, where the average is equal to 100, are 66 for no major risk factors; 98 for cigarette smoking; 136 for a combination of cigarettes and elevated blood cholesterol; and 202 for a combination of cigarettes, elevated cholesterol and high blood pressure. For women in the Framingham Heart Study, comparable ratios are 63, 113, 175 and 288, respectively.

predict whether you will have a heart attack, you can estimate your odds by evaluating your risk factors. Take the "Are You At Risk" test in the activities section to determine your risk and how to reduce it.

Primary risk factors are linked directly to the development of CHD; they increase the possibility of having a heart attack. *All primary risk factors are controllable.*

Controllable

1. High blood pressure	**3.** Cigarette smoking
2. High blood lipid level	**4.** Inactivity

The **secondary risk factors** for heart disease contribute to the development of coronary heart disease, but not as directly as the primary risk factors.

Controllable

1. Obesity	**3.** Emotional behavior
2. Stress	

Uncontrollable

4. Age	**7.** Positive family history
5. Gender	**8.** Diabetes mellitus
6. Race	

Notice that some of these secondary risk factors are *controllable.* The choices you make or the way you live have a profound impact in reducing these risk factors. If you possess several uncontrollable risk factors, it is imperative that you adopt a healthy lifestyle.

Primary Risk Factors

1. High Blood Pressure (Hypertension)   Blood pressure is the force exerted by the heart while pumping blood through the body. It is also the pressure of blood against the arterial walls.

There are actually two blood pressure levels, recorded as two separate numbers in fraction form (example: 120/80). When the heart contracts and pumps blood into the arteries, the pressure increases. This is the **systolic,** or pumping, **pressure** which is recorded as the upper number. The **diastolic,** or resting, **pressure** is the force of the blood against the arteries when the heart relaxes between beats. It is recorded as the lower number. Average blood pressure is 120/80, and the acceptable range is 90/60 up to 140/90. **High blood pressure (hypertension)** is generally acknowledged as blood pressure equal to or greater than 140/90.

High blood pressure causes the heart to overwork. Over a period of time the overworked heart weakens, enlarges, and has a difficult time keeping up with the demands of the body. High blood pressure also causes blood vessels to become inelastic, severely reducing the amount of blood flow to the body's vital organs. As a result, decreased levels of oxygen and other nutrients can produce heart, brain, and kidney damage.

Have your blood pressure checked regularly.

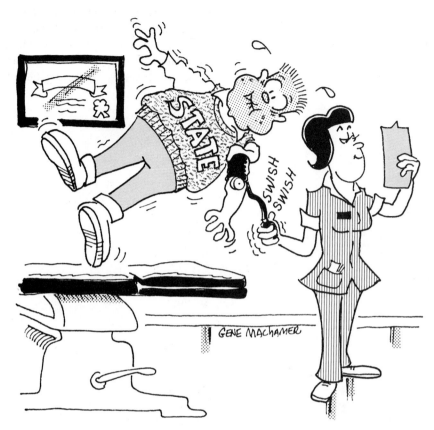

In 90 percent of the cases of high blood pressure there is no known cause. However, factors that can increase your chances of developing high blood pressure are heredity, cigarette smoking, male gender, age, black race, obesity, sensitivity to sodium, heavy alcohol consumption, use of oral contraceptives, and a sedentary lifestyle. In a small number of cases, hypertension is caused by a specific condition, such as kidney disease, tumor of the adrenal gland, or a defect of the aorta. This is called **secondary hypertension.** The cause of secondary hypertension can generally be identified and treated successfully.

How do you know if your blood pressure is too high? The only way of knowing is to have it checked. You cannot feel high blood pressure. High blood pressure has no symptoms, which is why it is so dangerous. You can be hypertensive for years and be unaware of the damage occurring. Of those with high blood pressure, over 46 percent do not know they have it.[9] It is imperative that you know your blood pressure, because high blood pressure, while it cannot be cured, can be controlled by reducing weight, increasing physical activity, eating a well-balanced diet, controlling sodium intake, and taking your medication, if prescribed. Studies by Dr. Herbert Benson at the Harvard Medical School found that patients' blood pressure remained significantly reduced 3 to 5 years after making lifestyle changes that included meditation, group support, diet, and exercise.[10]

2. High Blood Lipid Profile (Cholesterol and Triglycerides)   Research has firmly linked high levels of cholesterol and other blood fats to the development of arterial plaque, a major cause of atherosclerosis and coronary heart disease. **Cholesterol** is not a true fat, but a waxy substance found in the blood stream. It is manufactured in the liver and is also consumed in foods of animal origin.

Cholesterol is not all bad. It is needed by the body for cell structure and for the manufacture of hormones. The problem with cholesterol is that your body makes most of what it needs, and the normal American diet adds much more. As a result, one half of all adult Americans have cholesterol levels high enough to require treatment[11] (see fig. 6.5).

Figure 6.5

Estimated percentage of American adults with serum cholesterol of 200 mg/dl or more.

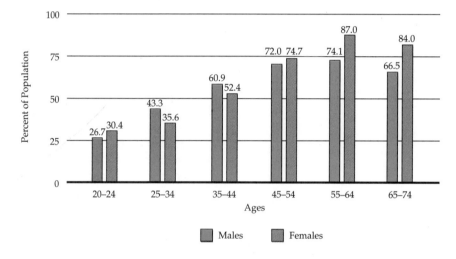

Ninety-five percent of the fats in the body are in the form of triglycerides, a true fat stored in the fat cells and found in the blood. Both high cholesterol and triglycerides increase the risk of developing atherosclerosis.

When evaluating your blood lipid profile for risk of heart disease, there are two factors to consider: (1) the total amount of cholesterol/triglycerides found in the blood, and (2) the way cholesterol/triglycerides are transported in the bloodstream.

Total Amount of Lipids. Knowing your total cholesterol level provides you with a rough estimate of your heart disease risk. Blood cholesterol is measured by analyzing a small blood sample in a laboratory. Total cholesterol level includes the amount of cholesterol carried by high-density lipoprotein, low-density lipoprotein, and very low-density lipoprotein. The National Heart, Lung, and Blood Institute relates cholesterol level to heart disease risk as illustrated in table 6.2.

Transportation of Lipids. Like oil and water, cholesterol and blood do not mix. So, cholesterol must attach itself to a protein molecule to be carried through the bloodstream. This combination is called a lipoprotein. There are two main types of lipoprotein:

HDL cholesterol clearing away plaque in arteries.

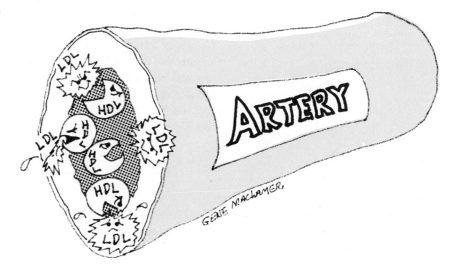

1. **Low-density lipoprotein (LDL).** LDLs are considered "bad" because they carry a large amount of cholesterol. The lower density of the lipoprotein allows it to easily attach to the inner wall of the blood vessel, thus accelerating the atherosclerotic process. A *high* LDL cholesterol level increases your risk for heart disease (see table 6.3). Cigarette smoking, emotional stressors, and diets high in saturated fat have been shown to increase the LDL level. Very low-density lipoproteins (VLDL) are even more dangerous.

2. **High-density lipoprotein (HDL).** HDL is considered to be a "good" form of cholesterol because of the dense structure of the lipoprotein. It is thought that HDL acts as a garbage collector in clearing away plaque and other debris as it flows through the blood stream to the liver to be excreted from the body. The higher your HDL-cholesterol level, the better, and the more protection from heart disease it provides. How can you increase your level of HDL? Exercise regularly, don't smoke, and maintain a normal weight. High fiber and low-fat diets may also increase the HDL cholesterol level.

   Alcohol consumption has received attention recently as a protective factor against heart attack because it is thought to raise HDL-cholesterol in the blood. Consuming one drink a day (12 oz. of beer, one glass of wine, or one shot of hard liquor) is the amount associated with a reduction in the rate of heart attacks. Consuming more than two drinks a day is known to damage the heart. It should be emphasized that a protective effect of alcohol consumption has not been proven, but many adverse effects are well documented. Besides the danger of automobile accidents and social disruption, excess intake of alcohol can raise blood pressure and triglyceride levels and cause diseases of the liver, pancreas, and nervous system. Even though alcohol consumption above moderate levels adversely affects blood pressure and triglycerides and can damage the heart, alcohol is currently not considered a primary or secondary heart disease risk factor, however.

Table 6.2

Total Blood Cholesterol Levels (mg/dl)

Source: National Heart, Lung, and Blood Institute, U.S. Department of Health and Human Services.

	Total Cholesterol (mg/dl)
Desirable	Under 200
Borderline High	200–239
High	240 or more

Note: The levels apply to anyone 20 years of age or older.
Recommended treatment: Reduce saturated fat and cholesterol in your diet. If your blood cholesterol goal is not reached, drug therapy may be needed.

Table 6.3

LDL-Cholesterol Levels

Source: National Heart, Lung, and Blood Institute, U.S. Department of Health and Human Services, National Institute of Health.

Desirable	Less than 130 mg/dl
Borderline High Risk	130 to 159 mg/dl
High Risk	160 mg/dl and above

Scientists now believe that the ratio of total cholesterol to HDL-cholesterol is a better indicator of risk for cardiovascular disease than the total value alone. To determine your ratio, take a laboratory blood test that will reveal your total cholesterol and HDL-cholesterol levels. Next, divide the total cholesterol level by the HDL-cholesterol level to find the ratio. For example, if the total cholesterol was measured to be 160 and the HDL-cholesterol 40, your ratio would be four (160 ÷ 40 = 4). This would place you at lower than average risk, as you can see in table 6.4. It is generally accepted that a 4.5 or lower ratio (total cholesterol/HDL-cholesterol) is excellent for men, and 4.0 or lower is best for women.[12]

Table 6.4

Ratio of Total Cholesterol and HDL-Cholesterol to Risk of CHD

Source: The Wellness Encyclopedia, University of California, Berkeley.

Risk of Heart Disease	Ratio of TC/HDL-C Men		Ratio of TC/HDL-C Women	
Very Low	under	3.43	under	3.27
Low		4.97		4.44
Moderate		9.55		7.05
High	more than	23.39	more than	11.04

Average HDL levels in adult Americans are about 45 to 65 mg/dl, with women averaging higher than men. Studies suggest that HDL levels above 70 may protect against heart disease, while those below 35 signal coronary risk.[13]

There is genetic variability in how efficiently (or inefficiently) a person metabolizes dietary saturated fat and cholesterol. Some people can eat almost anything and their blood cholesterol levels remain stable. Others find that even a small amount of dietary fat makes their blood cholesterol levels increase. Most of us are somewhere in between on this spectrum.

Drs. Michael Brown and Joseph Goldstein won the Nobel Prize in Medicine in 1985 for their discovery of **LDL cholesterol receptors.** Located primarily in liver cells, they bind and remove cholesterol from the blood. The more cholesterol receptors you have, the more efficiently you can remove cholesterol from the blood. The number of cholesterol receptors is, in part, genetically determined. Lifestyle factors also influence the number. A diet high in saturated fat and cholesterol produces what Drs. Brown and Goldstein termed "double trouble." It not only saturates the receptors, it also decreases their number—a bad combination. Only about 5 percent of the population have genetically high cholesterol levels that remain elevated regardless of lifestyle.[14] This condition is known as hypercholesterolemia.

Triglycerides are manufactured in the body to store excess fats. They are also known as free fatty acids, and in combination with cholesterol, they accelerate the formation of plaque. Triglycerides are carried in the bloodstream by very low density lipoprotein (VLDL). These fatty acids are found in poultry skin, lunch meats, and shellfish. However, they are mainly manufactured in the liver from refined sugars, starches, and alcohol. High intake of alcohol and sugars (honey included) will significantly increase triglyceride levels. Thus, they can be lowered by decreasing consumption of the above mentioned foods, along with weight reduction (if overweight) and aerobic exercise. As a general rule, you should keep your triglyceride level below 250 mg/dl of blood. However, some reports indicate triglyceride levels over 150 should be cause for concern.

You should know your cholesterol level and have it checked annually, especially if you have a positive family history of heart disease. The National Heart Savers Association states that only 8 percent of Americans know their cholesterol level and more than 50 percent have a level that is too high. A diet rich in cholesterol—or worse, one rich in saturated fat—can increase your blood cholesterol level. Keep fat consumption between 10 percent and 30 percent or less of total calories per day. This small modification in dietary fat can reduce cholesterol levels by 10 percent to 15 percent. (See chapter 9 for other dietary strategies that affect heart health.) To lower cholesterol, reduce body weight if overweight. Weight reduction alone can lower cholesterol and triglyceride levels. Lowering your stress level also helps offset high cholesterol. Finally, increase daily activity. Try to walk more, use escalators and cars less, be a participant rather than a spectator.

3. Cigarette Smoking   Cigarette smoking is a primary risk factor. Every cigarette package is required by law to carry a consumer warning. One such warning is, "Quitting Smoking Now Greatly Reduces Serious Risks to Your Health."

Numerous studies have proven that cigarette smoking causes oral cancer, lung cancer, emphysema, and in women it is linked to cervical cancer, early menopause, and damage to the fetus during pregnancy. It also leads to the development of wrinkles in both men and women. The number of Americans killed each year from smoking is greater than the number killed during World War II and the Vietnam War combined.[15] No level of smoking is safe!

The American Heart Association reports that smokers have more than twice the risk of heart attack as nonsmokers. Even limited smoking (4–5 cigarettes per day) increases CHD risk. Also, smoking increases the risk of developing peripheral vascular disease (narrowing blood vessels in the arms and legs), which may lead to the development of gangrene and eventually amputation.

Passive smoke, synonymous with secondhand smoke, is the cigarette smoke inhaled by nonsmokers from environmental air. Research has shown:

1. Heavy smoking in the same work place or study area gives the nonsmoker the equivalent of "mainstream" smoking 2–3 cigarettes a day.

2. Nonsmokers who live with smokers have a 20 percent to 30 percent higher risk of dying from heart disease than do other nonsmokers. Secondhand smoke is linked to 37,000 heart disease deaths annually.

3. The toxic agents (such as nicotine, ammonia, tar, and carbon monoxide) are found in greater concentration in sidestream smoke from the burning end of a cigarette than in mainstream smoke.

4. Secondhand smoke is a human carcinogen, killing about 3,000 non-smokers a year because of lung cancer. Smoking is everyone's business!

We also know:

1. Nicotine, the addictive element in tobacco, causes the heart to beat faster and is a heart muscle irritant. Smoking can cause disturbances in the heart rhythm, producing sudden death.

2. Heart rate and blood pressure are raised by cigarette smoking, causing the heart to work harder.

3. Carbon monoxide, a substance in cigarette smoke, damages the smooth inner lining of blood vessel walls. This accelerates the atherosclerotic buildup. Carbon monoxide, higher in the blood of smokers than in nonsmokers, also decreases the amount of oxygen carried in the blood.

4. Cigarette smoking *decreases* the HDL levels in the bloodstream (the "good" type of cholesterol).

Smoking promotes heart disease. A nonsmoker should not begin to smoke. Smokers should stop smoking *now*.

4. Inactivity   Countless studies have linked inactivity to coronary heart disease. The Centers for Disease Control (CDC) in Atlanta has found that 59 percent of Americans exercise less than three 20-minute sessions per week, and that our nation's most common cardiac threat is physical inactivity[16] (see fig. 6.6). The American life-style is very sedentary. We no longer have to hunt and grow our own food, build our own homes, or walk to school and work. Our ancestors did

Americans are ingenious at avoiding activity.

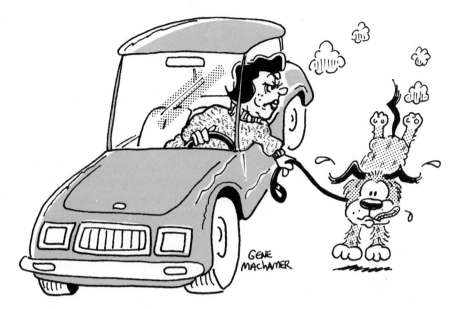

not have to build physical activity into their daily lives; it was a part of their lifestyle. A landmark study of 2,300 men and women, reported in the American Journal of Epidemiology, focused on the effects of alcohol consumption and exercise on the heart. Researchers found that while 31 percent of heart attacks among their subjects were associated with smoking (many drinkers smoke) and 22 percent could be attributed to hypertension (alcohol elevates blood pressure), an overwhelming 43 percent resulted from physical inactivity.[17]

In yet another ongoing inquiry into the relationship between physical activity and mortality, the Harvard Alumni Study produced results that led its director Dr. Ralph S. Paffenbarger to conclude that "There's no doubt whatever that

Figure 6.6

Estimated percentage of U.S. population having selected risk factors for coronary heart disease.

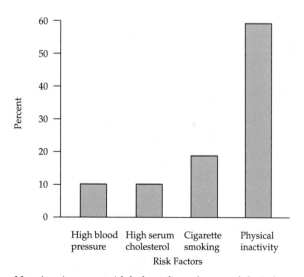

More Americans are at risk for heart disease because of physical inactivity than because of any other manageable risk factor.

insufficient activity will shorten your life." The results of this study suggest that longevity may be more closely tied to activity such as gardening or walking the dog than to strenuous exercise.[18] Modern conveniences and technology have virtually eliminated physical activity from our lifestyles. The culprits are the automobile, television (now with remote control), elevators, escalators, riding lawn mowers, and portable telephone. You can probably add more to this list.

Vigorous physical exercise is essential to a healthy cardiovascular system. Equally important, however, is overall lifestyle and how long you have been exercising. News from the University of Auckland School of Medicine in New Zealand indicates that the longer you have been exercising, the lower your risk of developing heart disease. The type of regular exercise they found to be protective included light activities as well as the intense variety. For example, they noted that the protection given by jogging was similar to that for light activities such as brisk walking, dancing, and calisthenics. It was reported that after 5 years of regular exercise, the risk of heart disease decreased sharply, indicating that the longer you adhere to an exercise program the healthier your heart will be.[19] The old saying "Use it or lose it!" is true. You don't have to run marathons to be physically active. Small increases in daily activity can significantly burn up excess calories, make the heart muscle stronger and a more efficient pump, lower blood pressure, alleviate stress, increase HDL levels, and build self-confidence.

The American Heart Association reports that regular vigorous exercise may protect against coronary heart disease and may even improve the survival rate after a heart attack.[20] That is life insurance that money cannot buy. The single most important thing you can do to improve your health and well-being is to *exercise!* What is the least amount of exercise you have to do to protect your heart? Significant benefit from exercise comes from expending an extra (beyond daily living requirements) 2,000 calories per week. Expending more calories in exercise than this is not going to change your risk appreciably. Thus, exercise burning approximately 300 calories a day, 7 days a week is sufficient—this is about 30 minutes to 45 minutes per day of exercise. Ride your bike, walk to school, play tennis instead of watching others doing these activities. Park at the back of the parking lot instead of right next to the building. There are many ways to add activity to your daily life.

Secondary Risk Factors
These are factors associated with increased risk of heart disease, though not as directly as the primary risk factors.

1. Obesity Obesity is uncomfortable and increases the burden on the vital organs, especially the heart. Research supports the link between obesity and coronary heart disease. Hypertension is nearly 6 times higher in overweight people aged 20 to 44.[21] Also, obese individuals have high blood cholesterol levels twice as often and develop diabetes three times more frequently than the nonobese. Gaining weight often precipitates diabetes. In addition, obesity puts women in particular at increased risk of heart disease. A study conducted by the Harvard Medical School of 115,000 women age 30 to 55 found that of all the women in the 8 year study who developed heart disease, 40 percent of them had no other risk factors except being 20 percent or more over their ideal weight.[22] Women who had been slim at age 18 and gained weight in adulthood seemed to be at increased risk. The first step in medical treatment for these conditions is usually weight reduction. Obesity is controllable and can be reversed. You can eliminate the obesity risk factor by maintaining reasonable weight (see chapter 10).

Physical inactivity is a major factor in the development of obesity in men, women, and children. Watching too much television is one of the main culprits. The average number of television hours per home, per day, has increased from 4:35 in 1950, 5:56 in 1970, to 6:55 in 1990. Americans should limit TV viewing to about one hour a day to prevent physical and mental inactivity.[23]

If over 35, you should have a tolerance test before an exercise program is started.

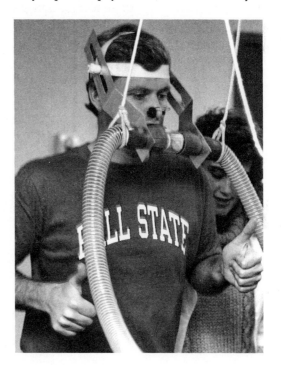

2. Stress Stress is unavoidable. It includes happy, wonderful, and positive events as well as sad, destructive, and negative ones. For example, the birth of a child produces stress just as does the death of a family member. Job stress may be particularly unhealthy. High blood pressure is 3 times more common among people who have jobs with high demands but little control (i.e., assembly line worker, waitress).[24] Stress has been found to cause a rise in heart rate, blood pressure, and blood cholesterol, and can lead to excessive smoking or eating—all linked to coronary heart disease. The type of stress is not that important.[25] Indianapolis 500 race car drivers have higher cholesterol levels after they raced than before. Tax accountants have increased cholesterol around April 15 when compared to the rest of the year. Students have higher cholesterol levels during exams. Stress causes chemical wear and tear on the body by releasing stress hormones into the blood stream (i.e., adrenalin). Large amounts of stress hormones are found in the blood stream of people who react to stressful situations with hostile and angry behavior. However, low levels of stress hormones are found in the blood streams of people who react normally to stressful events. How you react to stress seems to be the critical factor. You should recognize stress in your life (both the positive and the negative) and learn to handle the stressful situations in a healthful manner. Coping with stress successfully is vital in today's hectic, life-in-the-fast-lane lifestyle. Exercise and behavioral modification have been found to be excellent methods for reducing stress. We need to change the way we look at stressful situations. Problems are to be solved, not worried about! Read more about ways to reduce stress in chapter 7.

3. Emotional Behavior   Several studies have linked personality to increased risk of heart disease. There are basically three **personality patterns—Type A, Type B, and Type C.** The Type A individual exhibits hostility, aggressiveness, competitiveness, impatience, and is easily annoyed. Type As demonstrate a high degree of time urgency—a tendency to do two or three things at the same time. The Type B individual is more relaxed, noncompetitive, patient, and slow to anger. A third personality pattern, Type C, has been identified recently.[26] Type Cs are not as aggressive as Type As, nor as laid back as Type Bs. Type Cs learn to cope with emotional stress by using the five Cs: control, commitment, challenge, choices in lifestyle, and connectedness. Such a person welcomes change, considering it a challenge. They are committed to goals, gaining confidence as a result (see chapter 7).

Early studies identified the Type A personality as the one at greater risk of having a heart attack. However, more recent research indicates it is only when the Type A personality exhibits the behaviors of *hostility* and *anger* that a serious risk is apparent. These behaviors significantly elevate blood pressure and overstimulate the production of stress hormones. The other Type A behaviors do not seem to be as significant but may be a factor in overall poor health.

Learning to modify Type A personality behaviors, especially hostility and anger, is not difficult, and it may add years to your life. How does a "hostile heart" become less angry and cynical—and become a "trusting heart"?

Carry a notebook and record every time you feel angry and/or hostile. Once you do this for awhile, you will start to recognize the situations that provoke these reactions and be able to head off the troublesome behavior. Other suggestions include:

- *Stop cynical thoughts.* Every time you have a cynical thought, think to yourself, "STOP!" An effective behavior modification technique when practiced regularly.
- *Practice laughing at yourself.* Once you realize how silly your anger is in many situations, laughing quickly at yourself replaces fuming.
- *Be empathetic.* Put yourself in the other person's shoes. Often the other individual is a victim of circumstances, too.
- *Reasoning and understanding your anger.* There will be times when anyone would be angry

in that same situation, but you must say, "I have this trait, and it is bad for my health."

- *Practice patience and trust.* Instead of getting irritated while standing in a line, concentrate on a relaxing word (such as "quiet") until your anger subsides. Trust that others are not out to cheat you.

- *Become a good listener.* Pay attention to what others are saying and do not interrupt.

- *Live as if you have a serious disease.* You will soon see that the little problems that once riled you up aren't really so important.

- *Learn to forgive.* Compassion is the strongest medicine for anger.

4. Age   Being older has some advantages (wisdom and experience), but protection from CHD is not one of them. As you age, your risk for developing heart disease increases. This does not mean that coronary heart disease is *only* a disease of the old. You don't just suddenly drop dead one day at age 45 from a "heart attack." At any age and certainly at age 18, you have atherosclerotic plaque in your arteries. It accumulates over time, and by the time you've gained "age," you've also increased the private stash of cholesterol in your arteries. There is little that can be done to stop the calendar. Adopting a healthy lifestyle early in life may add years to your life, and life to your years.

5. Male Gender   Males have a higher risk of coronary heart disease and stroke throughout their lives than do females. Even after menopause, when women's death rate from heart disease increases, it is less than men's. The increased male risk is not clearly understood. Some credit the increased risk to the male sex hormone testosterone, which triggers production of low-density lipoproteins, thereby clogging blood vessels. Others say a male's lifestyle may be the culprit. We do know that a female's hormonal makeup is protective until menopause. Female hormones signal the liver to produce more "good" cholesterol (HDL) and make blood vessels more elastic than male's blood vessels, especially during childbearing years.[27]

It is imperative that males modify other risk factors to protect their cardiovascular systems.

6. Race   According to the American Heart Association, black Americans have approximately a 33-percent greater chance of having high blood pressure than whites (fig. 6.7). A hereditary intolerance to sodium may account for this danger. They have a higher prevalence of diabetes, smoke more than whites (however, heavy smoking is greater among whites), and obesity is more common in black women.[28] Consequently, black Americans have a greater risk of heart attack and stroke. Social and economic stresses may also contribute to increased risk. Being aware of these risks, black Americans should adopt a healthy lifestyle early.

7. Positive Family History   A family history of heart disease in brothers, sisters, parents, or grandparents increases your risk of developing coronary artery disease. Tendencies toward high blood pressure, stroke, peripheral blood vessel disease, rheumatic fever, high blood lipid levels, obesity, and early heart attack

Figure 6.7
Estimated percentage of population with hypertension by race and sex in U.S. adults.

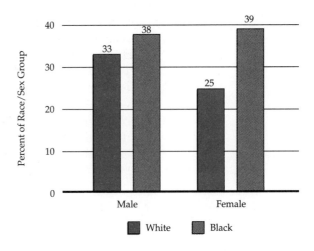

Hypertensives are defined as persons with a systolic level ≥140 and/or a diastolic level ≥90 or who reported using antihypertensive medication.

appear to be hereditary. This is why your physician is so interested in your family history. You should find out as much as possible about your family's medical history. You can be alerted early to a possible risk and take preventative measures.

8. Diabetes Mellitus **Diabetes mellitus** (which includes both Types I and II) is a condition characterized by the body's inability to produce enough insulin or to use it properly. In the normal digestive process, sugars, starches, and other foods are changed to a form of sugar called glucose. The blood stream carries glucose to the body cells. There, with the help of insulin, a hormone produced in the pancreas, it is converted to quick energy for immediate use or stored for future needs. In diabetes, this normal process is interrupted. Glucose accumulates in the blood until some of the surplus is eliminated by the kidneys, passing it off in the urine. Too much sugar in the urine and in the blood are classic signs of diabetes.

Diabetes is found in two forms. In insulin-dependent diabetes (IDDM), also known as Type I or juvenile-onset, the pancreas makes little or no insulin. The diabetic must receive insulin injections everyday to stay alive and must carefully watch their diet and exercise regularly. It occurs most often in children or young adults. Symptoms develop rapidly, usually within a period of months or even weeks.

More common (85%–90% of diabetics) is non-insulin-dependent diabetes (NIDDM), also known as Type II or adult-onset, in which the pancreas makes insulin but either the amount is insufficiently released or the body cannot properly utilize what is available. This type of diabetes can often be controlled without insulin injections through other medications, diet, and weight management. This form of the disease frequently occurs in people over 40 years old and is usually associated with aging and obesity. Because the onset of Type II is gradual, the disease may go undetected for years. Diabetes seriously increases risk of developing cardiovascular disease. In fact, more than 80 percent of people with diabetes die of some form of heart or blood vessel disease. Part of the reason is that diabetes affects cholesterol and triglycerides levels by producing a different kind of LDL that is even worse for the arteries than ordinary LDLs. This accelerates atherosclerosis.[29] Even so, Type II diabetes can be delayed or averted by weight management. Current theories suggest a genetic predisposition to both Type I and Type II diabetes.

Symptoms of both types can include excessive thirst, frequent urination, frequent hunger, and a weight loss or weight gain. Unless detected and controlled, diabetes can ultimately lead to stroke, heart disease, kidney failure, blindness, amputation of limbs, and death. According to the American Diabetes Association, the disease is a leading cause of death in this country and warns that diabetics are twice as prone to heart attack and stroke as nondiabetics.

Treatment for Blocked Coronary Arteries

As you have discovered, most of the risk factors linked to coronary heart disease can be controlled. The way you live, the choices you make, can have a profound impact on the health of your cardiorespiratory system. When coronary arteries do become blocked, usually the first treatments prescribed are diet modification (low fat) and exercise therapy. These are two major areas of one's life which if maximized can have positive results. When these methods are unsuccessful, the following procedures may be required.

Drug Therapy

This involves drug treatment affecting the supply of oxygen to the heart muscle or the heart's demand for oxygen. Some drugs (coronary vasodilators) cause the blood vessels to relax, enlarging the opening inside them. Blood flow then improves and more oxygen reaches the heart. Nitroglycerine is the most commonly used drug in this category. Another category of drugs slows down the heart rate or reduces blood pressure, thus decreasing the heart's need for oxygen, reducing its workload.

Angioplasty (or Balloon Angioplasty)

The American Heart Association describes this treatment as a nonsurgical procedure that improves the blood supply to the heart by dilating a narrowed coronary artery. The blocked part of the coronary artery must be identified before this technique is performed. During this process (cardiac catheterization) a doctor guides a thin plastic tube (catheter) through an artery from the arm or leg into the coronary arteries. A liquid dye, visible in X-rays, is injected into the catheter and X-ray movies are taken as the dye flows through the arteries. Doctors can identify obstructions in the arteries by tracing the flow of the dye. Once obstructions are identified, another catheter having a balloon tip is inserted inside the first; the balloon tip is inflated at the obstruction site. This compresses the plaque and enlarges the opening of the blood vessel. The balloon is deflated and both catheters are removed. About 25 percent of the people who have this technique have renarrowed arteries within 6 months.[30]

Coronary Bypass Surgery

This is a surgical technique in which doctors take a blood vessel from another part of the body (usually the leg) and use it to detour around a blockage in the coronary artery. Blood flow to the heart is restored.

New Techniques

New techniques under research and showing great promise:

1. Enzyme therapy, a nonsurgical process whereby enzymes are injected into the blockage, dissolving it.

2. Laser beam is a treatment used to break up the plaque, after which the particles of debris are vaporized.

3. A virus has been identified in the blocked arteries of heart patients during autopsy. This could mean that a vaccine might be given early in the life (such as the polio vaccine) to treat some forms of coronary artery disease.

The Future . . . Focus on Lifestyle

The cost of treating cardiovascular diseases in this country is staggering (see fig. 6.8). In order to reduce the cost and tragedy of these diseases, many scientists believe we will be more successful if we focus on prevention rather than rely on expensive, high-tech treatments. "An ounce of prevention is worth a pound of cure" will, in all likelihood, be the slogan of the twenty-second century. Heart disease prevention in our future will focus primarily on lifestyle changes and approaches that involve "mind and body" concepts. Many scientists are already substantiating these trends in their research and medical practices.

One example is Dr. Dean Ornish, cardiologist, clinical professor of medicine at the University of California at San Francisco, and pioneer in the treatment of coronary heart disease. He found that after treating his patients with the current, recommended medical procedures—medication, angioplasty (balloon technique), and coronary by-pass surgery, all expensive and dangerous—most did not stay well. Despite the procedures, some died and many returned for further treatment. He began to question the wisdom of such dramatic medical care for coronary heart disease. He found it interesting that lifestyle factors could trigger all mechanisms known to cause CHD. The lifestyle choices we make each day, such as, what we eat, how we respond to stress, how much we exercise, and whether or not we use tobacco, have a profound impact on our heart's health. With this concept in mind, he developed a plan that focused on lifestyle. His new program, "Reversing Heart Disease" is having significant success in reducing atherosclerosis without medication or surgical procedures. The program involves the following lifestyle changes:[31]

- Diet—The Reversal Diet is 10 percent fat, 70–75 percent carbohydrate, 15–20 percent protein and 5 milligrams of cholesterol per day. The typical American diet is 40–45 percent fat, 25–35 percent carbohydrate, 25 percent protein, and 400–500 milligrams of cholesterol per day. The diet allows but does

Figure 6.8

Estimated cost of major cardiovascular disease by expenditure.

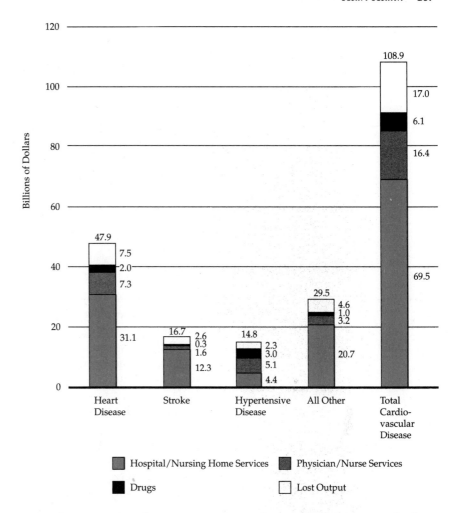

not encourage moderate alcohol consumption (less than 2 ounces per day). It excludes caffeine, allows moderate use of salt and sugar, and is not restricted in calories.

- Smoking is prohibited.
- Thirty minutes a day or one hour every other day of moderate exercise is prescribed.

- Stress management methods are prescribed everyday. These include yoga stretches, progressive relaxation, abdominal breathing, meditation, and imagery.
- The program also includes enhancement of communication skills and techniques for increasing intimacy.

By adhering to the five steps involved in the "Reversing Heart Disease" plan, Americans can save billions of dollars and thousands of lives every year. Can we afford *not* to stop smoking, dramatically reduce the fat in our diets, make commitment to life-time exercise and stress management and become more in tune with each other?

Mind and Body Connection

The traditional risk factors explain only a portion of the known causes of heart disease. Why do some people develop heart disease and others do not? Clearly, all the risk factors are important, but could there be something more? Are there common psychological—and perhaps even spiritual factors—that lead to or prevent coronary heart disease? Is there an unconscious connection between mind, body, and spirit that would explain the unknown causes of heart disease?

Scientists are beginning to examine these questions: Is laughter good for you? Can prayer bring down blood pressure? Does a bad marriage, or divorce, suppress your immune system? Does listening to others lower blood pressure? Is a cynic more likely to have heart trouble? To each of these questions there is a scientist able to answer "YES!" and provide data to back it up. There is a whole field of mind/body research tapping into the interaction between our immune system and our bodies, mind, moods, and spirit. Just as we learned the importance of exercise and nutrition to our health, we are now discovering ways to go deeper into inner wellness. Ponder these studies that support the mind/body concept:

- Norman Cousins, author, philosopher, and professor at the Department of Psychiatry and Bio-behavioral Sciences at UCLA Medical School (now deceased), found that laughter heals because it replaces fear and stress with serenity and homeostasis. His research confirmed that positive emotions boost health.[32]

- Larry Scherwitz, professor of psychology at the University of California, found that people who overuse the self-centered pronouns "I" or "me" are twice as likely to have heart attacks. These people put their own self-centered interests and pleasures ahead of all others.[33]

- Redford Williams of Duke University found that cynics, being full of contempt for other people, have more than their share of heart trouble.[34]

- Many psychologists have developed psychological tests to measure levels of anger that bring on heart attacks.[35]

- Studies linking social support (i.e., loving family, happy marriage, one or two close friends) to vitality, longevity, lowered blood pressure, and healthier immune systems[36, 37, 38]

- Dean Ornish, M.D., is convinced that one cause of blocked coronary arteries stems from three kinds of loneliness (or isolation): (1) we feel isolated from ourselves, (2) we lack "connectedness" and intimate relationships with others, (3) we have a cosmic loneliness of the spirit (or higher part of ourselves). He feels that isolation leads to chronic stress and to illnesses such as heart disease and that real intimacy and feelings of connectedness with others can be healing. That the ability to be intimate with ourselves, with others and to a higher spirit—within ourselves—is the key to emotional health and essential to the health of our hearts, as well.[39]

Summary

Heart disease is the number-one killer in the United States today. Extensive studies have identified several factors that increase the risk of developing coronary heart disease. These factors lead to the development of atherosclerosis. The most significant factors are high blood pressure, high blood lipid profile, cigarette smoking, and inactivity. These are labeled primary and can be controlled. Other contributing factors are obesity, stress, and emotional behavior. These are secondary risk factors that may also be controlled. Other secondary risk factors, which cannot be controlled, are age, male gender, race, positive family history, and diabetes. The more risk factors you have and the longer they are present, the greater the chance you have of developing heart disease. By age 20, fatty deposits are already present in the coronary arteries.

If the coronary arteries become blocked due to advanced atherosclerosis, there are several treatments available. These include exercise and diet modification, drug therapy, angioplasty, and coronary bypass surgery. The cost of treating CVD continues to spiral upward every year. To counter this trend, many scientists are convinced that preventing CVD through lifestyle change is the **key** to heart health.

As was stated earlier, adopting a healthy lifestyle early in life can add years to your life—and life to your years. In addition, great discoveries await us as the field of mind and body research gains wider acceptance in the quest for increased well-being.

References

1. *1992 Heart Facts.* American Heart Association National Center, 7272 Greenville Avenue, Dallas, TX 75231-4596.

2. *1992 Heart Facts.*

3. *1992 Heart Facts.*

4. *1992 Heart Facts.*

5. *1992 Heart Facts.*

6. Kavanagh, Terrence, M.D. "Does Exercise Training Improve Coronary Collateralization? A New Look at an Old Belief." *The Physician and Sports Medicine,* Vol. 17, No. 1, January 1989, pp. 96–113.

7. *1992 Heart Facts.*

8. *1992 Heart Facts.*

9. *1992 Heart Facts.*

10. Ornish, Dean, M.D. *Dr. Dean Ornish's Program for Reversing Heart Disease.* New York: Random House, 1990.

11. Sempos, C., Fulwood, R., Haines, C. et al. "The Prevalence of High Blood Cholesterol Levels Among Adults in the United States." *Journal of American Medical Association,* 1989, 262(1).

12. *The Wellness Encyclopedia,* from the Editors of the University of California, Berkeley Wellness Letter, Boston: Houghton Mifflin Company, 1991.

13. *The Wellness Encyclopedia,* 1991.

14. *1992 Heart Facts.*

15. "Fascinating Facts," *University of California, Berkeley Wellness Newsletter 6.* No. 3 (Dec. 1989): 1.

16. Hurley, Judith and Schlaadt, Richard. *The Wellness Lifestyle.* Guilford, Ct: The Dushkin Publishing Group, 1992.

17. Scragg, Robert. "Alcohol and Exercise in Myocardial Infarction and Sudden Coronary Death in Men and Women." *American Journal of Epidemiology,* Vol. 126, No.1, July 1987, pp. 77–85.

18. Raven, Peter B., Ph.D., and Judy Wilson, Ph.D. "Exercise for the Elderly." *Sportsmedicine Digest.* Vol. 10, No. 6, June 1988.

19. Scragg. "Alcohol and Exercise in Myocardial Infarction and Sudden Coronary Death in Men and Women."

20. *1992 Heart Facts.*

21. *The Wellness Encyclopedia.*

22. *The Wellness Encyclopedia.*

23. Tucker, Larry A., Ph.D., and Glenn Freidman, M.D., "Television Viewing and Obesity in Adult Males." *American Journal of Public Health,* 79(4): 516–518, 1989.

24. Schmall, Peter, M.D., Pieper, Carl, Ph.D., Schwartz, Joseph, Ph.D., Karasek, Robert, Ph.D., Schussel, Yvette, Ph.D., Devereaux, Richard, M.D., Ganau, Antonello, M.D., Alderman, Michael, M.D., Warren, Katherine, Pickering, Thomas, M.D. *JAMA* 263: 1929–1935, "The Relationship Between Job Stress; Work Place Diastolic Blood Pressure, and Left Ventricle Max Index," April 11, 1990.

25. Eliot, R. S. and Breo, D. L. *Is it Worth Dying For?* New York: Bantam Books, 1986.

26. Sweeting, Roger. *A Values Approach to Health Behavior.* Champaign, IL: Human Kinetics Books, 1990.

27. *The Wellness Encyclopedia.*

28. *The Heart Facts.*

29. Liebman, Bonnie. "The HDL/Triglycerides Trap." *Nutrition Action,* Vol. 17, No. 7, September 1990.

30. *1992 Heart Facts.*

31. Ornish, Dean, M.D. *Dr. Dean Ornish's Program For Reversing Heart Disease.*

32. Cousins, N. *The Healing Heart.* New York: Avon Books, 1983.

33. Scherwitz, L., Graham, L., Grandits, G., Billings, J. "Speech Characteristics and Behavior-Type Assessment in the Multiple Risk Factor Intervention Trial (MRFIT) Structured Interviews." *Journal of Behavioral Medicine,* 1987.

34. Williams, Redford. *The Trusting Heart.* New York: Times Books, 1989.

35. Blumenthal, J., Barefoot, J., et al. "Psychological Correlates of Hostility Among Patients Undergoing Coronary Angiography." *British Journal of Medical Psychology,* 1987.

36. Spiegal, David, Bloom, J., et al. "Effect of Psychosocial Treatment on Survival of Patients with Metastatic Breast Cancer. *Lancet,* 1989.

37. Syme, Leonard. "Social Determinants of Disease." *Annual of Clinical Research,* 1989.

38. Seeman, T., Syme, L. "Social Networks and Coronary Artery Disease: A Comparison of the Structure and Function of Social Relations as Predictors of Disease." *Psychomatic Medicine,* 1987.

39. Ornish, Dean, M.D., *Dr. Dean Ornish's Program for Reversing Heart Disease.*

Suggested Readings

Cooper, G. R., Myers, G. L., Smith, S. J., Schlant, R. C., March 25, 1992. "Blood Lipid Measurements: Variations and Practical Utility." *JAMA,* Vol. 267, No. 12.

Cooper, Kenneth H., M.D., M.P.H. 1988. *Dr. Kenneth Cooper's Preventive Medicine Program Controlling Cholesterol.* Bantam Books, New York.

Dooley, Denton, M.D., and Carolyn Moore, Ph.D. R.D. 1987. *Eat Smart for a Healthy Heart Cookbook.* Barron's Educational Series, Inc., 113 Crossways Park Drive, Woodbury, N.Y. 11797.

Healthy People 2000. Department of Health and Human Services No. (PHS) 91-502B Washington, DC 20201, 1990.

1993, Heart Facts. American Heart Association National Center, 7272 Greenville Avenue, Dallas, Texas 75231-4596.

Hoeger, Werner W. K. 1988. *Principles and Labs for Physical Fitness and Wellness.* Morton Publishing Company, 925 W. Kenyon Ave., Unit 4, Englewood, CO 80110.

Melby, Christopher, Roseann Lyle, and Geraod Hyner. "Beyond Blood Pressure Screening: A Rationale for Promoting the Primary Prevention of Hypertension." *American Journal of Health Promotion,* Fall 1988, Vol. 3, No. 2, pp. 5–11.

Ornish, Dean, M.D., *Dr. Dean Ornish's Program for Reversing Heart Disease.* New York, Random House, 1990.

Pickering, T. G. March 4, 1992. "Predicting the Response to Nonpharmacologie Treatment in Mild Hypertension." *JAMA.* Vol. 267, No. 9.

Report of the Expert Panel on Population Strategies for Blood Cholesterol Reduction, U.S. Department of Health and Human Services, PHS & National Institutes of Health, Nov. 1990.

Strube, Michael. *Type A Behavior,* Newbury Park, California. Sage Publications, 1991.

For More Information Contact:

American Heart Association
7272 Greenville Avenue
Dallas, TX 75231
(214) 750-5300

National Heart, Lung, and Blood Institute
Information Center
4733 Bethesda Avenue, Suite 530
Bethesda, MD 20814-4820
(301) 951-3260

National Stroke Association
1565 Clarkson Street
Denver, CO 80218
(303) 839-1992

American Diabetes Association, Inc.
Two Park Avenue
New York, NY 10016 (212) 683-7444

The Juvenile Diabetes Foundation International
23 East 26th Street
New York, NY 10010
(212) 889-7575

National Diabetes Information Clearinghouse
Box NDIC
Bethesda, MD 20205
(301) 496-7433

7
Coping with Stress

Chapter Objectives

After reading this chapter you will be able to:

1. Define the terms *stress*, *stressor*, and *stress response.*
2. Explain the three stages of the stress response.
3. Define and give examples of eustress, distress, and optimal stress.
4. Measure the amount of life changes on the Holmes and Rahe Life Event Scale you have encountered this year and be able to predict your susceptibility to a stress-related illness.
5. Explain the difference between daily hassles and daily uplifts and how each affects overall health.
6. Describe six harmful effects of too much stress.
7. Contrast Type A, Type B, and Type C behavior patterns.
8. List five Type A behavior modification techniques.
9. Explain how perception and control are involved in stress.
10. List five strategies for managing stress.
11. Describe two methods of relaxation that produce the relaxation response.
12. List three benefits of the relaxation response.
13. List seven positive lifestyle changes that reduce stress.
14. Explain the importance of exercise in the management of stress.

Terms

- Autogenic training and imagery
- Biofeedback training
- Daily hassles
- Daily uplifts
- Distress
- Eustress
- Fight-or-flight response
- General Adaptation Syndrome (GAS)
- Meditation
- Optimal stress
- Progressive relaxation
- Psychosomatic disease
- Reframing
- Relaxation response
- Stage of exhaustion
- Stage of resistance
- Stress
- Stressors
- Stress response
- Transcendental meditation (TM)
- Type A personality
- Type B personality
- Type C personality

*L*isa came to the university from a small rural farming community where the most exciting event of the year was the Covered Bridge Festival. Back home she was the girl voted "most likely to succeed," homecoming queen, president of the National Honor Society, editor of the yearbook, and in the upper 10 percent of the senior class. She was the oldest child of three and the first person in her family to go to college. College was wonderful—a roommate, sorority rush, football games, fraternity parties, open visitation in the residence hall, and no curfew hours. But lately, Lisa was feeling edgy, arguing with her roommate (who was borrowing her clothes too often), and having constant headaches. She had a cold that just would not clear up. Lisa was worried about making the "right" sorority, and Bill, her fraternity Big Brother, was pressuring her for more than "a few little kisses," and to join in on the beer-drinking fun after the football games. It was midterm exam time, and Lisa had just not been able to keep up with all the reading. She was convinced that her grades would not be as good as they were in high school, and this would be a terrible disappointment to her parents, who were having financial problems because of her college expenses. On top of this, her parents didn't seem to be getting along all that well. She wondered what was going on at home. Sleep? What was that? There never was enough of it, that was certain. The "action" never settled down in her hall until 12:30 or 1:00 A.M. Additionally, her jeans were getting so tight she could barely breathe. She had heard about the "Freshman Twenty," but thought she would never gain so much weight. Feeling depressed, she thought maybe she should try diet pills or eating only one meal a day. Maybe she would just stay in bed all weekend and hibernate. How could her life have gotten so out of control? College life was exciting, but there were some problems she would have to deal with.

The scene just described is not all that uncommon on the typical college campus. The many challenges faced by college students can be stressful and can cause feelings of anxiety. Stiff competition for grades, career choices, selection of classes, test anxiety, sense of loss of family and home, peer pressure, inadequate sleep, poor nutritional habits, low physical fitness levels, and increased social involvements all contribute to high levels of stress. Clearly, college is a stressful environment, one that makes demands on you physically, socially, intellectually, and emotionally. It's no wonder that you sometimes feel anxious, irritable, and "stressed out." Contrary to what many college students believe, stress does not "evaporate" after graduation. Improvement in the quality of your life is dependent on balancing stress and the demands made upon you. To do this it is essential that you increase your *knowledge* about stress, become *aware* of situations that may cause stress, *assess* the amount of stress in your life, and develop effective ways to *manage* stress.

What Is Stress?

Stress is the way your mind and body react to any demand made upon it. It is the response of the body to any new, threatening, or exciting situation. Both pleasant and unpleasant events can trigger stress. **Stressors,** factors causing stress, can be either real or imagined and can be of different types. For example *physical* stressors include such things as illness, accidents, injury, heat, cold, and noise. *Psychosocial* or *emotional* stressors involve deadlines, final exams, work

College students face many stresses

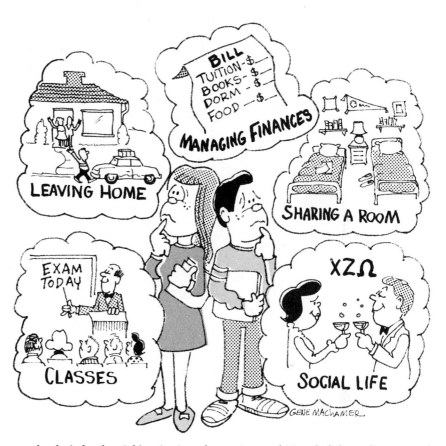

overloads (school or job), rejection, depression, ambition, holidays, divorce, and marriage. Stress mobilizes the body's defenses and allows human beings to adapt to the challenges of everyday life. The adaptation (reaction) to stress is both physiological and psychological and is called the **stress response.** No one is exempt from stress. This is good since a certain amount is beneficial for an optimal level of health and achievement, plus it helps us cope with emergency situations. Figure 7.1 illustrates how the "right" amount of stress improves health and performance, but our health and well-being can be adversely affected when stress becomes excessive. Too much stress ultimately exhausts the body's ability to adapt; vital organs wear out, and various illnesses may appear. Since stress is a normal part of life, why do so few people understand it or how to manage it?

In the 1920s, Dr. Hans Selye, the father of stress research, introduced the concept of stress to the medical community. Dr. Selye discovered that many different types of good and bad life events, thoughts, emotions, and changes (all stressors) caused the body to go through certain predictable internal changes, producing symptoms of stress. The body's reaction to "good stress" (Christmas, getting married, etc.) Dr. Selye termed **eustress** and to "bad stress" (flunking an exam, breakup of a relationship, etc.) he termed **distress.**[1] **Optimal stress** is a point at which the stress is intense enough to motivate and physically prepare us to perform optimally, yet not intense enough to cause the body to overreact or to sustain harmful effects.[2] Figure 7.1 illustrates this concept. Optimal stress gives the athlete the competitive edge and the public speaker the enthusiasm to project with charisma. Overstress results in poor performance, produces overreaction, poor concentration, test anxiety, and health problems.[3] Dr. Selye concluded that regardless of what caused stress (good or bad), the body reacted similarly. Dr. Selye labeled the entire stress response the **General Adaptation Syndrome (GAS).** Today, Selye's GAS is simply called the Stress Response.

Figure 7.1
Optimal stress

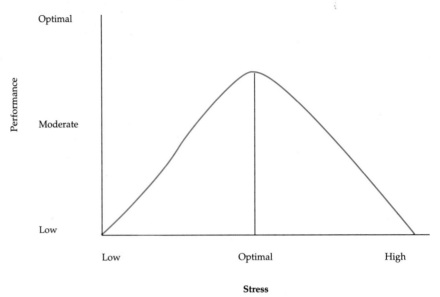

The Stress Response—A Three-Stage Process

Hans Selye summarized the Stress Response in a three-stage process:[4]

1. **Fight-or-flight response:** The body prepares itself to cope with a stressor. It is a warning signal that a stressor is present. Physiological and psychological responses appear.

2. **Stage of resistance:** The body actively resists and attempts to cope with the stressor. In this stage the stress response is channeled into the specific organ system most capable of suppressing it. It is this adaptation process that contributes to stress-related illness. The specific organ system becomes aroused and if prolonged it may fatigue and begin to malfunction. Headache, forgetfulness, colon spasms (constipation or diarrhea), asthma, anxiety attacks, and high blood pressure are examples of prolonged arousal.

3. **Stage of exhaustion:** Adaptation energy is exhausted and signs of fight-or-flight reappear. During the exhaustion phase, the organ system involved in the repeated stress response breaks down. Disease or malfunction of the organ system or even death may occur. For example, high blood pressure (caused by excessive stress) promotes kidney and heart damage, which can kill the individual if allowed to continue.

Fight-or-Flight   The body responds to stress, whether emotional or physical (real or perceived), by activating a series of mechanisms collectively known as the fight-or-flight response.[5] This response prepares us to either fight or to flee to safety by pumping powerful stress hormones and steroids into the blood stream (table 7.1). Early mankind, faced with daily life and death situations, relied heavily

Table 7.1
The Body Reacts to Stress

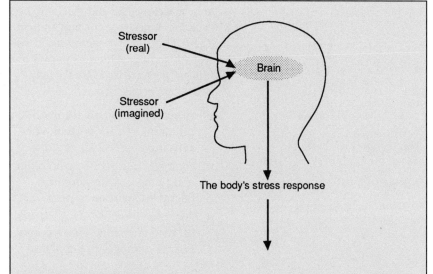

The body reacts to stressors

- Adrenalin and other stress hormones are pumped into the body causing the heart to beat faster; an increased rush of strength and energy is felt.
- Stored sugars and fats pour into the blood stream to provide quick energy.
- Blood pressure is elevated to ensure sufficient oxygen to muscles.
- Muscular tension increases in preparation for action.
- Breathing rate quickens to provide greater oxygen to muscles to do battle or to run from danger.
- Blood clots faster for protection should injury occur—less blood lost.
- Digestion ceases so blood may be shunted to the muscles and brain for quick physical and mental action.
- Other physiological responses include increased perspiration, serum cholesterol in blood, hydrochloric acid in the stomach, and changes in brain waves.
- Pupils of the eyes dilate, aiding vision. Other senses, such as hearing, also become heightened.
- Urge to urinate and move the bowels increases to reduce danger of infection if abdominal injury should occur.

on this response for survival. The caveman could escape the jaws of a hungry lion (stressor) by swiftly running (the fight-or-flight response in action). These mechanisms work best where the danger is clear, well-defined, and short-term (acute not chronic). Many examples of the fight-or-flight response can be found even in today's world. Imagine this scenario. . . You are crossing the street on your way home when suddenly you see a car fast approaching you. Instinctively your muscles tense, and you jump back on the curb with such force that you fall back into a newspaper stand and cut your head, which quickly stops bleeding. The fight-or-flight response saved your life (the quick backward jump/cut that stops bleeding). Other examples of the response, normally cited as "super-human" acts, are in reality the fight-or-flight response in action. Perhaps you can add others to this list.

- A person lifting an automobile off an injured individual when arriving at an accident scene
- A small child rescuing an older child who is drowning in a backyard swimming pool
- After having both arms ripped off by a farm machine, a young farmer manages to telephone for help by dialing 911 with a pencil clenched in his teeth
- A mother knocking down a locked bedroom door to rescue her children from a burning house
- Out-running a mugger on a dark corner of campus

These are only a few examples that have required action to prevent physical harm. A few minutes after the frightening event (acute stressor) you return to your normal physiological state. Other stressors, the kind you encounter every-day, such as noise, arguments, keys locked inside the car, missed deadlines, traffic tickets, or any new situation that causes us to adapt, have the same potential for eliciting the fight-or-flight response.

Physical and emotional stress (too much to do, breakup of a relationship, public speaking, etc.) may be either acute or chronic. We are designed to cope with acute stress much better than chronic stress.[6] Unfortunately, physical and emotional stress in modern times tends to be chronic rather than acute. The pace of life in the past ten years seems to be accelerating. Federal Express overnight service is no longer quick enough—the letter needs to be faxed immediately. Receiving one telephone call at a time is not enough; now, with call waiting two or more can be received. Even the traditional places of refuge in the twentieth century—the car and the home—are transformed into offices away from offices, with fax machines and computers at home, telephones in the car, fax machines for the car. With portable telephones and lap top computers, work stress never ends. We often do not have time to recover from one stressful situation before we face another one.

Physiological stress responses (table 7.1) have evolved over the centuries to help us survive danger and prepare us for swift action whether or not it is needed. However, the buildup of unused stress products produces excessive wear and tear on the body, which may increase the rate of aging. When stressors provoke the fight-or-flight reactions many times a day, the body repeatedly responds as if experiencing real emergencies. We need to learn how to avoid triggering the stress response except in real emergencies.

Stage of Resistance   The longer our bodies stay in a chronic "on guard" resistance stage, the more likely we are to experience ill effects. Today we don't have much opportunity to physically play out the fight-or-flight response, as is done in acute stress situations because today's stress is mostly chronic. As a result, the body remains in the resistance stage for longer periods. Our sedentary lifestyles decrease the outlets for fight-or-flight hormones that are pumped into the body. The length of time that a stressor is with you is an important factor. Stress becomes harmful when it is prolonged and perceived as negative to the recipient.

Learning stress management skills is important in coping with the stresses of life. People who have learned these skills may overreact to a stressor but will relax more quickly to their resting physiological state than people who have not learned these skills.

Stage of Exhaustion   The exhaustion stage of the stress response is not often reached. If our bodies are successful in resisting stress, exhaustion does not follow. We usually adapt to the stress and make whatever adjustments are necessary to cope, whether the stress is physical or psychological.

Perception and Control

Individuals may respond differently to the same stressor. Whether a particular stressor causes a negative reaction depends on whether or not the person perceives that stressor as being negative.[7] This concept was confirmed by the research of Dr. Richard Lazarus who asserted that we are, after all, thinking, cognitive creatures. We are able to assess the positive and negative consequences of any situation or threat. One may *perceive* a stressor as threatening, and as a result, experience a fight-or-flight response. Another may encounter the same event and not perceive it as a stressor. We are all different, and each of us perceives stressors in a different light. How do you perceive snakes, announcement of an exam, competition, a doctor's appointment, being called on to contribute to class discussion, a professor requesting to speak with you after class? These items do not bother some individuals but are agonizing to others. In reality, most people's problems have to do with *faulty perception*—that is, unnecessarily seeing a situation as hopeless, harmful, or negative. Fortunately, we each have the power to develop cognitive skills to cope with faulty perception. As Duke Ellington put it, "A problem is a chance to do your best." Before gearing up to fret, fight (or flee), ask yourself, "Does a threat really exist? Is the issue really important to me? Can I make a difference?" If the answer to any of these questions is "no," do not waste your energy. It is not worth it. Some situations are truly threatening and deserve high energy stress responses. When the threat you perceive in a situation is quite real, go ahead and gear up. You can then benefit from the energy generated by your natural stress response by applying it to the situation at hand.

We all perceive stressors differently.

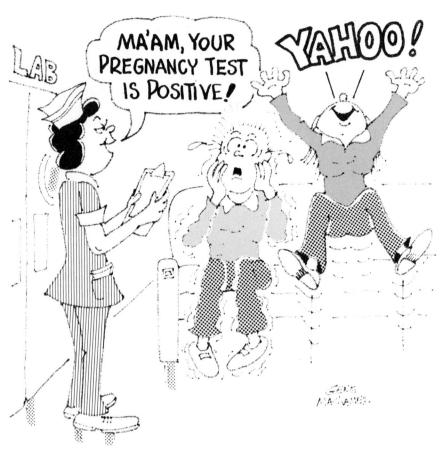

Control is another important factor in the total stress picture. You are in much greater control over your stress than you ever realized! Managing stress means taking control rather than relinquishing the control to events, to other people, to your environment, or to the calendar. People who handle stress best tend to control their lives and look for active solutions to the problems and circumstances of their lives. You are responsible for allowing stressful situations to raise your blood pressure and heart rate. We can all recount events that made us angry one time but did not even faze us the next. Why is this? It is because we *allowed* ourselves to become upset. Perhaps the situation was complicated by nasty weather, lack of sleep, or buildup of particular events. The bottom line is this particular time we *allowed* the event to provoke an angry response. This does not need to be the case. You cannot control what other people say or do, but you can change how you react to what others say or do. Whether or not to allow stressful events to provoke physiological reactions, such as increased muscle tension and nervous stomach, is your decision. By taking charge, you can decide whether or not to be an overstressed, nervous wreck or a calm, collected person. It is your decision to smoke or not smoke, to learn and implement time management skills, to exercise or not to exercise, to eat nutritionally or to gobble up beer, colas, and greasy junk food. You must decide when to take on added duties and assignments or when to say, "No, sorry, not at this time. I have too many irons in the fire right now." It is, likewise, your decision to regularly practice relaxation techniques or to find excuses for not incorporating these relaxing skills into your daily life. Often people say they would like to meditate but can't find the time. Nonsense! Why not make a *commitment* to taking control of your life and controlling your stress? Begin now to employ one or more of the stress coping strategies described in this chapter, restore a sense of control, and reduce symptoms of stress. Remember, only you can decide if you want to manage your stress. It is your responsibility to learn these skills, practice them, and incorporate them into your daily life. You will be a healthier person for it! The key to surviving and even thriving on stress is self control. Take charge of *you*—for *you*!

Measuring Your Stress

In 1967, two psychiatrists at the University of Washington School of Medicine, Thomas H. Holmes, M.D. and Richard H. Rahe, M.D., observed that certain life events coincided with illness.[8] After studying medical histories and personal biographies of patients, the doctors found a curious link between these life events and illnesses such as heart disease, ulcers, and psychiatric problems (depression, anxiety, etc.); thus, they developed a list of life changes that range from severe to minor, and assigned points to each one based on the amount of stress evoked (table 7.2). Another scale has been developed for college students.

How would you estimate your current stress level? Indicate your estimation by placing an "X" on the line below.

Totally free of stress	Usually not stressed	Average stress level	Usually stressed	Extremely highly stressed

Take a few moments to go down the Life Event Scale and identify those events that have occurred in your life during the past year. Add up your score (how did it compare to your estimate?) and evaluate your potential for developing a serious illness due to the amount of stress you have had to adapt to this year.

Perhaps you can adapt this list to include factors that concern you personally, then substitute them into this scale. Whether you use the original Holmes and Rahe scale or an adaptation of it, this is an excellent method of measuring the number of stressful events in your life. It can also be an effective tool when used to *anticipate* major life events that you can control. Scheduling predictable life events such as marriage or recreation provides you with some control over them and is helpful in reducing stress. Realizing there are certain life events you cannot control is equally important in stress reduction. Remember, change is

Table 7.2

Holmes and Rahe Life Event Scale

Source: Reprinted with permission from Journal of Psychosomatic Research *11:213–218. Thomas H. Holmes and Richard H. Rahe, "The Social Readjustment Rating Scale," 1967. Pergamon Press, Inc.*

Determine which of the following events you have experienced within the past year.

Mean value	Life Event
(100)	Death of spouse
(73)	Divorce
(65)	Marital separation
(63)	Jail term
(63)	Death of close family member
(53)	Personal injury or illness
(50)	Marriage
(47)	Fired at work
(45)	Marital reconciliation
(45)	Retirement
(44)	Change in health of family member
(40)	Pregnancy
(39)	Sex difficulties
(39)	Gain of new family member
(39)	Business readjustment
(38)	Change in financial state
(37)	Death of a close friend
(36)	Change to different line of work
(35)	Change in number of arguments with spouse
(31)	Mortgage or loan for major purchase (home, etc.)
(30)	Foreclosure of mortgage or loan
(29)	Change in responsibilities at work
(29)	Son or daughter leaving home
(29)	Trouble with in-laws
(28)	Outstanding personal achievement
(26)	Spouse begins or stops work
(25)	Change in living conditions
(24)	Revision of personal habits
(23)	Trouble with boss
(20)	Change in work hours or conditions
(20)	Change in residence
(19)	Change in recreation
(19)	Change in church activities
(18)	Change in social activities
(17)	Mortgage or loan for lesser purchase (car, TV, etc.)
(16)	Change in sleeping habits
(15)	Change in number of family get-togethers
(13)	Vacation
(12)	Christmas
(11)	Minor violations of the law

Table 7.2—*Continued*
Life Event Scale for the College Student

Determine which of the following events you have experienced within the past year.

Mean Value	Event
(87)	Death of a spouse
(77)	Death of a close family member
(77)	Married
(76)	Were divorced
(74)	Had a marital separation from your mate
(68)	Pregnancy or fathered a child
(68)	Death of a close friend
(65)	Had a major personal injury or illness
(62)	Were fired from work
(60)	Broke or had broken a marital engagement or a steady relationship
(58)	Had sexual difficulties
(58)	Had a marital reconciliation with your mate
(57)	Had a major change in self-concept or self-awareness
(57)	Had a major change in usual type and/or amount of recreation
(56)	Had a major change in the health or behavior of a family member
(54)	Were engaged to be married
(53)	Had a major change in financial state (a lot worse or a lot better off than usual)
(52)	Took a mortgage or loan less than $10,000 (such as purchase of a car, TV, school loan, etc.)
(50)	Changed to a different line of work
(50)	Had a major change in the number of arguments with spouse (either a lot more or a lot less than usual)
(50)	Entered college
(50)	Changed to a new school
(50)	Gained a new family member (through birth, adoption, older person moving in, etc.)
(50)	Had a major conflict in or change in values
(49)	Had a major change in the amount of independence and responsibility (for example for budgeting time)
(48)	Had a major change in social activities
(47)	Had a major change in responsibilities at work (promotion, demotion, lateral transfer)
(46)	Had a major change in the use of alcohol (a lot more or a lot less)
(45)	Had a revision of your personal habits (friends, dress, manners, associations, etc.)
(44)	Had trouble with school administration (instructors, advisors, class scheduling)
(43)	Held a job while attending school
(42)	Had trouble with in-laws
(42)	Changed your residence or living conditions
(41)	Had your spouse begin or cease work outside the home
(41)	Made a change in choice of a major field of study
(41)	Changed dating habits

Table 7.2—*Continued*
Life Event Scale for the College Student

Mean Value	Event
(40)	Have had an outstanding personal achievement
(38)	Had a major change in the amount of participation in school activities
(36)	Had a major change in church activities (a lot more or a lot less than usual)
(34)	Experienced a major change in sleeping habits (sleeping a lot more or a lot less, or a change in part of the day when asleep)
(33)	Took a trip or vacation
(30)	Experienced a major change in eating habits (a lot more or a lot less food intake, or very different meal hours or surroundings)
(26)	Had a major change in the number of family get-togethers (a lot more or a lot less)
(22)	Have been found guilty of minor violations of the law (traffic tickets, jaywalking, etc.)

Directions for Life Event Scales

To obtain your score, multiply the number of times an event occurred by its mean value. Then total all of the scores. Your score is termed your **life change units (LCU).** This is a measure of the amount of significant changes in your life to which you have had to adjust. In other words, your LCU is a measure of the stressors you have encountered this past year.

Rating	Score	Implications for Illness
Low stress	150/less	This indicates that a person has a 37 percent chance of getting a stress-related disease in the next year or two.
Moderate	151–300	51 percent chance of getting a stress illness in the next year.
High stress	301/more	80 percent chance of getting a stress illness in the next year.

Source: G. E. Anderson, Unpublished Masters Thesis, 1972. Department of Education, North Dakota State University, Fargo, North Dakota.

inevitable; that's what living is all about. But keep in mind that you can plan ahead for change and regulate the timing of many events (stressors) that would have otherwise drained much of your adaptation energy. Spread change out over a period of time. When you feel in control, stressful situations are perceived as much less stressful; thus, there is less chance of provoking a stress-related illness. Change in life situations alone may not be enough to cause illness. When these changes are perceived as distressing, and result in chronic and prolonged emotional and physiological wear and tear, your risk of illness increases. Some people are more vulnerable to certain types of stress than others. If you would like to find out what type of stress you are most susceptible to, take the stress test in the activities section. This test also measures coping skills for dealing with stress.

Establishing coping techniques is a positive way to block the development of a stress illness. Well-timed social support is probably the best coping mechanism we have. When you are experiencing many life changes but have family and friends with whom you can discuss your problems, you probably will avoid a stress illness. Another individual with fewer life changes may become ill because they lacked social support. Ponder the wisdom of Alvin Toffler, *Future Shock,* "To survive (today), the individual must become infinitely more adaptable and capable than ever before. He must search out totally new ways to anchor himself. . . . "[9]

Daily Hassles and Uplifts

Studies by Richard Lazarus and colleagues suggest that perhaps too much emphasis was placed on the "life events" approach (which focused on change) and that there may be other factors involved in the complicated stress/health picture. In an effort to identify these factors, they developed a Hassles Scale and an Uplifts Scale. Their studies demonstrate how the little hassles of everyday life may be even more harmful to your health than major life changes.[10] They found that the greatest toll from stress may not come from a divorce, loss of a job, or other traumatic changes, but from an accumulation of the minor, frequent annoyances we experience daily. **Daily hassles** are the events or interactions in your daily life that you find bothersome, annoying, or negative in some way. These irritating demands include practical problems such as losing things, traffic jams, arguments, inclement weather, and family concerns. Having too many things to do, roommate problems, not enough sleep, parking on campus, and money problems were the most frequently reported hassles of our college students. Examine the top ten hassles that most of the people interviewed (by researchers) seemed to mention (table 7.3).

Table 7.3

National List of Top Ten Hassles and Uplifts[11]

Hassles	Uplifts
1. Misplacing or losing things	1. Being visited, phoned, or sent a letter
2. Troubling thoughts about your future	2. Visiting, phoning, or writing someone
3. Not getting enough sleep	3. Having fun (socializing . . . partying, being with friends)
4. Filling out forms	4. Completing a task
5. Money problems	5. Recreation (sports, games, etc.)
6. Social obligations	6. Making a friend
7. Concerns about weight and physical appearance	7. Hugging and/or kissing (relating well with spouse or lover)
8. Too many things to do	8. Getting enough sleep
9. Concerns about meeting high standards (not living up to expectations)	9. Being complimented
10. Being lonely	10. Having someone to listen to you
	11. Eating out

Everyday hassles can be the "straw that broke the camel's back" when they are added to your life at a time when it is already overloaded with stressful events. In fact, the average person is as likely to be "nibbled to death" by everyday hassles as to be overwhelmed by tragedies. The way you handle daily hassles to a large degree depends on your score on the Life Event Scales.[12] When scores are high (i.e., you are overstressed) you are more likely to react to daily hassles with less tolerance and a shorter fuse. For example, after Sue's mother died of cancer, she had to leave college in her first year and enroll at the local community college in her home town because she was needed at home to care for her younger brothers. On top of all this, she lost her billfold (with driver's license, credit cards, etc.) on the very first day of classes at the new school. Now, the hassles of too many things to do, losing the billfold, caring for the home and her brothers, and keeping up at school were overwhelming. She became ill. As with any stressor, the way you perceive it is critical. What constitutes a hassle or an uplift varies greatly from person to person. Concern about weight may not be a hassle to you but may be a real problem to another who places physical appearance as a top priority.

Everyday hassles won't end with college.

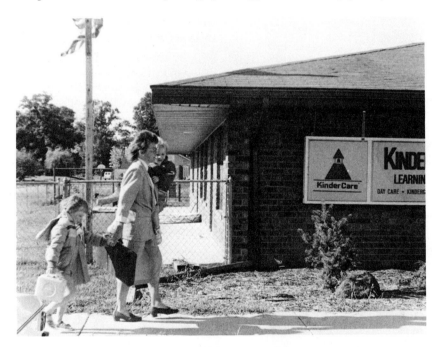

The counterpart to daily hassles is the **daily uplift.** These are positive events that make us feel good. Fridays, payday, going shopping, and having a date were the uplifts most often listed by our college students (see table 7.3). Research has shown that these little daily uplifts can actually reverse the negative effects of daily hassles. An appropriate balance between hassles and uplifts may be the important ingredient in your overall health and well-being. These daily uplifts may actually protect you from stress-related illnesses.

List the events in your everyday life that you find bothersome. How many of them can you eliminate? How many will you simply have to deal with in some manner? List the daily uplifts you find enjoyable. Can you find ways to add to this list?

Type A Behavior and Stress

We all know people who have the "hurry-up-itis" syndrome. They never have enough time, need more than eight hours a day to complete a day's work, could not survive without their car phone or lap top computer, and appear to be doing four or five things at one time. The woman who impatiently pushes ahead of you in line at the grocery, the young man who honks the horn of his automobile indicating for you to hurry up, or the person who constantly looks at his watch all exhibit Type A behavior.

The **Type A personality** is described as competitive, cynical, ambitious, driven, impatient, a workaholic, and always in a hurry. Type As often exhibit hostility and anger. They put big demands on themselves to accomplish more and more in less and less time. They have little time for or interest in hobbies or leisure pursuits and have few intimate friends. **Type B personality** is the opposite—relaxed, noncompetitive, unaggressive, and patient. Most Type Bs build time in the day for absorbing activities such as exercise, hobbies, and friendship. They speak more softly, are less obsessed with success, and tend to deal more effectively with stressful situations. Type A behavior was identified and named in the late 1950s by two cardiologists, Drs. Meyer Freidman and Ray Rosenman. Their research led many to believe that the individual who exhibits Type A behavior is prone to developing coronary heart disease, with increased risk of suffering a heart attack. However, recent research suggests that it may be the personality behaviors of *hostility* and *anger* that are the real culprits that increase the risk of heart disease.[13] People exhibiting hostility and anger in response to stress produce stress hormones (norepinephrine) that damage the cardiorespiratory system. These traits are also related to atherosclerosis and higher diastolic blood pressure. Type Bs exhibiting anger and hostility suffer from the same negative effects of these behaviors as do the Type A individuals. Do you become enraged when a car in front of you cuts you off? Do you find it intolerable to wait in lines? Do you react with gestures, raised voice, and increased heart rate, when someone does something that seems incompetent, messy, selfish, or inconsiderate to you? These are examples of angry, hostile behavior. While the debate continues connecting Type A and illness, the evidence is stacking up in favor of a positive connection—even without the hostility and anger. This means that just being a Type A person may have some health risks attached.

Constant stress causes many people to bristle with aggressiveness, hostility, and anger. Our increasingly complex world fosters the development of the Type A personality. We reward the student who excels in the classroom, the winning athlete, the "superwoman" (with career and family), the youngest-ever CEO, the secretary who never takes a break, the executives (women and men) who discuss business over lunch, and the college coed who is president of her sorority, homecoming queen, an A student, and on the tennis team. Our society provides a rich environment for Type A personality development. You should recognize your own behavior pattern. Are you a Type A person or a Type B? This brief quiz (table 7.4) will help you answer the question.

Table 7.4
Type A Quiz

Answer "agree" or "disagree" to the following statements.

1. I hate to wait in lines.
2. When driving, I get irritated at drivers who cut me off or drive too slowly. I frequently blow my horn and try to pass them.
3. I often interrupt others when they are speaking.
4. I am usually rushed. There's never enough time in the day.
5. I feel guilty when I have nothing to do or when I play.
6. I often use loud and accentuated words when I speak.
7. I get impatient when others perform tasks that I can do faster.
8. I eat faster than most of my friends.
9. I would find it difficult to read a complicated novel, walk through the woods and marvel at the wonders of nature, or spend an afternoon at a museum or art gallery.
10. I think about other things during conversations.

If you agreed to three or more of the statements, you probably fall into the Type A behavior category. Have a friend or loved one who knows you also check the statements that apply to you.

You should also be aware of the *amount* of stress in your life. Remember, you can take charge and be in control of your life. How do you respond to hassles and stress as they bombard you daily? Is it with hostility and anger? Then beware, you could be heading for trouble. Take the Hostility Quiz (table 7.5) to assess your behavior.

Table 7.5
Type H Quiz: Measure Your Hostility

1. Do you think you have to lash out at roommates or family members when they mess up?
2. Do you assume cashiers will shortchange you if they can?
3. If someone spills something on your new clothes, do you lash out at them?
4. After an irritating encounter, do you feel shaky or breathless?
5. Do you feel your anger is justified? Do you feel an urge to punish people—plot to get back at them?
6. Do you get irritated every time you stand in line? Get behind the wheel?

Any "yes" answer shows some hostile behavior—number six shows the highest level of hostility and that it has become a habit. How many of your responses were "yeses"?

Type A Behavior Modification

Okay, so you are a Type A. What can you do about it? We now know that even the most severe Type As can learn to modify their behavior and successfully control their reaction to stress in a more healthful way. Try these suggestions for behavior modification.

1. Take fifteen minutes a day to reflect on happy memories.
2. Be a good listener. Listen to others without interrupting.
3. Learn to savor food instead of grabbing fast food and eating "on the run."
4. Purposely choose the longest line in which to do your business (at the bank, at the checkout in the grocery store, in a fast food restaurant, or in a discount department store).
5. Discontinue polyphasic behavior (doing two or more things at once).
6. Practice smiling for a whole day.
7. Practice relaxation techniques daily.
8. Live by the calendar and not by the stopwatch.
9. Avoid irritating, competitive people.
10. Build a time each day for exercise or another absorbing activity.
11. Read a good book.
12. Spend an entire afternoon in a museum or art gallery.
13. Spend more time with friends and make these friendships more intimate.
14. Anticipate stresses and regulate their number and timing when possible.
15. Maintain a flexible schedule. Don't schedule appointments and activities unnecessarily.
16. Learn to say no and to protect your precious time. When possible, leave details to someone else.
17. Develop a sense of humor about life. *He who laughs lasts.*

Harmful Effects of Stress

All events, emotions, or situations, good or bad, cause you to react and force you to adapt. We are all constantly adapting to new things, things we like and things we don't like. This adaptation isn't harmful unless you are overloaded with too much in a short period of time—too many life change events and hassles, especially the ones perceived as undesirable or uncontrollable. It is part of being alive. In today's society, stress has increased dramatically. Having more stress than one can cope with can lead to a psychosomatic disease (see below) or to dysfunctional behavior (i.e., worry, neurosis, aggressive behavior, depression, domestic violence—even homicide or suicide). Controlling stress means adapting and changing as circumstances demand. There are a number of common signs of stress (table 7.6).

If you are experiencing five or more of these symptoms, you may be headed toward developing a psychosomatic disease and need to practice the antistress measures in this chapter.

Table 7.6
Common Signs of Stress

(Check the ones that you have experienced lately.)	
___ Disorganization (losing things, making dumb mistakes)	___ Flu (that lingers)
	___ Acne flare-up
___ Feelings of depression	___ Excessive dryness of hair or skin
___ Feelings of nervousness, anxiety	___ Frequent colds
___ Trouble getting along with others	___ Overeating/overdrinking
	___ Increased craving (tobacco, sweets, caffeine, drugs)
___ Daydreaming about escaping	___ Sleep disorders (sleeping too much, restless)
___ Feelings of "burnout"	___ Chest pain
___ Difficulty making small decisions	___ Upset stomach, nausea, or vomiting
___ Feeling like life is out of control	___ Neck, back, or shoulder pain
___ Increased irritability	___ Hands trembling
___ Increased feelings of being rushed	___ Excess perspiration
___ Headaches	___ Allergy flare-up and/or rashes
___ Often feel tired, or experience the "blahs"	___ Focus on unimportant details while not completing more important jobs
___ Heart pounding, racing, or beating erratically	___ Find yourself questioning your personal worth
___ Asthma attack	___ Feel more sensitive to criticism
___ Constipation and/or diarrhea	___ Often feel suspicious
___ Abdominal pains	
___ Muscle twitches, or eye twitches	

A **psychosomatic disease** involves the mind and the body. These diseases are not "all in the mind" as some people believe; they are real (i.e., physiological changes *do* occur) and can be diagnosed. When stress is prolonged, it can depress the immunological system and lower the body's resistance to disease. The mind and the body are an interrelated whole—what affects one ultimately affects the other. Examples of psychosomatic conditions are hypertension, stroke, coronary heart disease, ulcers, life-threatening gastrointestinal problems, migraine headaches, tension headaches, cancer, allergies, asthma, hay fever, rheumatoid arthritis, and backache. Stress is responsible for two-thirds of all doctor's visits and plays a role in two major killers—heart disease and cancer.[14] How is stress related to cancer? In addition to depressing the immune system, according to some studies, stress increases the incidence of smoking, alcohol consumption, and promiscuous sexual behavior, all of which have been associated with increased risk for developing certain kinds of cancer.[15]

The Stress-Resistant Hardy Person

Have you ever imagined what George Washington or any of our other founding fathers would think about our modern, high-tech, fast-paced world of today? Computers, fax machines, television with global news, heart transplants . . . as well as overcrowded calendars, never-ending deadlines, and chronic shortages of time! I'm sure they would agree that we have just cause to feel overwhelmed by our daily schedules and are glad not to be participating in the twentieth century with us. Yet, we all know some people, who, in spite of it all, seem relatively insulated from the potential negative effects of their hectic pace. Their lives are as full as ours, but they seem to carry on, taking "everything in stride"—often with a sense of enjoyment and fun. Who are these effective copers? Are they born this way or are they bred—learning strategies for coping with stress that protect them from being overwhelmed and feeling "stressed-out"?

Two psychologists (Dr. R. Flannery of Harvard University Medical School and Dr. S. Kabasa) independently researching these questions discovered that even when highly stressed many individuals manage to cope with lower incidence of physical illness, lower amounts of anxiety and depression, and increased longevity.[16] These stress-resistant, *"hardy"* individuals they found possessed the following skills for adapting to life stress. We call these skills *The Five Cs.* They are:

- *Control*—The hardy person is in control of life. They have a sense of internal control (influence) over the events and outcomes in life. They take daily hassles in stride. They think ahead, plan, and make lists of what needs to be done. They seek active solutions to problems. Do you feel "in control" of your life? If not, what plan can you implement that will help you gain more control?

- *Commitment*—The hardy person is committed to something that is important and meaningful to them. They have a sense of purpose in life and set short- and long-term goals. Rearing one's children, fraternity, community projects, religious values, reaching career goals, and working to complete "your degree" are examples of personal commitments that help us unstress. List one or two goals to which you have made a commitment.

- *Challenge*—The hardy person perceives life change as an opportunity and a challenge. They do not feel threatened by change. They accept setbacks as a part of life and as an opportunity for growth.

- *Choices in Lifestyle*—Hardy individuals make lifestyle choices that enhance health and reduce stress. They reduce use of caffeine, nicotine, alcohol, sugar, and incorporate aerobic exercise and relaxation activities into their lives. How much caffeine do you consume everyday? Do you practice any of the relaxation techniques found in this chapter? Sydney J. Harris said it best, "The time to relax is when you don't have time for it."

- *Connectedness*—Hardy people develop a social network that includes helping and being helped by others. They have developed a sense of "connectedness" to others. They are actively involved with others. Studies show that social interaction is important. It may lower pulse rate and blood pressure, enhance the immune system and boost the production of endorphins. When you're in a caring relationship with another person all these health benefits accrue. Do you have one or more close friends to whom you feel "connected" (i.e., sharing troubles, ambitions, and desires)?

The concept of the **Type C personality** emerged from research on the "hardy" personality.[18] It is based on the way certain individuals cope with stress. If you recall, Type As respond to stress with impatience and often with hostility and anger; Type B's responses are more relaxed. Type Cs, when stressed, accept challenges, feel in control of their lives, have feelings of connectedness, and have a strong commitment or purpose in life. There is a spirit of accomplishment and a spirit of self-confidence that comes from being a hardy, Type-C individual. All three personality types can benefit from the Stress Management strategies in this chapter—especially the Type As. Type Bs and Cs have probably already incorporated several of these strategies into their daily routine.

Research on the hardy, stress-resistant personality has made it clear that the five interrelated traits of control, commitment/challenge, lifestyle choices (personal health practices), and connectedness (social support) are important factors that buffer us from the ravages of our modern lifestyles and help us to adapt and even flourish in the face of it.[19, 20] How many of these hardiness traits do you possess? The "Becoming Stress Resistant and Hardy" exercise in the Activities section will help you strengthen these traits in your own life. Can you think of two ways you can apply the knowledge of these five traits to your life and in turn bolster your "hardiness" rating?

Building Skills for Stress Management

Your mind and body function most efficiently and effectively when you are relaxed. Performance and work decline when you feel "stressed out." You can learn to relax, to quiet down the mind and body (so you can get "in touch" or "connected to" your inner thoughts, feelings, goals, and values) and be successful in managing the stress in your life. Learn to identify the early warning signs of too much stress. This may include tight neck and shoulder muscles, clenched teeth, headaches, or feelings of "too much to do and not enough time to do it," etc. When these early warning signs are noticed, it is time to pay attention to your stress level and use one of the relaxation techniques mentioned in this chapter. Practice each of the relaxation techniques to find the ones that you feel most comfortable using and which works best for you. For best results, set aside some time every day for relaxation. By following the simple strategies in this chapter, you will be well on your way to becoming a stress hardy person. Enjoy!

Strategy #1 Exercise

An excellent method for reducing stress and aggressive feelings is regular aerobic exercise. Exercise allows us to play out the instinctive fight-or-flight response, to use the muscles that are tensed for action, and to reduce the adrenalin being pumped into the bloodstream. A number of studies suggest that exercise reduces the intensity of the stress response, shortens the time it takes to recover from stress, and can even help ward off illness in people who are experiencing stress.[21]

Exercise is a natural way to relax and renew energy. When hassles and problems begin to pile up in the office or at school, change into your workout clothes and take a vigorous run, a swim, or a brisk walk. The effect is amazing. Headaches, tension, anxiety, aggressiveness, and irritability are all diminished. Because research supports the value of exercise in reducing stress, physicians now recommend exercise to their patients instead of medications such as tranquilizers. Vigorous exercise increases the release of endorphins, brain chemicals that may alleviate harmful effects of stressors by producing a more relaxed state. Besides better stress management, other psychological benefits of exercise, documented by research, include increased self-esteem, increased alertness, and decreased depression and anxiety. Although vigorous exercise is best, even a relaxing walk can do wonders to relieve tension. Play tennis, racquetball, golf, bowl, swim, rake leaves, garden, bike, or whatever. Enjoy physical activity. It is the healthiest thing you can do for yourself, and it's inexpensive!

Strategy #2 Relaxation Techniques

2.1 Meditation   **Meditation** is a mental exercise that affects body processes, producing physical benefits. The purpose of meditation is to gain control over your attention—to internally quiet down, allowing **you** to choose what to focus upon and to block out distracting thoughts.

Meditation originated in the Eastern cultures of India and Tibet and was exported to the Western world by the Maharishi Mahesh Yogi. The Maharishi popularized the **transcendental meditation (TM)** method. In recent years, TM, as well as other forms of meditation, have been subjected to a battery of scientific studies. The findings have been revealing and conclusive. Meditation is a simple and valuable stress-management technique. It produces certain physiological changes, called the **relaxation response,** which we can employ to counteract stress. Specific benefits include:

- Decreased oxygen consumption and metabolic rate, thus less strain on the body's energy resources
- Increase in intensity and frequency of alpha brain waves associated with deep relaxation
- Reduced blood lactates (substances in the blood associated with anxiety)
- Significant decreases in blood pressure in hypertensive individuals (which remained lowered throughout the day)
- Reduced heart rate and slower respiration
- Decreased muscle tension
- Increased blood flow to arms and legs

- Decreased anxiety, fears, and phobias, and increased positive mental health (i.e., less anxious and greater self-actualization)

- Improved quality of sleep

Elements essential to meditation:

1. A quiet, comfortable environment. A place where you won't be disturbed. However, once you become experienced you will be able to meditate almost anywhere.

2. A mental device (unchanging object) or mantra (silently repeated word or phrase). This will help you shut out outside stimuli and keep you calm. A word or phrase is probably easiest to use. Any word will do (it doesn't have to be a secret one) as long as it is used consistently.

3. A passive attitude. Your attention should be focused on repeating the mantra and not on how you feel. Do not "try" to become relaxed. Let it happen. Disregard outside noise and thoughts, and return focus to the slow steady repetition of the mantra.

4. A comfortable position. This is necessary to avoid any undue muscular tension. Lying down or sitting in an over-stuffed chair may cause you to break the mantra and fall asleep. How to meditate is described in table 7.7.

Table 7.7

How to Meditate and Produce the Relaxation Response

1. Find a quiet room, and sit in a comfortable chair. A straight-back chair is best because you don't want to be so comfortable that you fall asleep. Rest your arms on the arms of the chair or in your lap.

2. Relax all your muscles as best you can, without forcing it. Assume a passive attitude, and focus on your breathing.

3. Close your eyes; there should be no tension in the forehead or eyes. Breathe easily and naturally through the nose. Repeat your mantra in your mind, very, very slowly, without a break. Many like to use the word "one." Remember, do not watch yourself relax. The rhythm of the mantra will be interrupted, and so will your relaxation period.

4. Continue to do this approximately twenty minutes. It is recommended that you meditate twice a day for twenty minutes each time.

5. When you stop meditating, give your body time to adjust. Open the eyes; focus on objects in the room. Take several deep breaths. Stretch while seated. When you feel ready, stand and stretch.

Helpful meditation guidelines are:

1. The best times to meditate are before breakfast and before dinner. Do not meditate directly after a meal. After eating, the blood is diverted toward the stomach area, aiding the digestive process. This diversion inhibits complete relaxation.

2. Wear nonrestrictive clothing while meditating, or loosen the clothes you happen to be wearing at the time.

3. Don't worry about meditating for a full 20 minutes at first. As you become more comfortable with the process, you will be able to progress up to 20 minutes or more, twice a day.

4. Do not smoke cigarettes or drink coffee, tea, or colas before meditating. These substances are stimulants and will not promote relaxation.

5. It would be helpful to disconnect the telephone. Also, definitely do *not* set the alarm clock for 20 minutes.

6. Relax and enjoy this time. Your problems will be there when you're finished. They will seem less distressing to you after meditation if you commit yourself to the time necessary to do it.

7. Don't come out of the meditative state too abruptly.

8. Practice regularly. It takes practice to learn to sit still, meditate, relax, and calm the mind. Be patient. You won't discover the benefits unless you practice every day.

2.2 Autogenic Training and Imagery   **Autogenic** means self-generating or self-induced. This relaxation technique uses exercises to bring about the sensations of warmth and heaviness in the limbs and torso, then uses relaxing images to expand the relaxed state. Both meditation and autogenic training lead to the relaxation response. Many who find meditation too easy and boring enjoy autogenic training because of the switches of focus from one part of the body to another and the use of imagery. Autogenic training has been found to be very successful in the treatment of chronic and lower back pain. Otherwise the physiological and psychological benefits are similar to meditation.

Autogenic training can be done lying down or in a seated position. Whatever position you choose, be sure that you are relaxed and comfortable. Eliminate muscle tension in any part of the body by changing position slightly. Practice 10 to 30 minutes, one or two times a day to become skillful at this technique.

The six steps to autogenic training are:

1. Concentrate on heaviness of arms and legs, beginning with the dominant side.

2. Concentrate on warmth of the arms and legs, beginning with the dominant side.

3. Concentrate on warmth and heaviness of heart and chest.

4. Concentrate on the breathing rhythm.

5. Concentrate on warmth of the abdominal area.

6. Concentrate on coolness of the forehead.

After the six stages of autogenic training have been mastered, body relaxation is transferred to mind relaxation by the use of images of relaxing scenes such as these:

- Sinking into a mattress
- A sack of sugar melting away in the rain
- Floating out to sea
- A feather floating in the sky
- A soaring bird

- Clouds drifting by
- Ocean surf splashing on the sand
- A warm, relaxing fire in the fireplace
- A sailboat on a calm lake

You should use images you find relaxing. They may be quite different than those of your friends.

2.3 Jacobson's Progressive Relaxation   Edmund Jacobson, a physician, designed a series of exercises to be used by his tense patients. He taught his patients exercises that required them to contract a muscle group, then relax it, progressing from one muscle group to another until the total body was relaxed. The idea was to learn to recognize tenseness and be able to consciously relax whenever it was needed. This method of relaxation, named after its developer, does not produce the relaxation response. However, if practiced regularly, it is very beneficial in helping people relax. It has been used in the treatment of insomnia and psychological conditions such as poor self-concept, depression, and anxiety.

There are many routines of contract-relax exercises for progressive relaxation. Try the progressive relaxation routine in this chapter (table 7.8) that begins at the head and ends at the feet, or develop your own routine. With practice, you will be able to eliminate the contraction phase and focus totally on relaxation.

2.4 Abdominal Breathing   Most of us breathe in short shallow breaths, expanding only the chest especially when we're under stress. This is called thoracic breathing and is really not the proper way to breathe. It does not allow the lungs to fill and empty completely, and it can increase muscle tension.

During stressful situations it is even more important to breathe from the abdomen. This method allows more oxygen to enter the body and relaxes the muscles. You can practice the simple steps described in this chapter almost any time or place, even on the telephone, in class, or at a meeting. Practice at least once a day so that it becomes natural when involved in stressful or fatiguing situations. This simple procedure has produced excellent results for many (table 7.9).

2.5 Hatha Yoga   Hatha Yoga is a discipline that involves the use of various exercises or postures (called asanas) in combination with proper breathing rhythm, to remove tension and inflexibility in the body. It also attempts to improve muscular strength, muscular endurance, and body alignment. Hatha Yoga should not be associated with religious or spiritual groups. The physiological and psychological benefits of Hatha Yoga have been thoroughly researched, confirming it to be an excellent form of exercise and an aid to improving the health and well-being of those who practice it.

Table 7.8
Progressive Relaxation Routine

1. Lie on your back on the floor in a quiet place with the lights dimmed. Remove the shoes. Let the feet relax and rotate outward. Arms should be beside the body, palms turned upward.
2. Proceed slowly over the body, tensing a muscle group, then relaxing it. Stop if cramping or pain develops.
3. Face: Squint your eyes, wrinkle your nose, make a face, and then relax. Open the mouth very wide, stick out your tongue. Close mouth and clench your teeth. Now relax.
4. Neck: Nod head downward to touch chin to chest. Relax.
5. Head: Try to touch the right ear to the right shoulder, and left ear to the left shoulder. Relax and center head over torso.
6. Shoulders: Shrug shoulders up toward ears: pull shoulders down from ears; press hard against the floor. One at a time. Relax.
7. Hands and arms: Squeeze fingers together, making a fist. Relax. Raise right arm, bending at the elbow and "make a muscle" with the biceps. Relax. Repeat with left arm. Relax. With arms on floor, stiffen both arms, making a fist. Relax.
8. Back: Try to squeeze shoulder blades together. Relax. Press lower back area into the floor. Relax.
9. Abdomen: Suck in abdominal muscles. Relax.
10. Buttocks: Contract buttock muscles. Relax.
11. Thighs: Contract thigh muscles, one at a time, then both at the same time. Relax.
12. Calves: Flex toes back toward head, then extend or point toes away from head, using the right leg, then the left leg. Relax.
13. Toes: Curl toes under, first the right foot, then the left foot. Relax.
14. Be aware of the relaxed state of your body.

Table 7.9
Abdominal Breathing

1. Inhale and exhale fully through your mouth.
2. Inhale very slowly and push out your abdomen (stomach) as though it was a balloon inflating. Move your chest as little as possible.
3. Exhale *slowly* and allow the stomach to flatten.
4. Repeat the pattern. On each "in" breath let the belly inflate, and on each "out" breath let it flatten.
5. Each "out" breath is an opportunity to rid the body of tension.

2.6 Massage   When you are bombarded with too much stress, the muscles in the neck, shoulders, and back can become tight and stiff to the point of pain. Without relaxation these muscles can become chronically tight and can cause much distress. One of the most enjoyable ways to relieve this condition is to have a massage.

These are two popular forms of massage.

1. *Shiatsu,* originating in Japan and China, is a technique that is actually a form of acupressure. Pressure is applied with the thumbs or fingers along acupuncture meridians. The idea is to restore balance so that the "chi" energy (an energy believed to be linked to the life force) flows freely and in a balanced manner.

2. *Swedish massage,* the most familiar form, involves kneading and rubbing the muscles to increase relaxation and circulation.

Massage given by a spouse or friend can be just as pleasant. You can even massage yourself when tight neck and shoulder muscles are tense. Put on your favorite music and enjoy.

2.7 Biofeedback Training   **Biofeedback training** is a technique in which machines measure certain physiological processes of the body. The machine then converts this information to an understandable form and feeds it back to the individual. This process allows a person access to biological information not usually available to one's consciousness. It is essentially a method of teaching people to regulate physiological responses, such as heart rates, electrical activity to muscles, peripheral skin temperature, blood pressure, headaches, and asthma attacks. With feedback training, stressors themselves are not removed, but the response to them is controlled. Control of physiological arousal is an important step in stress management. A major drawback of biofeedback is the cost and availability of the machines and the lack of trained professionals to operate them.

2.8 Relaxation (Floatation) Tanks   A floatation tank is one of the newest stress management devices. It is merely an oversized bathtub (or shell) (fig. 7.2) filled with body-temperature water, placed in a small room. The shell is light-proof and sound insulated. The idea is to reduce sensory stimuli, thereby providing complete relaxation. Epsom salts are dissolved in the water to help you float. The warm water, the quiet, and the darkness combine to create a pleasant sensation of floating in space. You just lie there, body and water becoming one, and relax. The distractions of the everyday world are left behind. Research supports the use of floatation tanks in the management of stress. They are now found in many health clubs in larger cities in the United States.

Strategy #3 Lifestyle Change

3.1 The Impact of Diet   Proper diet is an important part of your stress management program. A nutritious diet will help you look and feel good. Many feel that poor diet can increase your susceptibility to stress by causing fatigue and irritability. This is especially true for individuals who are eating too many meals

Figure 7.2
A flotation tank is a beneficial way to reduce stress.

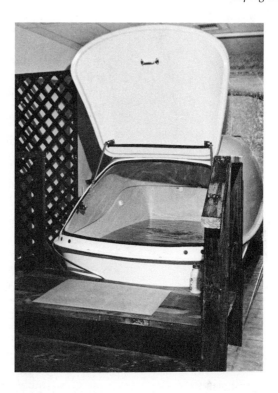

away from home, missing meals, or eating on the run. Follow these guidelines to help keep you from feeling irritable and uptight. Here is another area where you can take charge.

1. Reduce (below 250 milligrams per day) or eliminate the caffeine in your diet. Caffeine is a stimulant and magnifies the effects of stress (see "caffeine" in chapter 10).

2. Limit foods containing sugar, especially if you have been skipping meals. It robs the body of B-complex vitamins and may induce anxiety and failure to cope with stressful situations.

3. Limit your intake of sodium because excessive fluid build-up leads to discomfort and increased stress. Too much sodium (salt) can also increase blood pressure due to the fluid build-up.

3.2 Time Management   Insufficient time appears to be the plague of the twentieth century. How well you manage your time plays a large role in how much pressure you feel. Time management experts suggest these time-saving tips:

1. Analyze how you spend time, then evaluate that use of time. Keep a diary. You may find you are wasting too much time.

2. Learn to set goals. Write them down. This helps you plan for today and for the future.

3. Learn how to set priorities. Not everything you do is number one on your list of importance. With goals in mind, you will know how to prioritize your activities. Items on the "Do" list must get done, items on the "Maybe" list are those you would like to take care of today, if possible, and those on the "If Possible" list are those you would like to do if all the activities of the first and second lists are completed.

4. Schedule your priorities into your day. This may involve setting up a specific schedule—a time for homework, a time for play (or to watch TV), and a time for sleep. Learn to balance work and play.

5. Learn how to stop being inefficient. This is an art that anyone can learn. Go through mail one time only. Start a task with an intention of completing it now. Don't look it over and put it aside for later. You have wasted time looking it over the first time.

6. Don't allow too many demands to be made "on your time." You can say, "No!" Learn to delegate certain activities to others when possible.

7. Practice quick relaxation tricks frequently throughout the day. Get up and go for a drink of water. Give yourself a massage to the neck, shoulders, and forehead. This energizes you to complete tasks more efficiently.

College students have many demands on their time and must plan wisely.

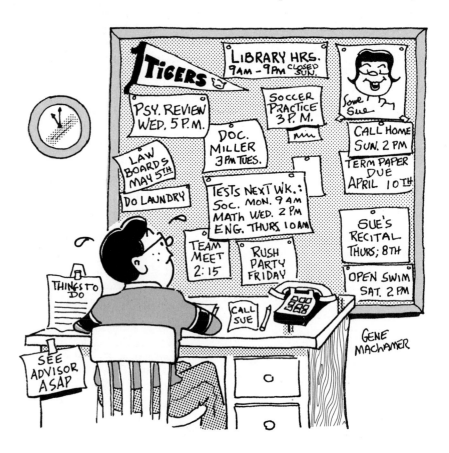

3.3 Alcohol, Drugs, and Cigarettes   Alcohol is a powerful depressant drug that temporally masks, but won't solve, your problems. In fact, it can increase stress by creating new problems—hangovers, arrests, traffic violations, fights, and accidents. Taking illegal drugs can only increase your stress. Why risk ruining your physical and mental health and the stress of being arrested? Do not smoke cigarettes or use other tobacco products (snuff, chewing tobacco). Nicotine is a stimulant that increases stress.

3.4 Get Plenty of Restful Sleep   Most people need 7 to 8 hours of restful sleep each night. Getting enough sleep can make you more alert, less irritable, and better able to cope with stressful situations. Don't lose sleep over things that you cannot control.

3.5 Develop Satisfying Relationships   Having close friends to share the joys and sorrows of living is a huge asset in protecting your health. It has been shown that unhappiness, depression, and feelings of isolation can be caused by lack of close emotional bonds with friends, a spouse, or family members. Intimate relationships and social support can be healing. Social support can both directly provide reinforcement for healthy behaviors and indirectly buffer disappointments that would otherwise lead to excessive stress.[22] You have to *be a friend to have a friend.* Make the effort. It's good health and happiness insurance.

3.6 Learn When to Seek the Help and Support of Others   There will be stressful situations you will not be able to deal with alone. Don't be embarrassed to seek professional help. Developing a variety of support groups such as family, friends, coaches, counselors, or physicians can be very helpful.

3.7 Balance Work and Play   Plan for regular recreation (or a time for yourself) and make that time inviolate. It is your special time. Let nothing else interfere. This can include learning to do nothing (loafing) at times and feeling okay about it.

Strategy #4 Reframing

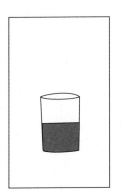

Reframing: Is the glass half empty or half full?

Reframing is a way of looking at life in a positive manner. Is the glass half empty or half full? Viewing yourself as a sick person because you have asthma is very different, for example, than perceiving yourself as a healthy person who also happens to have asthma. See if you can learn to "reframe" life's stumbling blocks into challenges. Look at the bright side of each situation. Remember, you are in control of you. Positive emotions and laughter play an important role in keeping well and fit. Optimists have higher hardiness scores, whereas pessimists are more likely to resort to anger and hostility. Laughing is like "internal jogging"—it causes endorphins (pain-relieving chemicals) to be released in the brain. Laughter is like a tranquilizer with no negative side effects. Scientific evidence is beginning to support the biblical axiom that "a merry heart doeth good like a medicine."

Strategy #5 Create a Memory Bank

Appreciate and take advantage of opportunities to savor a special experience each day. Store these in your memory bank. When you look back over your life, what special memories do you fondly recall? Roasting marshmallows over a campfire, watching the sunset, the smelling of a rose, the glow after a satisfying workout, a hug that said "I care" . . . What can you do today to increase your store of pleasant memories?

Summary

Stress is unavoidable. Optimal levels of stress improve health and performance, but excess levels, especially when chronic and perceived as negative, can be hazardous to your health. Major life events are significant stressors—death of a spouse, marriage, and divorce, for example. Other more frequent stressors are daily hassles (i.e., missed sleep, rush-hour traffic, losing things, etc.). We learn to cope with major life events and daily hassles in a variety of ways. Some are healthy; some are not. Healthy stress management strategies include exercise, relaxation techniques, lifestyle changes, reframing, and creating a memory bank. Hassles can be countered by the giving and receiving of daily uplifts (i.e., compliments, hugs, and getting enough sleep).

Three personality categories have been labeled as Types A, B, and C, according to how they cope with stress. Those who are impatient and become angry or hostile when stress builds up are classified as Type As. Type Bs are more relaxed than Type As. Type Cs are often referred to as "hardy." They accept challenges, feel they are in control of their lives, and have a strong commitment or purpose in life.

Your wellness is dependent on how well you balance the stress in your life, how well you can modify your angry and hostile behavior, and how successfully you take charge of your life. As one wise person said, "If you can't fight, and you can't flee . . . flow."

References

1. Selye, Hans. *Stress Without Distress*. J.B. Lippincott, New York, 1984.

2. Girdano, D. A., Everly, G. S., and Dusek, Dorothy. *Controlling Stress and Tension: A Holistic Approach* 3rd Ed., Englewood Cliffs, NJ: Prentice-Hall, 1990.

3. Girdano, D. A., et al. *Controlling Stress and Tension: A Holistic Approach*.

4. Selye, Hans. *The Stress of Life*. New York: McGraw-Hill, 1956.

5. Ornish, Dean. *Dr. Dean Ornish's Program for Reversing Heart Disease*. New York: Random House, 1990.

6. Ornish, Dean. *Dr. Dean Ornish's Program for Reversing Heart Disease*.

7. Lazarus, R. *Psychological Stress and the Coping Process*. New York: McGraw-Hill, 1966.

8. Holmes, T. H., and Rahe, R. H. "The Social Readjustment Rating Scale." *Journal of Psychosomatic Research*, November, 1967.

9. Toffler, Alvin. *Future Shock*. New York: Random House, Inc., 1970.

10. Delongis, A., and others. "Relationship of Daily Hassles, Uplifts and Major Life Events to Health Status." *Health Psychology*, January, 1982.

11. Miles, G. T. "Daily Hassles and Uplifts—Short Form: Item Selection and Cross Validation." Masters Thesis, Pennsylvania State University, University Park, 1986.

12. Kanner, Allen, James Coyne, Catherine Schaefer, and Richard Lazarus. "Comparison of Two Modes of Stress Measurement: Daily Hassles and Uplifts Versus Major Life Events." *Journal of Behavior Medicine* 4 (January 1981).

13. "How Anger Affects Your Health." University of California at Berkeley Newsletter, Vol. 8, Issue 4, January, 1992.

14. Sweeting, Roger L. *A Values Approach to Health Behavior*. Champaign, IL: Human Kinetics Books, 1990.

15. Sweeting, Roger L. *A Values Approach to Health Behavior*.

16. Flannery, R., Jr. "Towards Stress Resistant Persons: A Stress Management Approach to the Treatment of Anxiety." *American Journal of Preventive Medicine*, 3 (Jan. 1987).

17. Kobasa, S. C. "The Hardy Personality: Toward a Social Psychology of Stress and Health." *Social Psychology of Health and Illness,* Sanders, R. S., and Suls, J. (Eds.). Hillsdale, NJ: Erlbaum (1982).

18. Kriegel, R., and Kriegel, M. H. *The C Zone: Peak Performance Under Pressure.* New York: Doubleday, 1984.

19. Flannery, R., Jr. "Towards Stress Resistant Persons: A Stress/Management Approach to the Treatment of Anxiety."

20. De Benedetti, Valerie. "Getting Fit for Life: Can Exercise Reduce Stress?" *The Physician and Sportsmedicine* 16 (June 1988): 185–200.

21. Kobasa, S. C. "The Hardy Personality: Toward a Social Psychology of Stress and Health."

22. Sweeting, Roger. *A Values Approach to Health Behavior.*

Suggested Readings

Birkel, Dee Ann. 1991. *Hatha Yoga: Developing The Body, Mind and Inner Self.* Dubuque, IA: Eddie Bowers Publishing, Inc.

Delongis, A., Folkman, S., and Lazarus, R. "The Impact of Daily Stress on Health and Mood: Psychological and Social Resources as Mediators." *Journal of Personality and Social Psychology,* 1988, 54, 486–495.

Delongis, A., and others. "Relationship of Daily Hassles, Uplifts, and Major Life Events to Health Status." *Health Psychology,* 1982, 1, 119–136.

Donatelle, Rebecca, and Michele Hawkins. "Stress Management, Employee Stress Claims: Increasing Implications for Health Promotion." *American Journal of Health Promotion* (Winter 1989), Vol. 3, No. 3:19–25.

Eckenrode, John and Gore, Susan, eds. 1990. *Stress Between Work and Family.* New York: Plenum Press.

Ginter, Gary, John West, and John Zarski. "Learned Resourcefulness and Situation-Specific Coping With Stress." *The Journal of Psychology* (May 1989), Vol. 123, No. 3:295–304.

Girdano, Daniel, George Every, and Dusek, Dorothy. 1990. *Controlling Stress and Tension: A Holistic Approach,* 3rd Ed. Englewood Cliffs, NJ: Prentice-Hall.

Greenberg, Jerrold. 1992. *Comprehensive Stress Management.* Dubuque, IA: Brown & Benchmark Publishers.

Greenberg, Jerrold. 1992. *Your Personal Profile and Activity Workbook.* Dubuque, IA: Brown & Benchmark Publishers.

Holmes, Thomas, and Richard Rahe. "The Social Readjustment Rating Scale." *Journal of Psychosomatic Research* 11 (1967):213–18.

Jacobson, Edmund. 1938. *Progressive Relaxation,* 2d ed. Chicago, IL: Chicago Press.

Jones, Graham & Lew Hardy, eds. 1990. *Stress and Performance in Sport.* New York: J. Wiley & Sons.

Kagan, Dona, and Kris Berg. "The Relationship Between Aerobic Activity and Cognitive Performance Under Stress." *The Journal of Psychology* (September 1988), Vol. 122, No. 5:451–462.

Kanner, A. D., Coyne, J. C., Schaefer, C., and Lazarus, R. S. "Comparison of Two Models of Stress Measurement: Daily Hassles and Uplifts Versus Major Life Events." *Journal of Behavioral Medicine,* 1981, 4, 1–39.

Lazarus, R. 1966. *Psychological Stress and the Coping Process.* New York: McGraw-Hill.

Lazarus, Richard, and Susan Folkman. 1984. *Stress, Appraisal and Coping.* Springer Publishing Company, Inc., 200 Park Avenue South, New York, NY.

Matheny, Kenneth. 1992. *Stress and Strategies for Lifestyle Management.* Georgia State University Press.

Pennebaker, James. 1990. *Opening Up: The Healing Power of Confiding in Others.* New York: W. Morrow.

Powell, Trevor. 1990. *Anxiety and Stress Management.* New York: Routledge.

Quick, James, ed., 1992. *Stress and Well-Being at Work: Assessments and Interventions for Occupational Mental Health.* American Psychological Association.

Sarason, Barbara, Sarason, Irwin, and Pierce, Gregory, eds., 1990. *Social Support: An Interactional View.* New York: J. Wiley & Sons.

Schafer, Walt. 1987. *Stress Management for Wellness.* New York: Holt, Rinehart and Winston.

Schneider, Sharon K. "The Effect of Personality Variables as Stress Buffers." *Journal of Psychological Type* 14:51–56, 1988.

Selye, Hans. 1956. *"The Stress of Life."* New York: McGraw-Hill.

Smith, Jonathon. 1990. *Cognitive-Behavioral Relaxation Training.* New York: Springer Publishing Co.

Thoren, P. J., Floras, J., Hoffman, P., and Seals, D. 1990. "Endorphins and Exercise: Physiological Mechanisms and Clinical Implications." *Medicine and Science in Sports and Exercise* 22.

Tubesing, Donald. 1989. *Kicking Your Stress Habits.* Duluth, MN: Whole Person Associates.

Wagner, B., Compas, B., and Howell, D. "Daily and Major Life Events: A Test of an Integrative Model of Psychosocial Stress." *American Journal of Community Psychology,* 1988, 16, 189–205.

Resources

The American Association for Therapeutic Humor, 1163 Shermer Road, Northbrook, Illinois, 60062 (708-291-0211) can supply bibliographies on various aspects of humor-as-therapy and newsletter, *Laugh It Up.*

The Humor Project, 110 Spring Street, Saratoga Springs, New York, 12866 (518-587-8770). Supplies workshops, courses, free information packet on positive power of humor and magazine, *Laughing Matter.*

8

Special Exercise Considerations

Chapter Objectives

After reading this chapter, you will be able to:

1. Identify the physiological bases for differences in men's and women's exercise performance levels.
2. List the similarities in men's and women's responses to exercise.
3. Define amenorrhea, Kegel exercise, and stress incontinence.
4. Identify correct recommendations for exercise during pregnancy.
5. Identify recommendations for safe exercise in hot and cold weather.
6. Identify the best replacement fluid to prevent dehydration during exercise in hot weather.
7. Identify the safe exercises from a list of safe and contraindicated exercises.
8. Recognize the effect of aging on exercise performance.
9. Identify the effects of a regular program of exercise on the aging process.

Terms

- Amenorrhea
- Dysmenorrhea
- Endorphin
- Estrogen
- Hemoglobin
- Kegel exercise
- Menarche
- Stress incontinence

*T*his chapter brings together several different concerns related to exercise participation. Six major areas are addressed: females and exercise, males and exercise, environmental considerations, fluid replacement, contraindicated exercises, and aging.

Similarities and Differences in Men's and Women's Exercise Performance

While performance levels may differ, both men and women respond to exercise in a similar manner. Although women have approximately 20 percent lower maximal oxygen uptake than men, with exercise they show similar rates of improvement. Performance levels differ for several reasons. Due to hormonal changes during puberty, a woman adds fat, while a man's muscle mass doubles. The average male has 12 percent to 16 percent body fat and 40 percent muscle tissue, while the average female has 20 percent to 24 percent body fat and 23 percent lean tissue.[1] Therefore, women have half as much muscle tissue to move their weight and more inactive fat weight to carry. In addition, men's greater muscle mass gives them 30 percent to 40 percent greater strength. Women have fewer red blood cells than men and about 10 percent to 15 percent less **hemoglobin** (the oxygen-carrying component of red blood cells), so their blood has less oxygen-carrying capacity, which may limit endurance. Even though women are at a disadvantage in terms of physical performance, they benefit equally from aerobic exercise in terms of fitness improvement.[2] Training effect benefits, such as loss of fat from deposit areas, increased bone density, and decreased exercise heart rates, are similar for men and women. When differences in body size are taken into account, fitness gains for men and women are essentially the same.

Women often fear that exercise will make them develop large or bulky muscles or a masculine appearance. This is not likely unless a woman is using anabolic steroids and spending many hours in extremely strenuous weight training. Potential for muscular development is genetically determined by levels of the sex hormone testosterone, and women generally have only one-tenth as much of this hormone as men. While women, like men, vary in their potential for muscular size development, what most women want from exercise is exactly what they will gain—decreased fat, increased lean body tissue, and firmer, toned muscles.

Females and Exercise

Once, the sight of a female training on the road or competing in a race was sufficiently unusual that people would often stop and stare. As the interest in fitness as a lifestyle has grown, so has the number of women participants in aerobic activities and athletics. Now that large numbers of females have adopted a physically active lifestyle, research has provided us with new information concerning topics of special interest to women.

Menstruation

Is it all right to exercise during menstruation? Yes. Menstruation is just one small part of the ongoing female reproductive cycle. In the past, women sometimes used this as an excuse to avoid exercise, but now women are encouraged to lead a normal routine during all parts of the reproductive cycle. Menstrual cycle hormones affect heart rate, ventilation rate, basal body temperature, and blood hematocrit, the red cell portion of the total blood volume.[3] How women experience menstruation varies greatly. Some feel no different than usual; some may

More women are discovering the joys of physical activity.

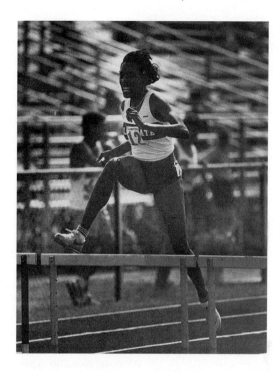

experience abdominal and leg cramps, backache, or mood swings, particularly during the first two days of the menstrual flow. **Dysmenorrhea,** or painful menstruation, is probably neither caused nor cured by exercise.

There is some evidence that enhanced fitness generally leads to a reduction in menstrual complaints, although this is still being researched. Some studies indicate that exercise decreases mood swings and relieves depression, anxiety, and irritability.[4] Excess body water lost through perspiration can reduce weight gain due to water retention, relieving premenstrual bloating and edema.[5] While there are no specific exercises that cure severe cramps, participation in a program of regular exercise has been shown to decrease the frequency of minor menstrual cramps. This is perhaps due to increased abdominal tone, increased circulation to the uterus, or increased levels of pain-relieving **endorphins.**[6]

Menstruation should be treated as a normal physiological function, not an illness. As long as she is comfortable, a woman should continue her regular exercise program. For women who want to look and feel their best, exercise is beneficial at any time of the month.

Effects of Exercise on the Menstrual Cycle   Recent studies indicate that young girls who exercise vigorously may experience a delay in **menarche,** the start of their menstrual cycle, decreasing their risk of cancer later in life.[7] While the average American girl experiences menarche between 11 and 12 years of age, those who train vigorously experience their first menstrual cycle at an average age of 15 1/2, the same as it was one hundred years ago.[8] This delay may be natural and even desirable, because it reduces the body's exposure to **estrogen,** a female sex hormone. The more menstrual cycles a woman has over her lifetime, the longer her exposure to estrogen and the greater her risk of cancer of the breast and reproductive organs. In addition, women who exercise tend to be leaner, thus producing less potent estrogen. In one study, women who had been athletic in college and high school as compared to sedentary women had half the incidence of breast and reproductive cancer in later life.[9] The role of exercise in reducing cancer risk is controversial and still under study.

After menarche, the stress of heavy athletic training and competition may cause irregular or infrequent menstruation, or even secondary **amenorrhea,** the cessation of a previously normal menstrual cycle (primary amenorrhea is never having had a menstrual cycle). Athletic amenorrhea (cessation of menstruation in athletes) has occurred in distance runners, dancers, swimmers, and gymnasts. It is rare in women doing moderate amounts of exercise as part of a fitness program. It is more frequent among those whose menstrual cycles started late, past age 15. Although the precise cause of this form of secondary amenorrhea has not been identified, a number of theories have been proposed, including: decreased intake of calories, protein, and fat; increased exercise intensity and volume of training; increased levels of psychological stress; and excessive losses of body weight (with extremely low body fat).[10] Although no specific body fat percentage has been associated with the development of athletic amenorrhea, the evidence suggests that decreased fat levels may lead to a decreased production of one form of estrogen. Thus, as fat percentages decrease, estrogen levels decline and the evidence of secondary amenorrhea increases. The focus of research is upon how all of the factors mentioned may affect the hypothalamus, thereby influencing the production of important regulatory hormones relative to menstruation and metabolism, including estrogen, epinephrine, and corticoids. Whatever the cause, exercise-induced (athletic) amenorrhea is generally considered reversible. Normal menstrual cycles resume with as minor a change in lifestyle as a 10 percent decrease in exercise, improved nutrition, or weight gain of 4 to 5 pounds.[11] Also, exercise-induced amenorrhea does not seem to affect long-term fertility.[12] In fact, while a woman with amenorrhea does not experience a regular menstrual cycle, it is still possible for her to ovulate and become pregnant. She should not rely on this for birth control and should continue her regular birth control method if pregnancy is not desired. Any active woman should be aware of her normal menstrual cycle and should discuss any irregularities with her physician to rule out such conditions as thyroid disorders, ovarian cysts, brain tumors, and pregnancy.

There is concern that low estrogen levels during amenorrhea accelerate bone mineral loss, increasing the risk of osteoporosis. Estrogen, exercise, and calcium must all be present in order for a woman to build or maintain bone mass. An excess of one element will not make up for an absence of another. While people who exercise tend to have greater bone densities than nonexercisers, loss of estrogen, regardless of age, may cause an irreversible loss of bone strength. A 20-year-old amenorrheic athlete can have the bone density of a 50-year-old.[13] While bone density does increase with a resumption in normal estrogen levels, it does not appear to recover fully. If an amenorrheic athlete has a low estrogen level, lifestyle

Exercise during and after pregnancy has many advantages.

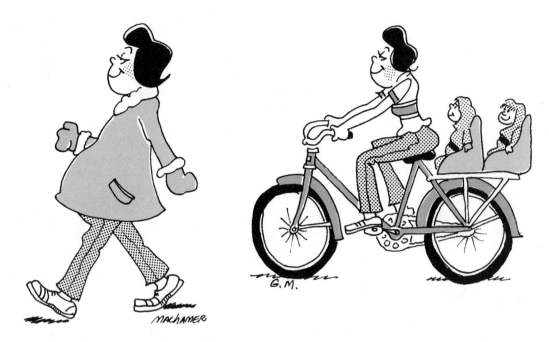

change and/or low-dose estrogen replacement therapy to prevent bone mineral loss should be discussed with a physician. In addition, a calcium intake of 1,500 mg/day (about 5 cups of milk) is recommended.

Pregnancy and Exercise

Is exercise advisable during pregnancy? How much? What are the benefits? Are there any limitations or cautions to keep in mind? Are some exercises better than others? Pregnancy is a natural and normal physiological function, not an illness. A pregnant woman is not fragile. She will be healthier and the pregnancy safer if she remains active. Of course, any pregnant woman should obtain medical clearance from her physician before beginning or continuing an exercise program. General advice for a healthy woman having an uncomplicated pregnancy is to continue her regular exercise program, being careful not to get overtired. If she has not been exercising before pregnancy, this is not a time to begin a crash program. A 20-minute to 30-minute walk, three to four days per week, is a program a doctor might approve. Throughout pregnancy, to keep the effort aerobic, a woman should use the "talk test." She should be able to carry on a conversation while exercising without getting out of breath. In early pregnancy, if exercising seems to require more effort, decrease intensity and duration. Particular care should be taken to avoid overheating, which has been linked to increased risk of central nervous system abnormalities (such as, spinal bifida) in the baby.[14] A gradual weight gain, which is natural and desirable, is likely to increase stress to joints, ligaments, and muscles. Also, muscles and connective tissues become more lax as they gradually undergo hormonal changes. This will facilitate the baby's birth but makes the pregnant woman more susceptible to strains and sprains. Therefore, good supportive shoes at this time are important for comfort and safety during exercise.

In the fifth to sixth months of pregnancy, due to increasing weight and joint flexibility, impact activities may become uncomfortable. At this time, many women switch to low- or no-impact exercises such as walking, swimming, or stationary cycling. While some women continue their normal exercise program right to the day of delivery with no ill effects, don't feel guilty if you feel a need to cut back. Toward the end of pregnancy, if you fatigue easily and exercise seems to require more effort, it is natural to decrease the activity level. After the fourth month it is not advised to do exercises that require lying on your back. This position can block the blood supply to the uterus and depress the fetal heart rate.[15] Throughout pregnancy, a woman needs to listen to her body and adjust exercise to maintain comfort. Note specific pregnancy exercise guidelines from the American College of Obstetricians and Gynecologists, in table 8.1.

There are many reasons why exercise is important during pregnancy. The physiological changes of pregnancy place a great demand on the body. Labor and delivery are perhaps the most physically demanding events a woman will ever experience. Exercise can maintain optimal fitness, enabling a woman to control weight gain, improve muscle tone, improve posture, decrease backache, and decrease constipation. Exercise can also aid in increasing energy, managing stress, enhancing sleep at night, and regaining prepregnancy figure.

While fitness is no guarantee of a quick labor or easy delivery, endurance and increased capacity to deal with the physical stress of childbirth are assets. A fit mother can enjoy a quicker recovery from childbirth than the unfit and can regain her normal fitness and activity levels in less time.

Stress Incontinence

Stress incontinence, an involuntary leakage of urine when you laugh, cough, sneeze, or jog, is a common problem, particularly in women over 30 who have given birth. During pregnancy and birth, these muscles become weakened and stretched. One solution is to wear a sanitary pad, but a better approach is to strengthen the perineal muscles that control this function. The pelvic floor is a hammocklike muscle layer attached at the front and back of the pelvis. It supports the pelvic organs, including the bladder, uterus, and rectum. Kegel exercises, named after the Los Angeles physician who developed them, strengthen the pelvic floor muscles, and may prevent or cure stress incontinence. As a side benefit, many women report increased pleasure during intercourse.

Kegel Exercise

Kegel exercises are done by contracting perineal muscles, which surround the bladder neck and vagina. To learn the exercise try this: when urinating, stop and start the flow. This is the muscle action. You can do these exercises anytime—contract hard, then release. Do ten in a row, and work up to five sets of ten daily. These exercises should be done before, during, and after pregnancy.

Table 8.1

ACOG Guidelines for Exercise during Pregnancy and Postpartum

Pregnancy and Postpartum

1. Regular exercise (at least 3 times per week) is preferable to intermittent activity. Competitive activities should be discouraged.
2. Vigorous exercise should not be performed in hot, humid weather or when you have a fever.
3. Ballistic movements (jerky, bouncy motions) should be avoided. Exercise should be done on a wooden floor or a tightly carpeted surface to reduce shock and provide a sure footing.
4. Deep flexion or extension of joints should be avoided because of connective tissue laxity. Activities that require jumping, jarring motions, or rapid changes in direction should be avoided because of joint instability.
5. Vigorous exercise should be preceded by a 5-minute period of muscle warm-up. This can be accomplished by slow walking or stationary cycling with low resistance.
6. Vigorous exercise should be followed by a period of gradually declining activity that includes gentle stationary stretching. Because connective tissue laxity increases the risk of joint injury, stretches should not be taken to the point of maximum resistance.
7. Heart rate should be measured at times of peak activity. Target heart rates and limits established in consultation with the physician should not be exceeded.
8. Care should be taken to gradually rise from the floor to avoid a sudden drop in blood pressure. Some form of activity involving the legs should be continued for a brief period.
9. Liquids should be taken liberally before and after exercise to prevent dehydration. If necessary, activity should be interrupted to replenish fluids.
10. Women who have led sedentary lifestyles should begin with physical activity of very low intensity and advance activity levels very gradually.
11. Activity should be stopped and the physician consulted if any unusual symptoms appear.

Pregnancy Only

1. Maternal heart rate should not exceed 140 beats per minute.
2. Strenuous activities should not exceed 15 minutes in duration.
3. No exercise should be performed lying on the back after the fourth month of gestation is completed.
4. Exercises that employ the Valsalva maneuver should be avoided.
5. Caloric intake should be adequate to meet not only the extra energy needs of pregnancy, but also of the exercise performed.
6. Maternal core temperature should not exceed 38° C.

Source: American College of Obstetricians and Gynecologists. Exercise during Pregnancy and the Postnatal Period (ACOG Home Exercise Programs). *Washington, DC: ACOG, 1985, p. 4. Reprinted with permission.*

Postpartum: Getting Back into Shape

Giving birth and coping with the demands of a new baby are both joyful and stressful for a new mother. The main problem in resuming exercise is not fatigue or shortness of breath, which might be expected, but finding someone to watch the baby while mother takes a well-deserved break! Postpartum recovery times vary greatly. If the delivery has been normal, walking is encouraged in the hospital the day after delivery. This can be continued when the woman returns home. Rest, good nutrition, and a progressive walking program will speed recovery faster than complete inactivity or becoming exhausted by trying to resume prepregnancy activity levels too soon. You should not rush into impact activities such as jogging until you have given loosened joints a chance to recover—6 weeks to 16 weeks.[16] Abdominal curls are important for toning overstretched abdominal muscles and preventing back problems. Also, do Kegel exercises to strengthen pelvic floor muscles.

A nursing mother needs to avoid fatigue and dehydration, which may reduce milk production. Drink eight or more glasses of fluid a day, and nap when the baby does to ensure adequate rest. Wear a good supportive bra, with pads to control leaks, and nurse before exercise for greater comfort. There is no conflict between nursing a baby and moderate exercise. Both help a mother regain her prepregnancy figure.

Breast Support

Does bouncing cause breasts to sag? Some believe that breast movement stretches the skin and ligaments that support the breasts. There is no evidence to support this claim; the main culprits are genetics and pregnancy.[17] Still, a good bra makes exercise more comfortable by reducing breast movement during activity. The best designs flatten breasts to redistribute their mass across the chest wall. This results in less mass for gravity to affect. Racerback and crossback straps prevent slippage off the shoulder. Certain designs are more suited to small-breasted women, while others are more comfortable for large-breasted exercisers. A woman should try different styles to decide what is best for her. A good exercise bra should (1) limit breast movement; (2) have wide straps that do not slip off the shoulders; (3) have a wide band at the bottom to prevent the bra from riding up; (4) have no rough seams, no fasteners, or well-covered fasteners, to prevent chafing; and (5) be made of nonabrasive materials and be seamless, or at least have seams that do not cross the nipple area.

Males and Exercise

Participation in sports and physical activities no longer ends with graduation from high school or college. Large numbers of men are continuing or beginning lifetime exercise programs.

Exercise appears to lower the hormonal levels of males like it does females. In one study, testosterone levels of men who ran 40 miles a week averaged 30 percent less than the levels of nonexercisers.[18] The runners' levels were still in a normal range, and the effect was reversible. Sperm count and libido were not affected.

While it may lower hormonal levels, overtraining is not associated with decreased fertility in male athletes unless accompanied by anorexic behavior and a high-stress lifestyle.[19, 20]

A more common male fertility problem results from constantly wearing tight undershorts. In order for the testicles to maintain normal sperm production, they must be a few degrees cooler than normal body temperature. Their position outside and slightly away from the body accomplishes this. When the testicles are overheated by consistently being held close to the body, sperm production temporarily decreases. A switch to boxer shorts solves the problem.

Environmental Considerations

Exercising in the Cold

True, all your friends think you're crazy, sharing a narrowed roadway with cars that spray you with slush as you exercise on a chilly winter day. Walking, running, and cycling are more complicated in the winter. Still, there is something liberating about a good workout on an icy winter day. Cold weather workouts can be invigorating, comfortable, and safe if you follow these tips:

1. Dress in several thin layers so you can remove or add a layer as needed. Wool and polypropylene clothing wick moisture away from the skin to keep you dry. Be sure to wear a cap and mittens. Don't overdress, however, or you'll overheat. You should feel a little cool until you warm up. Do take the windchill factor into account when preparing for your workout (fig. 8.1).

2. While frostbite *is* a possibility if you don't dress properly, there is *no* possibility that you will freeze your lungs or throat. If cold air bothers you, breathe through a bandana.

3. Waffled or ridged shoe soles provide extra traction on icy roads.

4. Exercise at midday as often as possible.

5. Plan out-and-back workouts, heading into the wind on the way out so you can return with the wind to your back. Not only will you appreciate the push when you're tired, but you'll avoid a chilling headwind when you've worked up a sweat.

6. Avoid patches of ice.

7. Don't worry about your pace. Between the slick footing and the heavy clothing, it's prudent to run relaxed. Just go fast enough to stay warm.

8. Tell someone your route and when you expect to be back. Better yet, go with a friend.

Don't hesitate to mix your usual exercise with other activities—cross-country skiing or sledding in snow country, aerobics, stair climbing, indoor cycling, or water exercise if you crave a break from the cold. Your heart will benefit as long as you stay in your training zone, and the cross-training will work new muscle groups.

Temperature (Fahrenheit)

Equivalent Chill Temperature

Wind Speed	40	35	30	25	20	15	10	5	0	-5	-10	-15	-20	-25	-30	-35	-40	-45	-50	-55	-60
Calm	40	35	30	25	20	15	10	5	0	-5	-10	-15	-20	-25	-30	-35	-40	-45	-50	-55	-60
5	35	30	25	20	15	10	5	0	-5	-10	-15	-20	-25	-30	-35	-45	-60	-65	-55	-65	-70
10	30	20	15	10	5	0	-10	-15	-20	-25	-35	-40	-45	-50	-60	-55	-70	-75	-80	-90	-95
15	25	15	10	0	-5	-10	-20	-25	-30	-40	-45	-50	-60	-65	-70	-80	-85	-90	-100	-105	-110
20	20	10	5	0	-10	-15	-25	-30	-35	-45	-50	-60	-65	-75	-80	-85	-95	-100	-110	-115	-120
25	15	10	0	-5	-15	-20	-30	-35	-45	-50	-60	-65	-75	-80	-90	-95	-105	-110	-120	-125	-135
30	10	5	0	-10	-20	-25	-30	-40	-50	-56	-65	-70	-80	-85	-95	-100	-105	-115	-120	-130	-140
35	10	5	-5	-10	-20	-25	-35	-40	-55	-60	-65	-75	-80	-90	-100	-105	-115	-120	-130	-135	-145
40*	10	0	-5	-15	-20	-30	-35	-45	-55	-60	-70	-75	-85	-95	-100	-110	-115	-125	-130	-140	-150

Little Danger

Increasing Danger (Flesh may freeze within one minute)

Greater Danger (Flesh may freeze within 30 seconds)

Figure 8.1
Windchill readings

Exercising in the Heat

Given a couple of weeks and plenty of water, the human body can adapt quite well to exercise in the heat. Hot weather workouts make the body work harder than in cool weather. The heart must pump enough blood not only to fuel working muscles but also to carry heat to the skin to be dissipated, reducing work capacity. Drinking plenty of water is critical in order to maintain sweating, your body's air conditioning system. The body can acclimatize to heat but not to dehydration. Overexertion in hot weather, particularly when coupled with dehydration, can lead to heat cramps, heat exhaustion, or heatstroke. Particularly susceptible are people who are over 40, out of shape, overweight, have heart disease, or have experienced heat injury.

To exercise safely in hot weather, follow these guidelines:

1. Respect the heat. Hot, humid, sunny weather poses a potentially life-threatening challenge to your body.

2. Monitor environmental conditions before exercising and adjust your workout accordingly. Exercise in the coolest parts of the day: early morning or after sundown. Avoid the hours between 10:00 A.M. and 4:00 P.M. Postpone the workout when the heat-safety index is in the danger zone or above (see fig. 8.2).

3. Avoid dehydration by drinking plenty of water before, during,

Figure 8.2
Heat-safety index

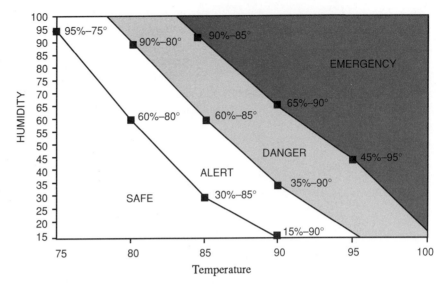

and after a workout. Alcohol and caffeinated drinks are poor choices because they promote water loss through the urine, increasing dehydration.

4. Weigh yourself before and after a workout. A loss of more than 2 percent to 3 percent of body weight is a health risk. You lose about a pint of fluid for every pound of weight you lose. Drink enough water to regain lost fluid. Thirty minutes before exercise, drink as much water as is comfortable, up to one pint. A good rule of thumb for fluid replacement is to drink one cup every 20 minutes during exercise. Afterward, drink even if you are not thirsty, because you will quench your thirst long before you replenish your body's fluids.

5. Wear loose-fitting clothing that allows air to circulate to your body, and expose as much skin to the air as possible to promote sweat evaporation. Light colors are best because they reflect rather than absorb sunlight. Vinyl or rubber sweat suits worn to lose body weight are definitely contraindicated. They can lead to dehydration and even death.

6. When becoming acclimated to warmer weather in the spring, decrease exercise intensity and duration. Allow two weeks to gradually increase the workload to normal levels.

7. Ask your doctor about the effects of any medications you take, because some can reduce heat tolerance.

8. Stop exercising at the first sign of heat illness (exhaustion, dizziness, nausea, headache, or shortness of breath).

Heavy Sweating during Exercise One of the hazards of exercising in hot, humid weather is dehydration caused by excessive loss of body water in the form of sweat. Dehydration disturbs cellular fluid and electrolyte balance, thus interfering with muscular contraction. Water losses of as little as 2 percent to 3 percent of body weight have been shown to impair exercise performance, reduce the amount of time a person can exercise, reduce cardiac stroke volume (volume of blood pushed out with each heartbeat), and reduce cardiac output (the amount of blood pumped by the heart over time).[21] Water loss can also interfere with the body's ability to regulate internal temperature, resulting in overheating.

Sweat is primarily water, but a number of major electrolytes (essential minerals in the form of salts), and other nutrients may be found in varying amounts. Sodium, chloride, and potassium are the predominant electrolytes found in sweat. They help to maintain normal body fluid volume and are involved in nerve impulse transmission and muscle contraction.

Electrolyte Replacement   Is profuse sweating likely to create an electrolyte deficiency? Studies over the years have shown this will not occur, even during prolonged exercise, such as marathon running. This is not to say that electrolyte replacement is not important. After prolonged exercise with heavy sweating, the body's stores of electrolytes are diminished and could eventually become deficient. However, with a normal diet, it is difficult to create an electrolyte deficiency.

Salt tablets are generally not recommended to replace lost sodium and chloride since these electrolytes are abundant in a normal diet. They may be prescribed for those who cannot replace them through normal dietary means. Keep in mind diets high in sodium have been associated with high blood pressure. Citrus fruits, fruit juices, and bananas are foods recommended for electrolyte replacement.

Fluid Replacement   Drink water. The most critical problem in heavy sweating is fluid replacement, since an electrolyte deficiency rarely occurs.

In the past decade many drinks have been advertised as replacing electrolytes lost through sweat. They are commonly known as glucose-electrolyte replacement solutions (GES) or sports drinks. Other than water, the major ingredients in these solutions are carbohydrates in the form of glucose and/or sucrose and some of the major electrolytes. The glucose/sucrose content varies with the different brands ranging from 1 percent to over 10 percent.

Are these sport drink solutions essential to replace lost fluids, electrolytes or glucose? No! Studies on these drinks show that both water and sports drinks (GES) rehydrate the body.[22, 23] Since rehydration is the main concern, water works just fine (and is free!). On the other hand, sports drinks containing carbohydrates will enhance performance by giving you a boost of energy that helps delay fatigue.[24]

If you prefer a sports drink, select it carefully. Drinks with high carbohydrate concentrations are slow to empty from the stomach, interfering with rehydration, and can cause bloating and nausea. It is best to avoid sports drinks containing carbohydrate concentrations higher than 8 percent (4%–8% works best).[25, 26] People often do not drink enough to replace the fluids they lose exercising. Due to this, sports drinks offer one advantage. Their taste may entice exercisers to consume more fluids than plain water does. Experiment during training to find out if you can handle one of these drinks. You should drink early and frequently during your workouts. Don't do anything new for competitive events.

Most experts agree, the fluids of choice for most effective rehydration or prevention of dehydration are water, sport drinks (made according to directions: not to exceed 8 percent carbohydrate concentration), or fruit juices diluted 50 percent with water. All three are preferable to caffeinated sodas.[27] Caffeine acts as a diuretic, and the carbonation gives you a feeling of being fuller than you are.

Contraindicated Exercises

A few stretching and toning exercises added to an aerobic program can promote balanced fitness by increasing flexibility in tight muscles and by strengthening weak ones. However, not all conditioning exercises commonly done in classes or seen on videotapes are good for you.

By studying people with aches and injuries, fitness experts have learned that some common stretching and toning exercises should be avoided. Others should be modified for safety and effectiveness. Be aware of commonly-done high-risk movements to avoid, and high-benefit, low-risk exercises to substitute. Here are some examples.

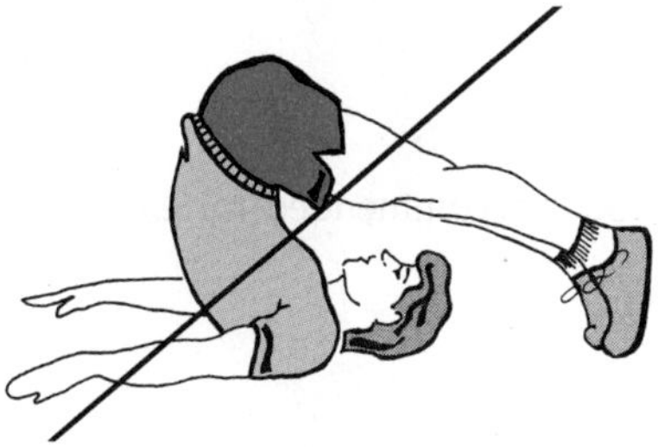

Don't

Yoga Plow

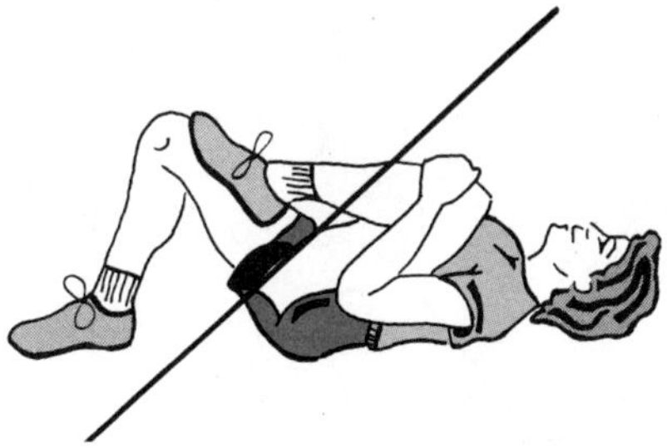

Don't

Single-knee tuck to chest

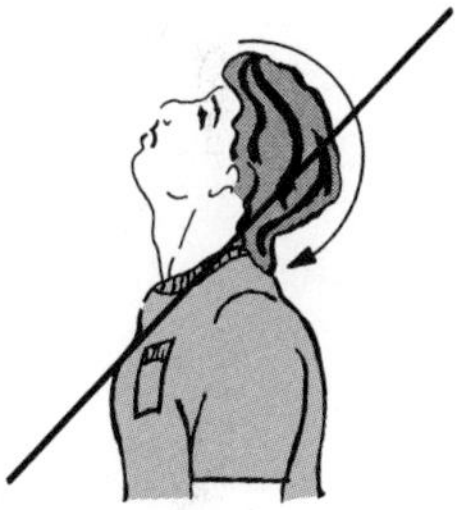

Don't

Head rolls

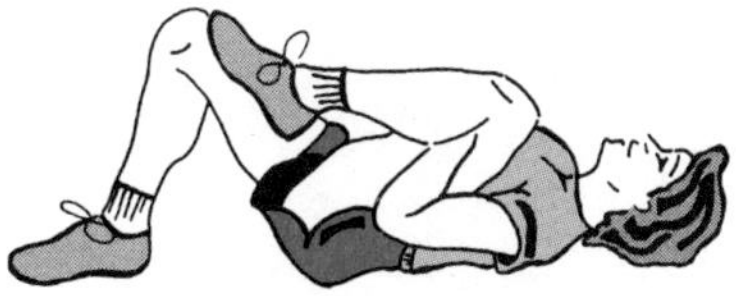

Do

Single-knee tuck to chest

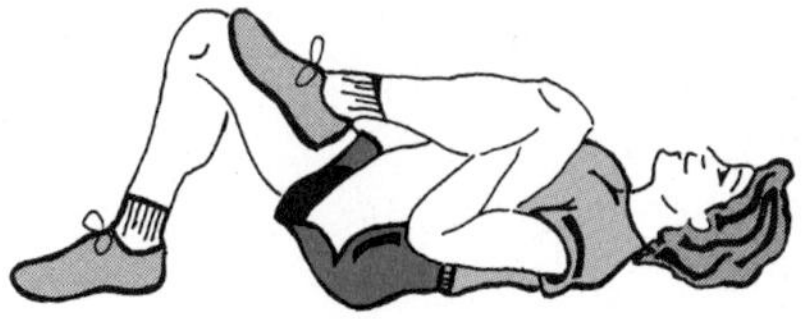

Do

Single-knee tuck to chest

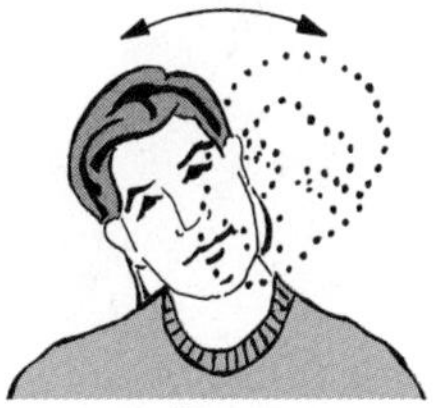

Do

Half-head rolls

1. A yoga plow, sometimes done as a back stretch, can injure discs, ligaments, and nerves in the neck and back.

A better back stretch is a single- or double-knee tuck to the chest.

2. Knee tuck to chest: hyperflexing the knee by pulling it to the body with the arms or hands placed on top of the tibia places undue stress on the knee joint. The hand position should be changed to hug the thigh rather than the shin.

3. Head rolls: Hyperextension can injure discs in the neck.

Safer neck stretches include half-head rolls to the front, turning the head side to side so that the chin touches the right and left shoulders, or touching an ear to each shoulder.

4. Hurdler's stretch can cause groin pull, injure knee cartilage, and overstretch the medial collateral ligament—the one that helps stabilize the knee. It may also cause hip joint discomfort because the femur of the leg that is tucked behind is in a position of extreme rotation in the joint capsule. Alternate hurdler stretch safely stretches hamstrings.

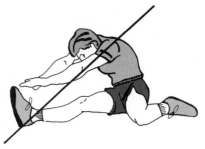

Don't

Hurdler stretch

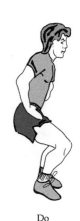

Do

Alternate hurdler stretch

5. Avoid excessive hyperflexion or hyperextension of the knee joint.
    To strengthen the quadriceps substitute half-knee bends for full squats, duckwalk, deep lunges, and squat thrusts. Deep knee flexion exercises overstress knee ligaments and cartilage.

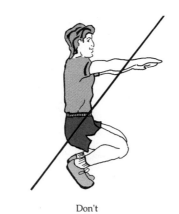

Don't

Full squat

Do

Half-knee bend

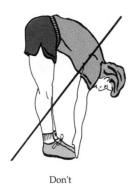

Don't

Standing toe touch

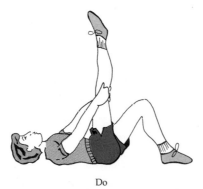

Do

Lying hamstring stretch

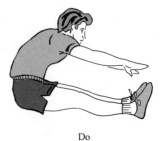

Do

Sitting hamstring stretch

6. Standing toe touches risk straining back ligaments. Limit forward flexion in a standing position. As your trunk dips below a 25 degree to 45 degree angle, the lower back muscles cease to work, and the posterior ligaments joining bone to bone must support the load.

7. Leg stretches at a ballet bar (or other high object) may be potentially harmful. When the extended leg is raised 90° or more and the trunk is bent over the leg, it may lead to sciatica problems, especially when the exerciser has limited flexibility.

Substitute the back and hamstring stretches suggested in numbers 1, 4, and 6.

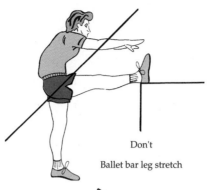

Don't

Ballet bar leg stretch

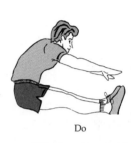

Do

Single-knee tuck to chest

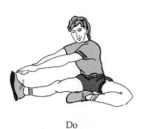

Do

Alternate hurdler stretch

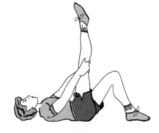

Do

Lying hamstring stretch

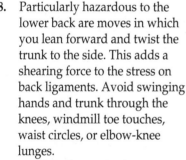

Do

Sitting hamstring stretch

8. Particularly hazardous to the lower back are moves in which you lean forward and twist the trunk to the side. This adds a shearing force to the stress on back ligaments. Avoid swinging hands and trunk through the knees, windmill toe touches, waist circles, or elbow-knee lunges.

There is no exercise you can do standing to tone your waist. The most effective exercise for reducing your waist is aerobic exercise and sensible nutrition. To tone oblique abdominals, the muscles that underlie the waist area, use twisting bent-knee abdominal curls. Lying on your back with heels next to buttocks and hands behind the shoulders, curl the shoulders first toward the right knee, then toward the left knee.

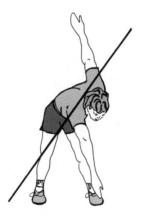

Don't

Windmill toe touches

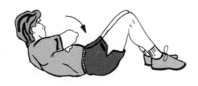

Do

Oblique abdominal curls

9. Double-leg lifts, straight-leg sit-ups, and low leg scissors do little or nothing to tone the abdominals. They tighten hip flexors, which in most people are too tight already, causing lordosis (swayback). They may also cause lower back strain.

The most effective exercise for toning abdominals is bent-knee abdominal curls in which the lower back stays on the ground while the shoulders curl forward about three inches. To avoid jerking on the head or neck, cross the arms across the chest or behind the head with a hand touching each shoulder.

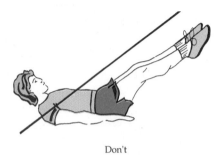

Don't

Double-leg lifts

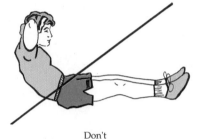

Don't

Straight-leg sit-ups

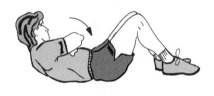

Do

Bent-knee abdominal curls

10. The swan arch, prone double-leg raises, and yoga cobra produce excessive back hyperextension and possible back strain.

In a prone position, raising right arm and opposite leg a few inches off the ground, then switching, strengthens the back safely.

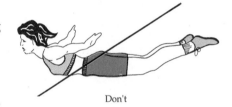

Don't

Swan arch

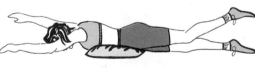

Do

Single arm/leg raises

11. Donkey kicks or fire hydrants, done on hands and knees with the back hyperextended may strain the lower back.

To protect the back, hold abdominals tight, round the back, and raise the leg no higher than 6 inches to 12 inches.

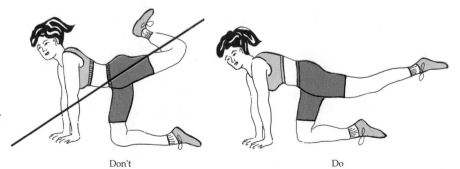

Don't

Donkey kicks

Do

Modified donkey kicks
(can be done with forearms on floor)

Your body is meant to move in many ways—to bend, twist, and stretch. Some people can do high-risk exercises for years with no ill effects. For others, after only a few repetitions, injury occurs. You may not know into which category you fit until it is too late. The problem is that some movements increase risks to muscles, joints, and connective tissue. While you may need to do deep squats if you are a competitive weightlifter, or a yoga plow if you are in a yoga class, these moves don't offer any special benefit for the fitness exerciser. Low-benefit, high-risk exercises should be minimized in programs designed to emphasize personal fitness. Follow these general rules when exercising.[28]

1. Do not hyperflex the knee.

2. Do not hyperextend the knee, neck, or lower back.

3. Do not apply a twisting or lateral force to the knee.

4. Avoid holding the breath during exercise.

5. Avoid stretching long/weak muscles (i.e., abdominals) and avoid shortening already short/strong muscles (i.e., hip flexors). See chapter 5, table 5.1.

   a. Most people should avoid aggravating common postural faults: forward head, dorsal kyphosis (rounded upper back), medial rotation of the thigh, and pronation of the foot.

   b. Most people need to stretch the chest muscles, hip flexors, calves, hamstrings, lower back, and medial thigh rotators.

6. Avoid stretching any joint to the point of pain.

7. Be especially careful when using passive stretches with another person (unless it is a therapist).

8. Avoid movements that place acute compressional forces on spinal discs, such as extending and rotating the spine simultaneously (i.e., trunk and neck circling and double-leg lifts).

9. Avoid movements that cause joint impingements or cartilage damage, such as arm circles in palm-down position.

10. If the nature of your sport regularly requires the violation of good mechanics (baseball catcher assuming a deep squat position or gymnast performing double leg lifts) make certain that the muscles are as strong as possible to endure the stress.

Aging and Physical Activity

Is your body older than you are? Physical educator T. K. Cureton estimated that middle age begins for the average person at age 26, because at that age he has the physical capacity our ancestors did when they were 40.[29] When we retire, we are expected to slow down and take it easy. This often produces disastrous results as atrophy and disuse take their toll. Disorders like cardiovascular disease, hypertension, and adult onset diabetes don't have to be the natural consequences of aging. We now feel that they are more related to physical inactivity. The body adapts to whatever load is placed on it, and the ability to do work is reduced if the load lessens. Thankfully, attitudes are changing. Older adults, encouraged by their doctors and by research revealing the benefits of exercise, are biking, swimming, jogging, and walking in ever-increasing numbers. We know that older adults (even up to 100) are remarkably responsive to exercise (positive health benefits). As the health-conscious baby-boom generation matures, they are likely to redefine the concept of aging.

Aging and Performance

Some say, "Growing old isn't so bad, if you consider the alternative." James Dean's "Live fast, die young, and leave a good-looking corpse" does have its proponents, but they are quickly weeded out of the genetic pool. I think a lot more of us would choose to die young, as late as possible. At birth, we each have a 70-plus-year warranty, but the maintenance is up to us. Just like any machine, the human body grows less efficient as it ages. The decline in max VO_2 among the sedentary is about 1 percent for every year after 25.[30] Decreases in strength, flexibility, and endurance, and increased body fat proportion as one grows older are often accepted as a natural part of the aging process. This may be common, but it is not inevitable. The most significant factor contributing to declines in physiological capacity at any age is the lack of regular exercise. The "use it or lose it" rule applies here. Unused muscles atrophy, lose elasticity, and grow weak. Ligaments and tendons shorten and tighten, decreasing range of motion and causing aches and pains as they pull across joints. As muscle tissue atrophies, basal metabolism drops, resulting in an increase in body fat even when a person is not eating enough to maintain adequate nutritional levels. Bones need the stress of weight-bearing exercise to absorb minerals. Inactivity accelerates bone mineral loss and increases risk of osteoporosis. Weight-bearing exercise is also crucial for bones of

Exercise is adult play

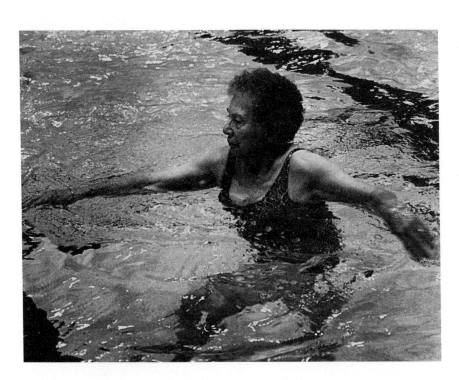

Exercise slows the aging process.

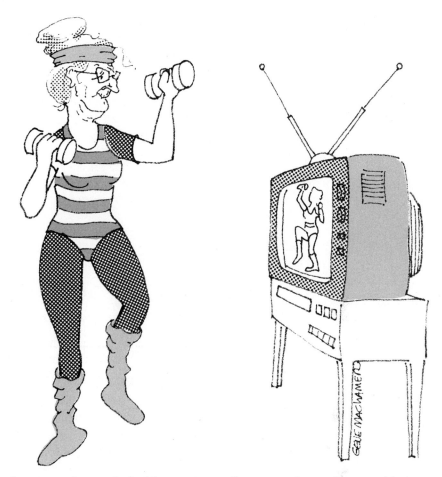

the arms and upper body. These areas usually are not adequately stressed by aerobic exercise. Recent studies show that men and women 60 and older who train with weights and resistance machines several times a week can quickly double their total body strength.[31] This helps fight osteoporosis by keeping skeletons sturdy. Also, such strength gains have major implications for maintaining independence in later years. While exercise alone cannot prevent osteoporosis, it may help premenopausal women build up their bone densities so they enter menopause ahead of the game. Lifelong exercise may also help protect the elderly against falls and the devastating effects of hip fractures. It's never too late to start exercising. Starting late in life is far preferable to not starting at all.

While aging is unavoidable, declines in functional capacity with age are not inevitable. How you age is largely up to you. Cardiologist George Sheehan has said that growing older isn't so bad; it is inactive people who give aging a bad name. Biological aging can be significantly slowed by regular exercise. As much as 50 percent of the functional decline seen in aging is related to disuse and can be prevented with regular aerobic exercise.[32] Older adults who engage in an aerobic exercise program can, however, slow this decline and may even have the same aerobic capacity

Table 8.2

Measurements in Exercising and NonExercising Men—A Longitudinal Study

Exercisers were followed from age 45 through 68, and the nonexercisers were measured while training at age 52 and again at age 70 after being detrained for 18 years. The data presents the value of regular aerobic exercise.

	Age (yr)		Height (cm)		Weight (kg)		Resting Heart Rate (bpm)		Resting Blood Pressure (min/Hg)		Average Body Fat
	I*	F**	I	F	I	F	I	F	I	F	F
Exercisers N=15	44.6	68.0	177.5	175.9	76.1	72.7	63.0	55.8	120/79	120/78	15.9%
Nonexercisers N=15	51.6	69.7	176.7	174.7	81.3	84.5	66.1	66	135/85	150/90	25.7%

* Initial data
** Final data

Source: "The Effect of Physical Activity and Inactivity on Aerobic Power in Older Men." Kasch, F., et al. The Physician and Sportsmedicine, Vol. 18, No. 4, April, 1990.

as that of a sedentary person 25 or more years younger.[33,34] Tables 8.2 and 8.3 confirm the fact that, as we age, VO_2 max values, as well as other measurable physical variables, decline. Notice, however, that those who stay physically active show an impressive delay in this decline.

As one physician observed, "So many things we think are linked to aging . . . actually have to do with lifestyle. Exercise produces a 40-year age offset. A fit person of 70 is the equal of an unfit person of 30 in regard to bones, muscles, heart, brain, sex, and everything else. I see an immense energy in old people who continue (exercise)."[35] Exercise intensity appears to be the key to greatest benefit. A group of master athletes (ages 40–75) studied over an 18-year period showed no significant decline in aerobic capacity if they maintained training intensity.[36] *For most elderly fitness exercisers, however, an exercise intensity of 40 percent to 50 percent maximal heart rate reserve is considered adequate.*

The effect of true nonpreventable aging involves a gradual loss of the speed and vigor with which we do activities, but it should not prevent us from doing them. As one older runner observed, "I can do everything I used to. It just takes longer to do it and longer to recover."

Exercise is adult play. At what point was our childhood eagerness to get out and romp replaced by hours of sitting in front of the TV watching others play? Whether aging is an extension of a full and active life or a gradual wasting away is determined by how you choose to live your life.

"We do not stop playing because we are old. We grow old because we stop playing."

Table 8.3

Decline in VO$_2$ Max with Age

VO$_2$ max declined 13% in 23 years in the exercisers, while the nonexercisers dropped 41% in 18 years. This is a threefold difference!
Source: "The Effect of Physical Activity and Inactivity on Aerobic Power in Older Men." Kasch, F., et al. The Physician and Sportsmedicine, *Vol. 18, No. 4, April, 1990.*

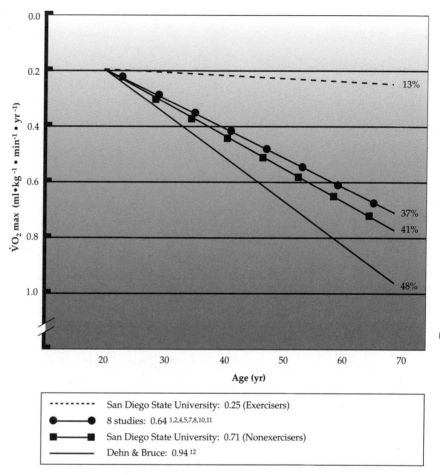

San Diego State University: 0.25 (Exercisers)
8 studies: 0.64 [1,2,4,5,7,8,10,11]
San Diego State University: 0.71 (Nonexercisers)
Dehn & Bruce: 0.94 [12]

Does Exercise Increase Lifespan?

While the length of your life may have a strong genetic component, research by Dr. Ralph Paffenbarger on Harvard alumni indicates that men who expend at least 2,000 calories a week in regular exercise can expect to add, on the average, about two years to their lives.[37] This is equivalent to walking 10 to 20 miles a week. For men between the ages of 35 and 54, this represents a return of 2 1/2 minutes for every minute spent exercising. Even men who expended 500 to 1,000 calories a week, about 5 to 10 miles of walking, experienced a 22 percent lower risk of death than sedentary men. While a healthful lifestyle can't guarantee a longer life, it does give you a better chance to live your years at their peak.

Table 8.4

Benefits of Exercise for Older Adults

1. Maintenance of a high level of physical and social activity increases the quality of life, enhancing social satisfaction.
2. Increased independence is enjoyed when fitness and health are maintained. Most Americans fear infirmity and dependence more than death.
3. A person has more energy and can perform daily routines with greater ease.
4. Increased muscle tone and flexibility improve balance, decreasing falls.
5. The more muscle tissue a person maintains, the higher his metabolism, making it easier to control weight.
6. Calories burned through exercise allow a person to take in more nutrients.
7. Exercise delays loss of bone mass.
8. A person's posture improves, decreasing backache and enhancing appearance.
9. Cardiorespiratory function is enhanced, improving peripheral circulation, decreasing risk of atherosclerosis, high blood pressure, and other circulatory problems.
10. Exercise improves the efficiency of elimination.
11. There is decreased depression and stress when a regular exercise program is followed.

Are you ever "too old" to begin exercise? No! While the overall impact you can make on the quality of your life is greater if you start exercising young and continue throughout life, there is no age at which the benefits of exercise stop. Frankly, the older you are, the more you need exercise. Table 8.4 shows the benefits of exercise for older adults.

Summary

Exercise is meant to be enjoyed throughout life. Regardless of gender or age, the body improves with use and degenerates with disuse. People don't wear out; they rust out! For greatest benefit from an exercise program, it is helpful to be aware of special concerns, such as overuse symptoms and high risk exercises. As you adjust to a physically active lifestyle, you will find that the benefits far outweigh the effort involved. Exercise will become a habit, and you will begin to look forward to your workout as an important part of your day.

Physical activity is important
at every age

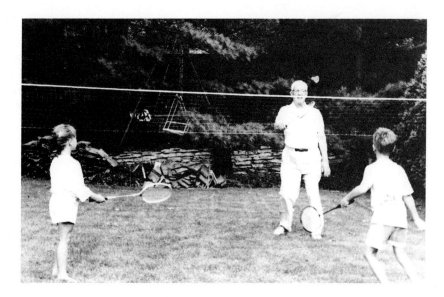

References

1. Costill, David L. *Inside Running: Basics of Sports Physiology.* Indianapolis: Benchmark Press, Inc., 1986.

2. Costill. *Inside Running: Basics of Sports Physiology.*

3. Seefeldt, Vern, ed. "Menstruation, Pregnancy and Menopause." *Physical Activity and Well Being.* Reston, VA: AAHPERD, 1986.

4. Cowart, Virginia S. "Can Exercise Help Women with PMS?" *The Physician and Sportsmedicine* 17 (April 1989): 168–78.

5. Seefeldt, Vern, ed. "Mental Health." *Physical Activity and Well Being.* Reston, VA: AAHPERD, 1986.

6. Johnson, Susan. "Solving the Mystery of Premenstrual Syndrome." *Reebok Instructor News* 1 (May–June 1988): 6.

7. *Cancer Facts And Figures—1992.* American Cancer Society.

8. Zimmerman, David R. "Maturation and Strenuous Training in Young Female Athletes." *The Physician and Sportsmedicine* 15 (June 1987): 219–22.

9. "Sweat Cure: Exercise May Prevent Cancer." *Time* 131 (February 29, 1988): 68.

10. Williams, Melvin H., *Nutrition for Fitness and Sport,* 3rd. ed. Dubuque, IA: Wm. C. Brown Publishers, 1992.

11. Munnings, Frances. "Exercise and Estrogen in Women's Health: Getting a Clearer Picture." *The Physician and Sportsmedicine* 16 (May 1988): 152–61.

12. Seefeldt, Vern, ed. "Menstruation, Pregnancy and Menopause."

13. Institute for Aerobics Research. "Young Women and Osteoporosis." *The Aerobics News* 3 (October 1988): 7.

14. McMurray and Katz, Vern. "Thermoregulation in Pregnancy Implication for Exercise." *Physician and Sports Medicine.* Vol. 10, No. 3 (146–158) Sept. 1990.

15. University of California, Berkeley. *The Wellness Encyclopedia.* Boston: Houghton Mifflin Co., 1991.

16. Cooper, Kenneth, and Mildred Cooper. *New Aerobics for Women.* New York: Bantam Books, 1988.

17. "What's New in Running Bras." *Runner's World* 21 (June 1986): 92–93.

18. Silberner, Joanne, and Erica E. Goode. "Should Women Stop Jogging?" *U.S. News and World Report* 104 (March 7, 1988): 72.

19. Groves, David. "Study: Hormone Levels in Ultramarathoners." *The Physician and Sportsmedicine* 15 (December 1987): 51.

20. Nash, Heyward L. "Can Exercise Suppress Reproductive Hormones in Men?" *The Physician and Sportsmedicine* 15 (January 1987): 180–86.

21. Hamilton, Marc; Gonzalez-Alonso, Jose; Montain, Scott, Coyle, Edward. "Fluid Replacement and Glucose Infusion During Exercise Prevent Cardiovascular Drift." *Journal of Applied Physiology*, Vol. 71, No. 3, 1991.

22. Presentation by Edward Coyle, Ph.D. and Colleagues at the University of Texas at Austin at the Annual Meeting of American College of Sports Medicine, May, 1991, Orlando, Florida.

23. Mitchell, J., Voss, K. "The Influence of Volume on Gastric Emptying and Fluid Balance During Prolonged Exercise." *Medicine and Science in Sport and Exercise*, Vol. 23, No. 3, March, 1991.

24. Mitchell, J. et al. "The Influence of Volume on Gastric Emptying and Fluid Balance During Prolonged Exercise."

25. Mitchell, J., et al. "The Influence of Volume on Gastric Emptying and Fluid Balance During Prolonged Exercise."

26. Murray, R., et. al. "Responses of Varying Rates of Carbohydrate Ingestion During Exercise." *Medicine and Science in Sport and Exercise*. Vol. 23, No. 6, June, 1991.

27. "Are Sports Drinks Better Than Water?" *The Physician and Sportsmedicine*, Vol. 20, No. 2, February, 1992.

28. Lindsey, Ruth and Charles Corbin. "Questionable Exercise—Their Safer Alternatives." *JOPERD*, October, 1989.

29. Allsen, P., et al. *Fitness for Life*, 4th ed., Dubuque, IA: Wm. C. Brown Publishers, 1989.

30. Kasch, F., et al. "The Effect of Physical Activity and Inactivity on Aerobic Power in Older Men (A Longitudinal Study). *The Physician and Sports Medicine*. Vol. 18, No. 4, April, 1990.

31. Sussman, Vic. "1992: Health Guide—No Pain and Lots of Gain: New Studies Show That Even Moderate Exercise Has Great Health Benefits." *U.S. News and World Report*, May 4, 1992.

32. Mullen, Kathleen, et al. "Aging: Adaptations for Wellness." *Connections for Health*. Dubuque, IA: Wm. C. Brown, Publishers, 1990.

33. Seefeldt, Vern, ed. "Physical Activity and the Prevention of Premature Aging." *Physical Activity and Well Being*. Reston, VA: AAHPERD, 1986.

34. Kasch, et al. "The Effects of Physical Activity and Inactivity on Aerobic Power in Older Men (A Longitudinal Study)."

35. Higdon, Hal. "Run for Your Life." *Runner's World* 24 (August 1989): 46–52.

36. Kavanaugh, Terence, and Roy Sheppard. "Can Regular Sports Participation Slow the Aging Process? Data on Master Athletes." *The Physician and Sports Medicine*, Vol. 18, No. 6, June, 1990.

37. Paffenbarger, R. S., R. T. Hyde, A. L. Wing, and C. H. Sieh. "Physical Activity, All Cause Mortality, and Longevity of College Alumni." *New England Journal of Medicine* 314 (1986): 605–13.

Suggested Readings

Birkel, Dee Ann, and Susan Freitag. 1992. *Forever Fit, A Step-by-Step Guide for Older Adults*. New York: Insight Books, Plenum Publishing Corp.

Costill, David L. 1986. *Inside Running; Basics of Sports Physiology*. Indianapolis, IN: Benchmark Press.

Holstein, Barbara. 1991. *Shaping Up For A Healthy Pregnancy*. Champaign, IL: Human Kinetics.

James and Pierre, Richard. 1992. *Healthful Aging*. Guilford, CT: The Dushkin Publishing Group, Inc.

Kavanaugh, Terence, and Roy Shephard. "Can Regular Sports Participation Slow the Aging Process? Data on Master Athletes." *The Physician and Sportsmedicine*, Vol. 18, No. 6, June, 1990.

Kime, Robert. 1992. *Pregnancy, Childbirth and Parenting*. Guilford, CT: The Dushkin Publishing Group, Inc. Potterfield.

Lubell, Adele. "Potentially Dangerous Exercises: Are They Harmful to All?" *The Physician and Sportsmedicine*, Vol. 17, No. 1, January, 1989.

Munnings, Frances. "Exercise and Estrogen in Women's Health: Getting a Clearer Picture." *The Physician and Sportsmedicine* 16 (May 1988): 152–61.

Munnings, Frances. June 1992. "Osteoporosis: What is the Role of Exercise?" *The Physician and Sportsmedicine*, Vol. 20, No. 6.

Myburgh, Kathryn, et al. "Are Risk Factors for Menstrual Dysfunction in Runners Cumulative?" *Physician and Sportsmedicine*, Vol. 20, No. 4, April, 1992.

Penner, Diane. 1990. *Elder Fit: A Health and Fitness Program for Older Adults*. Reston, VA: American Alliance for Health, Physical Education, Recreation and Dance.

Roberts, William. "Emergencies in Sports, Managing Heatstroke: On-Site Cooling." *The Physician and Sportsmedicine*, Vol. 20, No. 5, May 1992.

Robinson, William. "Emergencies in Sports, Competing with the Cold, Part II Hypothermia." *The Physician and Sportsmedicine*, Vol. 20, No. 1, Jan. 1992.

Seefeldt, Vern, ed. 1986. *Physical Activity and Well Being*. Reston, VA: AAHPERD.

Shepard, John and Pacelli, Lauren. "Why Your Patients Shouldn't Take Aging Sitting Down." *The Physician and Sportsmedicine*, Vol. 18, No. 11, Nov. 1990.

Sheppard, Roy. 1987. *Physical Activity and Aging*, 2nd ed. Rockville, MD: Aspen Publishers.

Stamford, Bryant. June 1992. "Keeping Cool During Hot Weather Workouts." *The Physician and Sportsmedicine*, Vol. 20, No. 6.

Stamford, Bryant. "How to Avoid Dehydration." *Physician and Sportsmedicine*, Vol. 18, No. 7, July 1990.

Thornton, James. "How Can You Tell When An Athlete Is Too Thin?" *Physician and Sportsmedicine*, Vol. 18, No. 12, December 1990.

White, Jacquline. "Exercising for Two, What's Safe for the Active Pregnant Women?" *Physician and Sportsmedicine*, Vol. 20, No. 5, May, 1992.

9

Nutrition

Chapter Objectives

After reading this chapter you will be able to:

1. Describe three ways dietary habits of Americans have changed in the past 75 years, and explain how these changes have affected our nutritional wellness.
2. Identify the percentages of calories recommended in the diet for carbohydrates, proteins, and fats.
3. List the seven dietary guidelines for Americans.
4. List the six major nutrients and describe their main function in the body.
5. Identify the health benefits of soluble and insoluble fiber, and list good food sources of each.
6. Differentiate between complex and simple carbohydrates.
7. Select the correct description of cholesterol, and identify the recommended limit of daily cholesterol consumption.
8. List three foods high in cholesterol.
9. Identify the correct descriptions of saturated, monounsaturated, and polyunsaturated fats, as well as list three examples of each.
10. Identify three preventive factors relating to osteoporosis.
11. Identify the recommended number of daily servings from the food groups in the Food Guide Pyramid.
12. Give seven specific examples of small changes that can be incorporated into daily food selections and preparations that could make a significant change in your nutritional wellness.
13. Look at a food label and identify the largest ingredient; calculate the percentage of calories that come from fat, carbohydrate, and protein; identify the sources of fat (including saturated fat); identify the sources of complex and simple carbohydrates.
14. Identify two ways to eat nutritiously in a fast food restaurant and as an athlete.

Terms

- Carbohydrate
- Cholesterol
- Complex carbohydrate
- Fat
- Fat soluble vitamin
- Fiber
- Glycogen
- Hydrogenation
- Insoluble fiber
- Ketone bodies (ketosis)
- Lacto-ovo-vegetarian
- Lactovegetarian
- Macrominerals
- Minerals
- Monounsaturated fat
- Omega-3
- Osteoporosis
- Polyunsaturated fat
- Protein
- Recommended Dietary Allowances (RDA)
- Saturated fat
- Semi-vegetarian
- Simple carbohydrate
- Soluble fiber
- Strict vegetarian (or vegan)
- Trace minerals
- Triglyceride
- U.S. Recommended Daily Allowances (U.S. RDA)
- Vitamins
- Water soluble vitamin

*F*undamental knowledge about nutrition can make a tremendous contribution to your level of wellness. It can help you make food choices that will enhance your health and vitality. This knowledge can also help you to decipher the social influences and messages related to eating and to understand the myths and quackery associated with food. This is just another step toward assuming self-responsibility for your own well-being and health. Learning about nutrition can be exciting! Since eating is a daily activity, you have many opportunities to affect your wellness in a positive way. We are fortunate to live in a country where food is plentiful; we have wide and varied choices.

We tend to see diet as affecting only the physical dimension of wellness. Actually, food can be easily associated with all of the dimensions. Much of our social life evolves around food. Providing food is an important sign of caring. Eating and being fed are intimately connected with our deepest feelings. Table 9.1 gives examples of how food relates to all six dimensions of wellness. Perhaps you can think of other connections.

After reading this chapter, you should be able to make responsible food choices in your pursuit of high-level wellness. You have heard it before, but it is remarkably true, "You are what you eat!"

Changing Times

In the agricultural lifestyle of the past, most people grew and prepared their own food. Foods were fresh and simple. As compared to today, early Americans consumed much greater amounts of fresh fruits, vegetables, and grains, and lesser amounts of salt, fats, and refined sugars. In those days, "eating out" meant eating out-of-doors—perhaps a picnic or a meal out in the field beside the plow. Today's fast-paced, technological society has contributed to drastic changes in the way we eat. Dual-career and single-parent families are commonplace. As parents juggle careers, child-care, social and professional meetings, education, and recreation, meals are often skipped, eaten on the run, or thrown together quickly. As a result, the food preparers are often McDonald's or manufacturers of frozen or processed food. After all, they tell us, "Have it your way!"; "Things go better

Table 9.1

Food Is Associated With Every
Dimension of Wellness

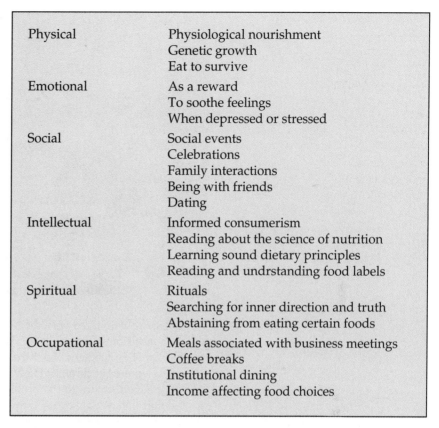

Physical	Physiological nourishment
	Genetic growth
	Eat to survive
Emotional	As a reward
	To soothe feelings
	When depressed or stressed
Social	Social events
	Celebrations
	Family interactions
	Being with friends
	Dating
Intellectual	Informed consumerism
	Reading about the science of nutrition
	Learning sound dietary principles
	Reading and undrstanding food labels
Spiritual	Rituals
	Searching for inner direction and truth
	Abstaining from eating certain foods
Occupational	Meals associated with business meetings
	Coffee breaks
	Institutional dining
	Income affecting food choices

with . . . !"; and "We do it all for you!" Realistically, this is done to sell products, not necessarily to enhance our nutrition. Supermarket shelves are lined with packaged food products bearing little resemblance to the original farm product. Most are highly processed. The result is a new form of malnutrition. Rather than a lack of food, we find ourselves eating too much of the wrong foods. As we progressed from eating nuts and berries to consuming hot dogs and Twinkies, the incidence of heart disease, stroke, hypertension, and cancer has increased. It has also cost us our vitality.

To complicate matters, there has been a blitz of nutrition advice in recent years—cut back on eggs, eat more oat bran, eliminate salt, forget red meat, don't consume too much iron, watch the caffeine. Overwhelmed by sometimes conflicting information, many throw up their hands in confusion or disregard nutrition advice entirely.

A survey[1] of the dietary habits and attitudes of American adults reveals that only 26 percent feel that nutrition is important and that they are careful about what they eat. The rest know that they are not doing much to manage their diet but are not interested in changing. Changing, they say, would mean giving up favorite foods and would take too much time. The survey also showed that most Americans have limited knowledge about dietary guidelines, and only 7 percent could identify the amount of fat recommended in our diet.

Many of our snacks are heavily processed.

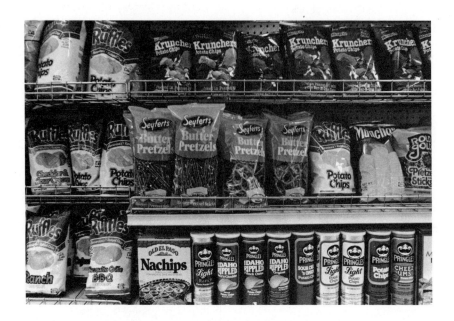

In college you are faced with the new responsibility of buying and preparing your own meals or making daily cafeteria selections. Data indicate that students are unaware of or apathetic about the implications of poor dietary habits on the future development of chronic diseases.[2]

Television contributes to the problem by presenting mixed messages about diet and nutrition. We are exposed to hundreds of commercials for sugary, high-fat snacks, often accompanied by enchanting music, jingles, and appealing characters. In prime-time programming, nutrition is anything but balanced—grabbing a snack is the norm. Yet, the models used in commercials are extremely thin, attractive, and seemingly healthy![3]

The Government Steps In

In 1988 *The Surgeon General's Report on Nutrition and Health* was released, giving attention to improved nutrition as a key to health maintenance and preventive medicine. This comprehensive, research-based report stated that for the 2 out of 3 Americans who neither smoke nor drink, eating patterns may shape their long-term health prospects more than any other personal choice.[4] *Healthy People 2000* followed by listing "improved nutrition" as one of its key objectives. As a service to the American people, the U.S. Department of Health and Human Services distributed a pamphlet entitled *Dietary Guidelines for Americans*. These guidelines (table 9.2) help answer the question "What should we eat to stay healthy?" The 7 guidelines reflect the newest research on diet and health relationships, with the purpose of giving *practical* suggestions on how to make healthy diet adjustments. It is impossible to specify the perfect diet for every individual. However, these guidelines give positive direction in making everyday food selections that can help you stay healthy.

Table 9.2

The 1990 Dietary Guidelines for Americans*

1. **Eat a variety of foods.**

   No one food contains all the nutrients in the amounts needed. These nutrients should come from a variety of foods, not from a few highly fortified foods or supplements. Include foods from the major food groups in your daily diet. Also select a variety of foods within each group. The content of your diet over a day or more is what counts!

2. **Maintain healthy weight.**

   If you are too fat or too thin, your chances of developing health problems are increased. Exercise, diet, and heredity all play a role in body size and shape. Whether your weight is "healthy" depends on how much of your weight is fat, where in your body the fat is located, and whether you have a weight-related medical problem.

3. **Choose a diet low in fat, saturated fat, and cholesterol.**

   Diets high in fat and cholesterol have been linked to heart disease, certain types of cancer, and obesity. Thirty percent or less of calories should come from fat, with less than 10 percent of calories from saturated fat. All adults are advised to have blood cholesterol levels checked.

4. **Choose a diet with plenty of vegetables, fruits, and grain products.**

   These foods provide complex carbohydrates, dietary fiber, and other components linked to good health. These foods are also generally low in fat.

5. **Use sugars only in moderation.**

   Sugars and many foods that contain large amounts of them supply calories but are limited in nutrients. It also contributes to tooth decay.

6. **Use salt and sodium only in moderation.**

   Most Americans eat more salt and sodium than they need, and using less will benefit those people whose blood pressure goes up with salt intake. Foods and beverages containing salt provide most of the sodium in our diets, much of it added during processing and manufacturing.

7. **If you drink alcoholic beverages, do so in moderation.**

   Drinking alcoholic beverages is linked to health problems, accidents, and addiction. They supply calories but little or no nutrients. Excessive use of alcohol can cause nutritional deficiencies and other serious diseases (i.e., accompanying poor eating habits, interferences with use and absorption of vitamins and minerals, liver dysfunction, damage to the brain and heart, and increased risk for some cancers).

*Recommendations for healthy Americans age 2 years and over.
Source: U.S. Department of Agriculture, U.S. Department of Health and Human Services. Nutrition and Your Health: Dietary Guidelines for Americans, *3rd edition, Home and Garden Bulletin No. 232, 1990.*

As you read these guidelines, some questions may be left unanswered. "The main challenge no longer is simply to determine what eating patterns to recommend . . . simply issuing and disseminating recommendations is insufficient to produce change in most peoples eating behavior."[5] As in making most lifestyle changes, we need *knowledge* (to identify problem diet behaviors and how to improve them), *motivation* (to make healthy changes), and a *supportive environment* (to maintain changes—restaurants, supermarkets, worksite and school food services, nutrition labeling, and nutrition education in the schools).

So how do you cut salt from your diet? What is a complex carbohydrate? How do you differentiate between a saturated and polyunsaturated fat? What is cholesterol? How do you eat out healthfully? These questions are addressed in the following sections, and we will give specific suggestions as to how to make daily food choices that will enhance your nutritional wellness.

Nutrition Basics

Your body is a priceless machine that needs fuel. This fuel should be composed of six major nutrients—carbohydrates, proteins, fats, vitamins, minerals, and water. These nutrients fulfill three main functions in the body:

> provide energy
> build and repair body tissues
> regulate body processes

Only the carbohydrates, fats, and proteins contribute energy or calories (kcal) to your diet. To function at optimal efficiency, you need a balance of each of the six essential nutrient groups.

RDA

The National Academy of Sciences–National Research Council periodically reviews current research on the nutritional needs of healthy Americans in order to establish recommended amounts of nutrients. These recommendations are called **Recommended Dietary Allowances (RDA).** The RDA are the amounts considered to be adequate to meet the nutritional needs of practically all healthy persons. In most cases, the RDA are higher than the amount needed to prevent nutritional diseases. For example, the body needs only 10 milligrams daily of vitamin C to prevent scurvy. The adult RDA for vitamin C is 60 milligrams. Since the RDA are established for healthy populations, they do not pertain to individuals who have special nutritional requirements as a result of special physical conditions or use of certain medications.

The RDA should not be confused with the **U.S. Recommended Daily Allowances (U.S. RDA).** The U.S. RDA are devised by the Food and Drug Administration for nutrition labeling. That is why your food labels show the U.S. RDA, rather than the RDA. The U.S. RDA for most nutrients approximate the highest RDA of all gender-age categories (excluding the allowances for pregnant and lactating females). For example, the RDA for vitamin C for children is only 45 milligrams. Since the adult RDA is 60 milligrams, the U.S. RDA for everyone is 60 milligrams because it is the highest RDA figure for vitamin C for any population group. Therefore, a product that furnishes 100 percent of the U.S. RDA for a nutrient will furnish the RDA for most people (and more for many). As you can see, all of these recommendations include a large margin of safety.

Let us look at each of the six nutrients and their specific roles.

Carbohydrates

Carbohydrates are the major source of energy for the body. In fact, they are the body's preferred form of energy. They provide 4 calories per gram. Carbohydrates are stored in the liver and in muscles in the form of **glycogen.** There is not an RDA for carbohydrate intake. Most dietitians, however, recommend that our daily caloric intake be 55 percent to 60 percent carbohydrate.[6] Carbohydrates have mistakenly earned the reputation of being "fattening." If we analyze the two types of carbohydrates, this unearned reputation can be understood. Carbohydrates, with the exception of milk sugar, come from plants. The two types are *sugars*—**simple carbohydrates** and *starches*—**complex carbohydrates.**

Sugars (Simple Carbohydrates)   When you see the suffix "-ose" as an ingredient on a package label (i.e., sucrose, fructose, dextrose, maltose), or see corn sweetener, corn syrup, sorghum, sorbitol, or honey, think *sugar.* The presence of these refined and processed sugars in our diet accounts for carbohydrate's "fattening" reputation. Instead of consuming the natural simple sugars found in fruits and vegetables, we consume too much of hidden processed sugars found in sweet desserts, soda, cookies, cereals, candy, jams, and condiments. These refined sugars have been extracted from their natural sources and have little nutritional value other than the calories they contain—thus the term "empty calories." Even if you profess not to eat sweets, you probably consume far more sugar than you realize because it is hidden in so many processed foods. For example, one can of Coke contains 10 teaspoons of sugar. Dannon blueberry yogurt is 14 percent sugar; Wishbone Russian salad dressing is 30 percent sugar; and Jell-O is 83 percent sugar. Check your breakfast cereal. Some are nothing more than "candy" fortified with vitamins.

Starches (Complex Carbohydrates)   The starches are potatoes, rice, whole grains, beans, fruits, and vegetables. These foods are low in calories. They are nutritionally dense, a rich source of vitamins and minerals that provide a steady amount of energy for many hours. What *is* fattening are the calorie-rich additives we often add to these foods (butter, sour cream, jams, gravies, sauces). Complex carbohydrates should comprise 45 percent to 50 percent of our total caloric intake, while simple sugars should be limited to 10 percent.[7] Carbohydrates supply many vital nutrients like vitamins, minerals, and water. In addition, they supply an important nonnutrient—dietary fiber. **Fiber** is the part of plant food that is not digested in the small intestine, where most other foods are digested and absorbed into the bloodstream. To many people, fiber is synonymous with oat bran. Actually, fiber is not a single substance, but a large group of widely different compounds with varied effects on the body. Formerly called roughage or bulk, fiber was once thought of primarily as a filler—it takes up room, leaving less space for high-fat, high-calorie items. That is still one of fiber's potential benefits, plus it is in foods rich in vitamins and minerals. But researchers now recognize that fiber plays a role in reducing the risk of heart disease, cancer, and diabetes.[8] There are two types of fiber—insoluble and soluble. Both play an important role in your nutritional health.

A fiber profile.

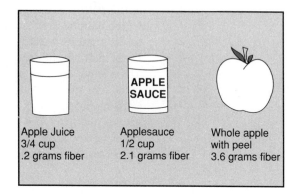

Apple Juice
3/4 cup
.2 grams fiber

Applesauce
1/2 cup
2.1 grams fiber

Whole apple
with peel
3.6 grams fiber

Insoluble fiber is from the cell walls of plants and is not digested by the body. Insoluble fiber absorbs water as it passes through the digestive tract, increasing fecal bulk. It quickens the passage of food through the system, helping to prevent constipation. This type of fiber acts as a deterrent to digestive disorders, including cancer of the colon and rectum, because it decreases the time in which your system is exposed to toxic substances in waste materials. Whole wheat bran is the richest source of insoluble fiber. This valuable bran is lost when whole wheat flour is refined to produce white flour. Lentils, skins of fruits and root vegetables, and leafy greens are other good sources of insoluble fiber.

Soluble fiber travels through the digestive tract in a gel-like form, pacing the absorption of carbohydrates. This prevents dramatic shifts in blood sugar levels and can help control diabetes. A diet rich in soluble fiber has also been shown to reduce blood cholesterol levels, especially the LDL, thus reducing the risk of cardiovascular diseases. However, this effect only occurs when coupled with a diet low in saturated fats.[9] Oat bran, beans, vegetables, and fruits are rich sources of soluble fiber, though most plant foods contain both types of fiber. Animal foods never contain fiber.

According to the National Cancer Institute (NCI), about one-third of all cancer deaths may be related to what we eat. Eating between 20 grams and 35 grams of fiber daily is recommended (about double the amount of the current American diet).[10] Since not enough is known about how each kind of fiber (soluble and insoluble) works, the NCI does not recommend any set dietary ratio for either type. Table 9.3 shows the fiber content of some common foods.

Proteins

Hundreds of different kinds of proteins make up the cells of your body. **Proteins** are the major substances used to build and repair tissue, maintain chemical balance, and regulate the formation of hormones, antibodies, and enzymes. Protein

Table 9.3

Dietary Fiber in Foods

Almost all fruits, vegetables, and whole-grain products contain some of both types of fiber. You should get your fiber from a variety of the following sources.

Good Source of Insoluble Fiber	Good Source of Soluble Fiber
More than 5 grams total fiber	
High-fiber wheat-bran cereal (1 oz)	Pinto, kidney, navy beans
Lentils (dried, cooked, 1/2 cup)	(dried, cooked, 1/2 cup)
2 to 5 grams total fiber	
Whole-wheat crackers (6)	Oat bran, oatmeal (dry, 1 oz)
Banana (medium)	Barley (dry, 1 oz)
Potato (medium, with skin)	Berries (1/2 cup)
Buckwheat groats (dry, 1 oz)	Apple, pear (medium, with skin)
Shredded-wheat cereal (1 oz)	Orange, grapefruit (medium)
Brown rice (cooked, 1/2 cup)	Figs, prunes, dried (3)
Brussels sprouts, broccoli, spinach (cooked, 1/2 cup)	Okra, cabbage, peas, turnips, sweet potato (cooked, 1/2 cup)
Wheat germ (3 Tbsp)	Chickpeas, split peas, lima
Whole-wheat flour (1 oz)	beans (cooked, 1/2 cup)
1 to 2 grams total fiber	
Whole-wheat bread (1 slice)	Carrots (cooked, 1/2 cup)
Pasta (cooked, 1 cup)	Peach, nectarine (medium)
Rye bread (1 slice)	Apricots (2)
Corn (1/2 cup)	
Low-fiber wheat cereal (1 oz)	
Cauliflower (cooked, 1/2 cup)	

can also be used as a source of energy, but only if there are not enough carbohydrates or fats available. It is not an efficient source of energy, however. When protein is broken down, the nitrogen part of the protein molecule is left over. The kidneys are overworked trying to excrete this excess nitrogen. Plus, if your body must rely on protein for energy, the protein is not available for building and repairing tissues—its real function.

Each gram of protein provides 4 calories of energy. We need protein daily, and most of us consume more than enough. Protein needs vary throughout the life cycle, due to different growth stages. Growing children need more protein per body weight than adults. Persons age 19 and older can approximate their daily protein need in grams by multiplying their weight (in pounds) by .36.[11]

Example: 130 lb. person × .36 = 46.8 or 47 grams of protein daily

To give you an idea of how little food this is, 47 grams of protein would be 4 ounces of meat (a piece roughly the size of your palm) plus 2 cups of skim milk.

Why do Americans consume
so much meat?

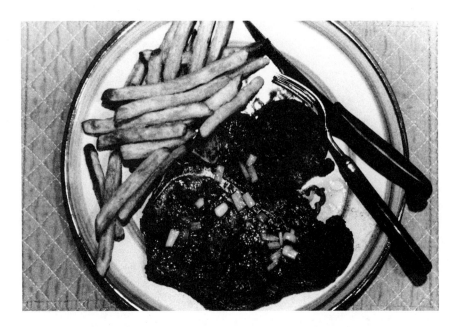

Good sources of protein are found in both animal and plant sources. Meat, poultry, fish, eggs, and milk products are good sources of animal protein. Since many of these sources also contain high amounts of fat and cholesterol, you are wise to select some plant sources of protein: legumes (beans and peas), whole grains, pastas, rice, and seeds. These plant proteins are also a great source of complex carbohydrates.

Fats

Fat is the most concentrated form of food energy, providing 9 calories per gram, more than twice the energy provided by carbohydrates and proteins. Fat adds texture and flavor to food. It helps satisfy the appetite because it is digested more slowly. Also known as lipids, fats are necessary for growth and healthy skin, and for transporting **fat soluble vitamins** in the body. Fats are also linked to hormone regulation. Because of their concentrated form, fats are an efficient way to store energy. Like protein, however, fats are not a good *single* source of energy. Fats burned for energy in the absence of carbohydrates produce a toxic waste

Changing the type of milk you drink
can reduce fat.

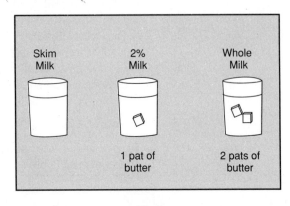

product called ketone bodies. A buildup of poisonous **ketone bodies (ketosis)** causes fatigue and nausea, and overtaxes the kidneys, resulting in brain damage. Fat is burned more completely in the presence of carbohydrates, another reason to have a diet high in complex carbohydrates.

An important distinction should be made among the three types of fatty acids. Ninety-five percent of all dietary fat consists of molecules called **triglycerides,** which are made up of fatty acids. The three types of fatty acids are classified according to the number of additional places available for atoms of hydrogen. Table 9.4 identifies and compares the three types of fats.

Table 9.4

Comparison of the Three Types of Fats

	Characteristics	**Examples**	
Saturated	No more room for hydrogen atoms	Coconut oil	Beef
		Palm oil	Bacon
H H H H		Butter	Lard
| | | |	In animal products and some	Cheese	Pork
H – C – C – C – C – H	vegetable products	Hot dogs	Lamb
| | | |		Chocolate	Veal
H H H H		Milk	Cream
	Raises cholesterol levels in the blood	Cocoa butter	
		Poultry skin	
		Luncheon meats	
	Solid at room temperature	Non-dairy cream substitutes	
Monounsaturated	Can accept 2 more hydrogen atoms	Peanut Oil	Olives
		Olive oil	Peanuts
H H H H H H		Avocados	Cashews
| | | | | |	No effect on cholesterol	Canola (rapeseed)	
H – C – C – C = C – C – C – H	levels in the blood	oil	
| | | |			
H H H H			
Polyunsaturated	Can accept 4 more hydrogen atoms	Corn oil	Fish
		Cottonseed oil	Pecans
H H H H H H H		Soybean oil	Walnuts
| | | | | | |	Lowers blood cholesterol	Safflower oil	
H – C – C = C – C – C = C – C – H		Sesame oil	
| | |		Sunflower oil	
H H H		Mayonnaise	
		Almonds	
		Most margarines	

C = Carbon Atom
H = Hydrogen Atom

Table 9.4 (continued)

Vegetable Oil Fat Comparison

Vegetable Oil Fat Comparison				
	Saturated Fat	Monounsaturated Fat	Polyunsaturated Fat	Cholesterol
Canola Oil	6%	62%	32%	0%
Safflower Oil	10%	13%	77%	0%
Sunflower Oil	11%	20%	69%	0%
Corn Oil	13%	25%	62%	0%
Olive Oil	14%	77%	9%	0%
Soybean Oil	15%	24%	61%	0%

An easy observation shows that with a few exceptions, animal fats are generally more saturated, whereas most vegetable fats are unsaturated. Additionally, all animal fats contain cholesterol, but vegetable foods have no natural presence of cholesterol. Diets high in fat, especially **saturated fats,** have a strong link to heart disease and stroke. They elevate blood cholesterol levels that, in turn, can lead to clogged arteries (atherosclerosis). **Polyunsaturated fats** are the healthier fats to consume.

We eat too much fat. Americans currently consume approximately 37 percent to 40 percent of their daily calories in fats—much of which is saturated.[12] It is recommended that our diet consist of no more than 30 percent fat (10% of each type).[13] Some nutritionists emphasize an even more prudent recommendation of only 10 percent to 20 percent of daily calories from fat. The excessive fat in our diet is the main reason America leads the world in heart disease deaths. Excess dietary fat is also linked to cancer of the colon, breast, and prostate.[14] The amount and type of dietary fat eaten—not the amount of cholesterol consumed—have the greatest impact on the blood cholesterol level. Dietary cholesterol also affects the level of blood cholesterol but to a lesser and more variable extent than does the fat content of the diet.[15]

Monounsaturated and polyunsaturated oils can be turned into solid saturated fats by a manufacturing process called **hydrogenation.** This technique adds hydrogen atoms to these fats as a way to prolong the shelf life of a product. Avoid completely and partially hydrogenated oils. Like saturated fats, they elevate your blood cholesterol level. Some margarines contain partially hydrogenated oils and may be acceptable if they contain twice as many polyunsaturated as saturated fats. As a rule, if the first ingredient listed on any product is "hydrogenated vegetable oil," avoid using it! Table 9.5 shows you how to figure your daily fat allowance in order to adhere to the 30 percent fat-calorie guidelines recommended in the *Dietary Guidelines for Americans.*

Table 9.5

Determining Your Fat Allowance

> For example, if you consume 2,000 calories a day:
> 30% × 2,000 calories = 600 calories
> 600 calories divided by 9 (calories per gram) = 66.6 or 67 grams of total fat recommended per day. (The saturated variety should *only* be 200 calories or 22.2 grams!)
> An easy way to *estimate* your fat gram limit per day is to divide your ideal weight in half. Keep your number of fat grams per day under this number. (Example: ideal weight is 140 pounds = fat gram limit of 70 grams per day)

Cholesterol   **Cholesterol** is not a true fat. It is a fat-like waxy substance found in animal tissue. It plays a vital role in the body's functioning. Your liver manufactures cholesterol, and you consume it by eating animal products (meat, egg yolks, cheese, dairy products, liver). Since a diet high in saturated fats and cholesterol has been linked to atherosclerosis, you are prudent to limit these in your diet. It is recommended that you reduce cholesterol consumption to 300 milligrams per day.[16] (Remember, vegetable foods contain no cholesterol, unless added in processing or food preparation.) Table 9.6 gives you an idea of the amount of saturated fat and cholesterol in selected foods.

Fish Oils   Studies of the diets of Eskimos and Oriental fishermen have revealed new information about fats. Their diets provide 40 percent of daily calories from fats. Yet Eskimos are listed among people with the lowest rates of heart disease in the world. Why? They eat lots of fish, and fish are rich in polyunsaturated fats called **omega-3s.** A diet rich in omega-3 fatty acids inhibits atherosclerosis in coronary arteries and can reduce the blood cholesterol level. The best omega-3 sources are salmon, mackerel, herring, tuna, and sardines. Therefore, eating fish once or twice a week is a sound dietary practice.

Vitamins

Vitamins are the organic catalysts necessary to initiate the body's complex metabolic functions. Because of our adequate food supply, symptoms of vitamin deficiencies are rare. Vitamins fall into two categories: fat soluble and water soluble. Vitamins A, D, E, and K are **fat soluble,** which means they are transported and stored by the body's fat cells. Extreme excesses may lead to toxicity, because they are not excreted and can accumulate in the body. Vitamin C and the B-complexes are **water soluble.** They are not stored in the body cells and need to be consumed daily. Excesses are excreted out of the body.

Are vitamin supplements necessary? It is important to remember that vitamins do not contain energy or calories. Therefore, extra vitamins will not provide more energy or power. Eating a variety of foods is a preferred way to maintain an adequate intake of vitamins. However, in today's lifestyle, some people may not be consuming a varied and balanced diet. Manufacturer's processing and preserving, food irradiation and chemical pollution, nutrient-depleted soil, and

Table 9.6

Fat and Cholesterol Checklist

Source: Adapted from Food 3, *1985. The American Dietetic Association and the United States Department of Agriculture.*

	Total Fat Grams	Saturated Fat Grams	Cholesterol Milligrams
Milk, whole, 1 cup	8.1	5.1	33
2% + milk solids, 1 cup	4.7	2.9	18
skim milk, 1 cup	.6	.4	5
Yogurt, plain, low fat, 8 oz.	3.5	2.3	14
Cottage cheese, 1%, 1/2 cup	1.1	.7	5
Cottage cheese, 4%, 1/2 cup	5.0	3.0	17
Cheddar cheese, 1 oz.	9.4	6.0	30
Mozzarella cheese, part-skim, 1 oz.	4.5	2.9	16
Sour cream, 1 tbs.	2.5	1.6	5
Half-&-Half, 1 tbs.	1.7	1.1	6
Coffee creamer, frozen, 1 tbs.	1.5	1.4	0
Vanilla ice cream, 1/2 cup	7.2	4.4	30
Frozen yogurt, 1/2 cup	1.5	1.0	6
Ground beef patty, cooked, 2 oz.			
regular	11.5	5.5	53
extra lean	3.5	1.7	52
Pork loin, lean, roasted, 2 oz.	8.0	2.9	50
Livers, chicken, cooked, 2 oz.	2.5	.6	423
Chicken, roasted, 2 oz.			
light meat with skin	6.2	1.7	48
light meat, no skin	2.6	.7	48
dark meat with skin	9.0	2.5	52
dark meat, no skin	5.6	1.5	53
Cod, broiled, 2 oz.	.5	.1	35
Tuna, oil pack, drained, 2 oz.	4.6	1.2	37
Shrimp, steamed, 2 oz.	.9	.1	117
Egg, large	5.6	1.7	274
Butter, 1 tbs.	11.5	7.2	31
Oil, corn, 1 tbs.	13.6	1.7	0
peanut	13.5	2.3	0
safflower	13.6	1.2	0
soybean	13.6	2.0	0
coconut	13.6	11.8	0
Lard, 1 tbs.	12.8	5.0	12
Margarine, 1 tbs. stick	11.4	2.1	0
soft	11.4	1.8	0
Mayonnaise, 1 tbs.	11.0	1.6	8

shipping and storage practices have significantly reduced the nutritional value of our foods. Other lifestyle practices, such as smoking, consuming alcohol, and using drugs such as aspirin and oral contraceptives, may increase the need for vitamin or mineral supplementation. Most medical authorities agree that a vitamin supplement containing 50 percent to 150 percent of the RDA will probably do no harm.[17] Familiarizing yourself with the RDA and the contents of your diet will help you decide whether you need a vitamin or mineral supplement (table 9.7). Consult your physician if you are in doubt.

Minerals

Minerals are inorganic substances critical to many enzyme functions in the body. Two groups of minerals are necessary to the diet—macrominerals and trace minerals. **Macrominerals** are needed in large doses (more than 100 mg daily). Examples are calcium, phosphorus, magnesium, potassium, and sodium. **Trace minerals** are needed in much smaller amounts. Examples are iron, zinc, copper, iodine, and fluoride.

Three minerals deserve special attention: calcium, iron, and sodium.

Calcium   Calcium is the body's most abundant mineral and is critical to many body functions. If the calcium supply in the blood is too low, the body withdraws calcium from the bones. This inadequate supply of calcium is a major factor contributing to **osteoporosis,** an age-related condition of insufficient bone mass. Healthy bone is living tissue that is continuously being replenished. In fact, an adult body replaces about 20 percent of its bone each year.[18] In osteoporosis, the formation of bone fails to keep pace with lost bone tissue. The result is porous, brittle bones susceptible to fracture. Women are more susceptible to osteoporosis because they have smaller, less dense bones. Women should ingest 1,200 milligrams of calcium daily. Since some bone loss is normal with aging in both males and females, it is important that you build strong bones now. Your present-day habits may determine your bone density later in life. There is growing evidence that the years from 11 to 24 are critical for bone growth, even though adult height is likely to be reached between age 16 and age 20.[19] Peak bone density is normally reached between ages 30 and 35.[20] The amount of bone mass you have at that age influences susceptibility to brittle bones in the future. To keep those bone "banks" filled:

1. Eat calcium-rich foods every day—low-fat dairy products, spinach, broccoli, fish with edible bones (salmon, sardines).

2. Get regular vigorous exercise (exercises that create muscular contraction and gravitational pull on the long bones, like walking and jogging, are most beneficial).

3. Do not smoke.

4. Avoid excesses of protein, alcohol, caffeine, and phosphates (in colas), which accelerate the excretion of calcium.

5. Be sure to consume foods rich in vitamins A and D to enhance absorption of calcium (no need to exceed the RDA, however).

6. If you have a lactose intolerance (i.e., you have trouble digesting dairy products), lactose-free products are available at some stores. Or, experiment with dairy foods lowest in lactose: ricotta, mozzarella, parmesan, American, and cheddar cheese; tofu; some yogurts; sherbet; 1% low-fat cottage cheese.

Table 9.7

Vitamins and Minerals

Vitamins Fat Soluble	Functions	Sources	Adult RDA*
A	Promotes growth and repair of body tissues; keeps skin cells moist; builds resistance to infection; promotes bone and tooth development; aids in vision	Green leafy vegetables, yellow fruits and vegetables, eggs, butter, margarine, cheese, milk, liver	800–1,000 RE
D	Regulates absorption of calcium and phosphorus; promotes normal growth of bone and teeth	Vitamin D fortified dairy products, fish, eggs, fortified margarines, sunlight (absorbed through the skin)	5–10 micrograms
E	Essential in preventing oxidation of other vitamins and fatty acids; maintains cell structure	Vegetable oil, green and leafy vegetables, whole grains, egg yolks, nuts, wheat germ	8–10 α-TE
K	Aids in blood clotting	Cabbage, cauliflower, spinach, green vegetables, liver, cereals	60-80 micrograms
Water Soluble			
C (Ascorbic Acid)	Builds resistance to infection; aids in tissue repair and healing; tooth and bone formation	Citrus fruits, strawberries, tomatoes, potatoes, melons, broccoli, peppers, cabbage	60 milligrams
B_1 (Thiamin)	Needed to convert carbohydrates into energy; promotes normal function of nervous system	Whole grains, fortified grain products, milk, pork, legumes, nuts, meats	1.0–1.5 milligrams
B_2 (Riboflavin)	Combines with proteins to make enzymes which affect function of eyes, skin, nervous system, and stomach	Meat, dairy products, whole grains, green leafy vegetables	1.2–1.7 milligrams
B_3 (Niacin)	Aids in energy production from fats and carbohydrates	Meat, poultry, fish, liver, nuts, whole grains, legumes	13-19 NE
B_6	Aids in protein metabolism and red blood cell formation	Whole grains, meat, fish, poultry, legumes, milk, green leafy vegetables	1.6–2.0 milligrams

Table 9.7 (continued)

Water Soluble (continued)	Functions	Sources	Adult RDA*
Folic acid (Folacin)	Aids in red blood cell formation; aids in synthesizing genetic material	Meat, poultry, fish, eggs, broccoli, asparagus, legumes	180-200 micrograms
B_{12}	Aids in function of all body cells and nervous tissue	Animal foods only: meat, poultry, fish, eggs, dairy products	2.0 micro-grams
Minerals Macrominerals			
Calcium	Bone and tooth formation; aids in utilization of phosphorus; helps muscle contraction and heart function	Dairy products, green leafy vegetables, broccoli, fish	800–1,200 milligrams
Phosphorus	Aids in all metabolism and energy production	Dairy products, eggs, meat, fish, poultry, legumes, whole grains	800–1,200 milligrams
Magnesium	Activates important enzyme reactions	Whole grains, nuts, legumes, green vegetables	280–350 milligrams
Potassium	Regulates body fluids and the transfer of nutrients across cell walls	Citrus fruits, juices, bananas, potatoes	2,000–5,000 milligrams
Sodium	Regulates body fluids in cells; aids in muscle contraction	Table salt, milk, seafood (abundant in most foods except fruits)	1,100–3,300 milligrams
Trace			
Iron	Essential for oxygen transport in the blood	Liver, meat, poultry, fish, dried fruit, whole grains, legumes, green vegetables	10–15 milligrams
Zinc	Aids in metabolism and growth of tissue	Seafood, poultry, eggs, whole grains, vegetables	12–15 milligrams
Copper	Involved with iron in the formation of red blood cells	Liver, nuts, shellfish, meat, poultry, vegetables	1.5–3.0 milligrams
Iodine	Forms thyroid hormone, affecting overall metabolism	Iodized salt, seafood	150 micrograms
Fluoride	Formation of bones and teeth	Fluoridated water, seafood, green vegetables	1.5–4.0 milligrams

*Adult RDA values from Recommended Dietary Allowances, 10th ed., 1989. Washington, DC 20418. National Academy of Sciences—National Research Council

Iron   A low intake of iron is a common nutritional problem for women. Due to menstruation, women need to ingest more iron than men (women need 15 milligrams daily; men need 10 milligrams).[21] Iron deficiency may cause chronic fatigue and listlessness. To increase your iron intake:

1. Eat foods rich in iron (lean meats, poultry, fish, fortified cereals and grains, green vegetables, beans, and peas).

2. Consume iron-rich foods together with foods high in vitamin C to triple iron absorption (a hamburger with tomato; cereal and orange juice).

3. Keep consumption of tea and coffee under 3 cups per day (caffeine reduces the absorption of iron).

4. Use cast-iron cookware (iron is absorbed into the food in a form that is readily assimilated into the body).

Sodium   Your body needs sodium to survive. The National Research Council recommends 1,100 milligrams to 3,300 milligrams of sodium a day as a safe and adequate range (about 1/2 tsp. to 1 1/2 tsp. of salt).[22] Many Americans consume much, much more than that daily—5,000–10,000 milligrams! We consume sodium most commonly in the form of table salt and in the processed foods we eat. Even if you never salt your food, 90 percent of all processed foods contain sodium—even milk! In this way, sodium becomes "hidden" in our diet. Sodium is also present in other popular condiments, such as monosodium glutamate (MSG), meat tenderizer, ketchup, onion salt, soy sauce, mustard, barbecue sauce, and baking soda. It is even present in many medications—antacids, for instance. Fast-food restaurants often add sodium to their products. Eating a Quarter Pounder cheeseburger, large fries, and a chocolate shake constitutes 1,590 milligrams of sodium. This is the recommended daily allotment of sodium consumed in one meal! Look at table 9.8 and compare the sodium content in processed and unprocessed foods. Which has more salt, a McDonald's apple pie or French fries? Were you right? "Hidden" salt is a problem in this age of processed foods. Since excess sodium consumption has been one factor linked to hypertension in some sodium sensitive individuals, be conscious of your sodium intake, and try to keep it within the recommended range.

Water

Water is often called the forgotten nutrient. However, it is *the most important* nutrient because it serves as the medium in which the other nutrients are transported. Almost all of the body's metabolic reactions occur in this medium. Water also helps rid the body of wastes, aids in metabolizing stored fat, and helps control body temperature. Water composes approximately two-thirds of your body weight. Your exact percentage of water weight varies depending on your body composition. Lean tissue contains more water than fat tissue. While you could survive for weeks without food, you can only last a few days without water. Some nutritionists claim that the average American is in a constant state of dehydration—that we fail to drink enough water. Drink plenty of fluids daily! The

Table 9.8
How Much Sodium Did You Eat Today?

Item/Amount	Sodium (mg)	Item Amount	Sodium (mg)
American processed cheese, 1 oz.	406	Milky Way, 1 bar	140
apple, 1	1	olives (green), 10	936
bacon, 2 strips	202	orange juice, 1 cup	2
banana, 1	1	peanuts, 1 cup	1187
bologna, 2 oz.	578	peanut butter , 2 tbls.	153
broccoli (frozen), 1 cup	40	peas (frozen), 1/2 cup	70
Budget Gourmet sirloin tips dinner	810	pickle (dill), 1	833
carrot, 1 (7" long)	25	pork & beans, 1 cup	1113
cheddar cheese, 2 oz.	352	potato (baked), 1	16
Cheerios, 3/4 cup	310	potato chips, 2 oz.	520
chicken breast, 1	64	pretzel twists, 10	966
chicken pot pie	810	salsa, 6 tbls.	480
cod, 3.5 oz.	78	sausage patty, 1	349
cottage cheese, 1 cup	960	tomato, 1	11
cream of chick soup, 1 cup	810	tomato juice, 1 cup	881
egg, 1	62	Totino sausage & pepperoni	
fish sticks, 4	330	pizza, 10.7 oz.	920
frankfurter, 1	639	tuna, 1/2 cup	620
ham lunch meat, 2 oz.	746	waffle (frozen), 1	250
Lean Cuisine sliced turkey dinner	590	whole wheat bread, 1 slice	180
macaroni & cheese, 3/4 cup	530	yeast donut, 1	222
milk, 1 cup	130		
McDONALD's		*TACO BELL*	
Quarter Pounder with Cheese	1150	Nachos Bell Grande	997
Large French fries	200	Chicken Meximelt	779
Chocolate Lowfat Shake	240	Mexican Pizza	1031
Apple Pie	240	Chilito	893
Filet of Fish	1030	Taco Salad	910
Hashbrown	330	Taco Salad without shell	680
Egg McMuffin	740	Taco	276
Biscuit with Sausage & Egg	1250	Taco Supreme	276
		Nachos	399
PIZZA HUT (2 slices of medium pizza unless otherwise noted)		Taco Sauce	126
		Nacho Cheese Sauce	393
Pepperoni—pan style	1127	Salsa	376
Pepperoni—thin 'n crispy	986		
Supreme—hand tossed	1470		
Super Supreme—hand tossed	1648		
Personal Pan Pizza (pepperoni— whole pizza)	1335		

minimum amount of water a healthy person should drink is 8-10 eight-ounce glasses a day. More is recommended if you are overweight, exercise a lot, or live in a hot climate. Water is also a component of many foods (i.e., apples, lettuce, melons, potatoes, green beans, fruit juices). Are you getting enough water? If so, your urine is clear, almost colorless.

The Well-Balanced Diet

Nutritious eating does not doom you to "nutrition martyrdom"—eating flavorless foods, counting grams, measuring portions, or passing up favorite desserts. Eating should remain as one of life's simple pleasures. Americans are fortunate to have food choices that are varied, plentiful, and safe to eat. Nutritionists often refer to three words when attempting to simplify the principles of good nutition: *variety, balance,* and *moderation.* Do you eat the same thing for breakfast every day? For lunch? For snacks? Despite our access to diverse foods, we have a tendency to consume relatively few types of foods and often become locked into standard meals that many times are culturally influenced. Why not have spaghetti, rice, chili, or pizza for breakfast rather than eggs, bacon, and donuts? Eating right means having a wide variety of foods, in moderation, throughout the week. There are no "forbidden" or "bad" foods—only bad eating habits! If you have a high-fat snack one day, make sure you balance it with restraint at other meals. The seven dietary guidelines provide a sound framework for helping us make food choices.

In 1956, the U.S. Department of Agriculture (USDA) introduced the "basic four food groups" to graphically convey healthy nutrition to Americans. For almost four decades the "basic four" (dairy products, meats, fruits and vegetables, breads and grains) has been drawn on school chalkboards and printed in nutrition booklets. As the science of nutrition grew more sophisticated, and the roles of fats and carbohydrates became better understood, the "basic four" design came under fire. Nutritionists argued that giving dairy products and meats equal emphasis with fruits, vegetables, and grains has caused heart disease and some cancers. In 1992, the USDA introduced "The Food Guide Pyramid" (fig. 9.1, table 9.9) with grains taking up the largest space on the bottom, thereby becoming the foundation of our diet. Fruits and vegetables are the next largest component. Meat, dairy, and fats occupy smaller spaces near the top. Eating according to this pyramid, with the greatest emphasis on grains, fruits, and vegetables, is the key to sound nutrition and is in harmony with the *Dietary Guidelines.* Look at table 9.10 for a concise summary of the recommendations for your daily diet.

Making Positive Changes

All of this information about nutrition can seem confusing and appear contradictory; for example, consume enough meat for iron, yet reduce saturated fat. Make sure you get plenty of calcium; yet watch out for those high-fat dairy products. You certainly hear enough about what *not* to eat. Since we believe in a positive approach to a wellness lifestyle, table 9.11 gives advice to help you eat more nutritiously in today's fast-paced world. These suggestions are ways to incorporate the dietary guidelines into sensible and simple practices. In fact, studies have

Fig. 9.1

Food Guide Pyramid: A Guide to Daily Food Choices

Source: U.S. Department of Agriculture, Human Nutrition Information Service, USDA's Food Guide Pyramid, Home and Garden Bulletin No. 249, 1992.

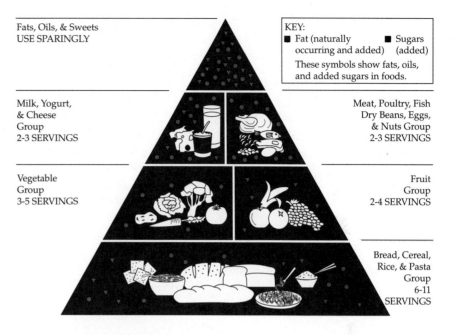

Fats, Oils, & Sweets
USE SPARINGLY

KEY:
■ Fat (naturally occurring and added)   ■ Sugars (added)
These symbols show fats, oils, and added sugars in foods.

Milk, Yogurt, & Cheese Group
2-3 SERVINGS

Meat, Poultry, Fish Dry Beans, Eggs, & Nuts Group
2-3 SERVINGS

Vegetable Group
3-5 SERVINGS

Fruit Group
2-4 SERVINGS

Bread, Cereal, Rice, & Pasta Group
6-11 SERVINGS

What is the Food Guide Pyramid?

The Pyramid is an outline of what to eat each day. It's not a rigid prescription, but a general guide that lets you choose a healthful diet that's right for you.

The Pyramid calls for eating a variety of foods to get the nutrients you need and at the same time the right amount of calories to maintain a healthy weight.

The Pyramid also focuses on fat because most American diets are too high in fat, especially saturated fat.

Fat

● In general, foods that come from animals (milk and meat groups) are naturally higher in fat than foods that come from plants. But there are many lowfat dairy and lean meat choices available, and these foods can be prepared in ways that lower fat.

Fruits, vegetables, and grain products are naturally low in fat. But many popular items are prepared with fat, like french-fried potatoes or croissants, making them higher fat choices.

Added Sugars

▼ These symbols represent sugars added to foods in processing or at the table, not the sugars found naturally in fruits and milk. It's the added sugars that provide calories with few vitamins and minerals.

Most of the added sugars in the typical American diet come from foods in the Pyramid tip—soft drinks, candy, jams, jellies, syrups, and table sugar we add to foods like coffee or cereal.

Added sugars in the food groups come from foods such as ice cream, sweetened yogurt, chocolate milk, canned or frozen fruit with heavy syrup, and sweetened bakery products like cakes and cookies.

shown that significant changes in your nutritional health can be accomplished with *simple* changes, without excluding commercially-prepared foods or drastically reducing the amount of food.[23]

It is not advisable or possible to do a complete overhaul of your diet. After reading this chapter, do not go to your refrigerator and throw everything out. It is easier, and usually more lasting, to make small and gradual changes. Realize that no one is perfect or eats perfectly all of the time. Just remember that you do

Table 9.9
What Counts as a Serving?

Milk, Yogurt and Cheese Group	Meat, Poultry, Fish, Dry Beans, Eggs, and Nuts Group	Vegetable Group	Fruit Group	Bread, Cereal, Rice, and Pasta Group
1 c. milk or yogurt	2–3 oz. cooked, lean meat, poultry or fish	1 c. raw leafy greens	1 medium apple, banana, orange	1 slice bread
1 1/2 oz. natural cheese	1/3 c. nuts	1/2 cup other kinds of vegetables (raw or cooked)	1/2 c. chopped, cooked, canned fruit	1/2 bun or bagel
2 oz. process cheese	(count 1/2 c. cooked dry beans, 1 egg, or 2 Tbls. peanut butter as 1 oz. of meat)	3/4 c. vegetable juice	3/4 cup juice	1 oz. dry cereal
1 c. frozen yogurt				1/2 c. cooked cereal, rice or pasta
1 1/2 c. ice cream				3–4 small plain crackers
2 c. cottage cheese				

Table 9.10
Daily Diet Recommendations

Calories from carbohydrates	58% or more (48+ from complex) (10 from simple)
Calories from protein	12%
Calories from fat	30% or less (10 from saturated) (10 from polyunsaturated) (10 from monounsaturated)
Cholesterol	under 300 milligrams
Fiber	20–35 grams
Sodium	1,100–3,300 milligrams

have choices. As you pursue wellness, try to do the best you can with the knowledge that you have about nutrition. Perhaps some of these suggestions could become a central goal for writing a wellness contract (as discussed in chapter 1).

A good way to assess your nutritional habits is to record everything you eat for 3 to 7 days in a log. By actually observing types and quantities of food consumed, you can best judge if your diet is nutritionally sound, that is, conforms to the *Dietary Guidelines,* RDA, and mimics the "food guide pyramid." Keeping a log can help you set goals for making positive dietary changes. You can write your own food log. (There is a sample food log form in the activities section at the end of the book.) You may prefer to use one of the many computer programs that are available for dietary assessment. It is not always practical to constantly count milligrams, calories, or ounces, but an analysis can show you where improvements in your diet can be made.

Table 9.11

23 Tips for Nutritional Wellness

1. Use fresh, unprocessed foods whenever possible.
2. Eat more poultry. Remove the skin (the source of most of the fat).
3. Eat low-fat dairy products. There are plenty of reduced fat cheeses available. Switch to skim or 1% milk.
4. Increase consumption of complex carbohydrates.
5. Trim all excess fat from meats; eat leaner cuts of red meats (i.e., "loin" or "round"). "Select" is lower in fat than "choice" or "prime".
6. Eat fish once or twice a week (baked or broiled, *not* fried or breaded).
7. Instead of focusing a meal around a meat, use a small amount of meat (diced, shaved, chopped, sliced) to mix in with other vegetables and rice or pasta.
8. Steam, bake, broil, or roast foods using a cooking rack to allow fat to drain from the food.
9. Select salad oils, cooking oils, and margarines made with unsaturated fats. Soft, tub margarines with liquid oil listed as the first ingredient are good choices.
10. Try bagels, muffins, or whole wheat toast with jam or apple butter (without butter or margarine), rather than croissants, donuts, sweet rolls, or biscuits.
11. Use a nonstick vegetable oil spray for sauteing.
12. Use deli luncheon meats such as shaved chicken breast and turkey instead of high-fat bologna, salami, beef, or hot dogs.
13. Remove the salt shaker from the table; experiment with recipes by substituting herbs and other seasoning for salt.
14. Make your own salad dressings and sauces using polyunsaturated oils.
15. Replace snack items such as potato chips, salted nuts, and crackers with fresh fruit, raw vegetables, unsalted unbuttered popcorn, pretzels, or rice cakes.
16. Use plain, low-fat yogurt as a substitute for sour cream in dips and on baked potatoes. Fat-free sour cream and cream cheese are now available.
17. Eat a meatless dinner one night a week.
18. Use ground turkey in casseroles, chili, spaghetti sauce, and skillet dinners that normally require ground beef.
19. When making scrambled eggs, separate the eggs, eliminating half of the yolks. If a recipe calls for one egg, substitute 2 egg whites to reduce the cholesterol.
20. After making soups and broths, chill; scrape off the congealed fat.
21. Substitute fruit juices or plain water for soft drinks.
22. Top off your meals with fresh fruit for a nutritionally "sweet" dessert. Try frozen yogurt, juice bars, vanilla wafers, fig newtons, or angel food cake to satisfy your sweet tooth.
23. Read labels; learn about what you are eating.

Nutrition Labeling

Now that you understand the basics of nutrition, how do you know the actual nutritional content of the foods you are eating? You do this by reading labels. Read about what you are eating! Part of self-responsibility is becoming a "nutrition-wise" consumer. The federal government regulates food labeling. In the past, nutrition labeling was voluntary. Only foods fortified with protein, vitamins or minerals, or making a nutrition claim had to be labeled. As a result, only about half of the processed foods regulated by the Food and Drug Administration were labeled. With a new era of health consciousness, consumers began demanding reliable information on food packages. In 1990, the President signed the "Nutrition Labeling and Education Act" into law. No longer are food producers and marketers able to mislead, confuse, or make false claims about foods. The goal of the new law is simple: to provide food labeling that the public can understand and count on, and that will bring them up-to-date with today's health concerns. It has three objectives: (1) to clear up confusion; (2) to help consumers make healthy choices; and (3) to encourage food companies to produce healthier foods (to make them work on the "insides" of the package, instead of merely tinkering with the words on the label).[24] The new rules require nutritional labeling on nearly all grocery items. Meat and poultry are exempt. Restaurants, bakeries, delis, and sidewalk vendors are also exempt from nutrition labeling, as are packages smaller than 12 square inches. All manufacturers have until May 1994 to comply with the new rules. Some points to remember when reading labels are:

1. Check serving size.
2. Ingredients are listed in order of concentration in a product, with the ingredient in the largest quantity listed first.
3. Watch for hidden sugars added to a product: syrup, sucrose, molasses, corn sweetener, dextrose, maltose, honey, etc. They are all sugars! The new labeling law requires all sweeteners in a product to be listed together in the ingredient list under the collective term "sweeteners."
4. Check fat content. Avoid hydrogenated fats.
5. Some crackers, pastries, cookies, candies, and instant cocoas are loaded with coconut and palm oil, which are more saturated than beef fat.
6. Select *whole* wheat bread ("wheat flour" means refined *white* flour—the bran and wheat germ have been removed). All whole wheat bread is brown, but not all brown bread is whole wheat!
7. Do not be deceived by advertising "mumbo jumbo." *Diet* entrees may have saturated fats and sodium, probably worse for you than the calories! *No cholesterol* can still contain saturated fat. *All natural, quick energy* may reflect extravagant claims. Also, there is no legal definition for *organic* or *natural*.
8. *Sugar free* means no sucrose (table sugar), but the item may have other sweeteners that contain the same caloric value as sucrose.
9. *Salt free* means no salt (sodium chloride), but may still contain sodium!
10. Fortified foods contain added vitamins and minerals that were

not originally in the food or were present in lower amounts. Breakfast cereals are commonly fortified. Can you name the vitamin milk is commonly fortified with?

11. Enriched foods have lost nutrients during processing and then had them replaced by the manufacturers. For instance, when wheat is turned into white flour, it loses at least 50 percent to 80 percent of many nutrients. Of these, iron, niacin, thiamin, and riboflavin are replaced; but other nutrients lost in the milling process, such as fiber, zinc, and copper, are not restored.

12. You can figure the nutrient source of the calories per serving by multiplying the gram amount of each nutrient by the calories per gram:

Example—suppose a product has 120 calories per serving:

Protein 2 grams per serving × 4 calories = 8 (8 ÷ 120 = 6%)

Carbohydrates 17 grams per serving × 4 calories = 68 (68 ÷ 120 = 56%)

Fat 5 grams per serving × 9 calories = 45 (45 ÷ 120 = 38%)

13. Milk is labeled by percent of fat by *weight*, not calories:
   - whole milk is 3.3% fat by weight, but *50% fat by calories*
   - 2% milk is 2% fat by weight, but *35% fat by calories*
   - 1% milk is 1% fat by weight, but *23% fat by calories*
   - skim milk has a trace of fat by weight, but *5% fat by calories*

One of the problems in food labeling has been the confusing descriptors that manufacturers put on food products, for which there have previously been no definitions. (Example: "lite" or "light" could have meant light in calories, color, texture, or weight!) Under the new labeling law, specific definitions will be assigned to ten core descriptors used on the label of any product (free, low, lean, lite or light, less, high, good source of, reduced more, percent fat free). Consistency in these terms will help shoppers who do not scrutinize all the numbers on food labels, but who want to pick up a "low sodium" or "fat free" version of foods as they walk through the supermarket. Look at the label in table 9.12 for further label-reading tips.

Fast Foods

One out of every 5 Americans eats at a fast-food restaurant daily. Eating out has become routine for many of us. Meal preparation time at home has decreased due to changing lifestyles, and it is evident this trend will not reverse. In fact, adults eat roughly 30 percent of their calories *away* from home, and fast-food restaurants serve 4 out of 10 meals eaten at away-from-home eating establishments.[25] Most fast-food chains now supply nutrient information on their food products. What has this information revealed about the nutrient value of fast-food? Are fast-foods "junk" foods? Nutritionists have found that fast-food items do have significant amounts of certain nutrients (especially protein), but many tend to be low in fiber and high in calories, sodium, and fat.[26] How often do you rely on these foods? What other foods are you eating during the day? Occasional

Table 9.12 How to Read a Label

A sample label for:

MACARONI
A N D
CHEESE

Nutrition Facts

Serving Size 1/2 cup (114g)
Servings Per Container 4

Serving sizes are standardized to reflect the amounts of foods people actually eat. They are also expressed in both common household and metric measures. (You should note whether you are consuming *more* than one serving.)

Amount Per Serving

Calories 260	Calories from Fat 120

	% Daily Value*
Total Fat 13g	**20%**
Saturated Fat 5g	**25%**
Cholesterol 30mg	**10%**
Sodium 660mg	**28%**
Total Carbohydrate 31g	**11%**
Sugars 5g	**
Dietary Fiber 0g	**0%**
Protein 5g	**

Vitamin A 4% • Vitamin C 2% • Calcium 15% • Iron 4%

This mandatory list of nutrients includes those most important to today's consumers. In the past, the concern was vitamin and mineral deficiencies. Now the worries pertain to fat, cholesterol, sodium, types of carbohydrates and protein amounts.

% Daily Values shows how a food fits into the overall daily diet. For each item, it shows the percentage or recommended daily consumption for a person eating 2,000 calories a day (e.g., the 5 grams of saturated fat is 25% of the *recommended* daily value of 20 grams).

Percentage of daily requirements for selected vitamins and minerals.

* Percents (%) of a Daily Value are based on a 2,000 calorie diet. Your Daily Values may vary higher or lower depending on your calorie needs:

Nutrient		2,000 Calories	2,500 Calories
Total Fat	Less than	65g	80g
Sat Fat	Less than	20g	25g
Cholesterol	Less than	300mg	300mg
Sodium	Less than	2,400mg	2,400mg
Total Carbohydrate		300g	375g
Fiber		25g	30g

Recommended daily amounts of each item for two average diets.

1g Fat = 9 calories
1g Carbohydrates = 4 calories
1g Protein = 4 calories

**No daily values have been determined for sugars and protein intake

This information can help you calculate what percentage of *calories* of this food comes from fat, carbohydrates, and protein.
e.g.:
TOTAL FAT = 13g
13g x 9 = 117 calories
117 ÷ 260 = .45
This macaroni and cheese is 45% fat.

TOTAL CARBOHYDRATE = 31g
31g x 4 = 124 calories
124 ÷ 260 = .476
This macaroni and cheese is 48% carbohydrate.

Voluntary components that will be allowed on labels are: calories from saturated fat; polyunsaturated fat; monounsaturated fat; potassium; soluble and insoluble fiber; sugar; alcohol; other carbohydrates, and other essential vitamins and minerals.

visits to fast-food restaurants will have little effect on the nutritive value of your total diet. In response to consumer demand, many chains have become quite diversified and have added many more items to their menus. Table 9.13 gives suggestions for healthy eating at fast-food restaurants.

Table 9.13

Fast Tips for Fast-Foods

1. Think about what else you have eaten or will eat that day. Fit this meal into your total fat, sodium, and calorie intake.
2. Salad bars are a wise choice for vitamins A and C and fiber; go easy on the dressings, high-fat cheeses, bacon, olives, sour cream, and refried beans.
3. Potato bars are another good choice if you avoid the heavy cheese and butter-type sauces, bacon, and sour cream.
4. Chicken and fish sound healthy, but many are coated with fat. Select the baked or grilled without breading or the skin.
5. Pizza is a great choice, especially if the toppings are vegetables; avoid the pepperoni, sausage, and olives.
6. Hamburgers—order the small one instead of the "jumbo" burger.
7. Drink low-fat milk or juice instead of a shake or soda.
8. If Mexican, emphasize soft tortillas, beans, chicken, and vegetables (easy on the cheese).
9. For breakfast avoid croissants, biscuits, sausage, bacon, butter, and the danish. Better choices are pancakes, English muffins, bagels, bran muffins, and whole grain cereals.

Special Nutritional Concerns

High-level wellness means adjusting to life changes as well as seeking information for special situations. This section discusses dietary considerations for vegetarians, pregnant mothers, the elderly, and those persons engaging in regular, vigorous exercise.

Vegetarian Diet

For a variety of health and moral reasons, many people prefer a vegetarian diet. A vegetarian diet can be very nutritious and healthy. Due to the lack of animal foods, vegetarians normally have lower body fat, blood cholesterol, blood pressure, and rates of coronary heart disease. Recent studies show that mortality rates are lower for vegetarians than for nonvegetarians.[27] There are different vegetarian diets, however. Careful planning and food selection is important to avoid nutritional deficiencies. All vegetarian diets emphasize the use of vegetables, fruits, and grains as main staples. Some diets exclude all animal products, while some include dairy products and eggs.

Types of vegetarian diets:

1. **Strict vegetarians** or **vegans** consume only plant foods. (Vitamin B_{12} supplementation is recommended since it is not in any plant foods.)

2. **Lactovegetarians** will consume plant foods and dairy products.

3. **Lacto-ovo-vegetarians** will consume plant foods, dairy products, and eggs.

4. **Semi-vegetarians** only exclude red meat.

Meat is not essential to your diet, but protein is. Therefore, following a vegetarian diet requires careful planning and food selection in order to consume sufficient vitamins and minerals (especially vitamin Bs, vitamin D, calcium, zinc, and iron). The vegetarian needs to search for good quality protein sources such as legumes (beans), nuts, grains, and seeds. A thorough knowledge of nutrition is essential to the vegetarian. For example, combining a good source of vitamin C with whole grains and legumes will greatly enhance iron absorption from grain and legumes. Drinking fortified soybean milk will help the vegetarian obtain calcium and vitamin B_{12}. (For more information on vegetarian eating, refer to the Suggested Readings.)

Pregnancy

Many women become more nutritionally aware and eat more wisely during pregnancy. This makes sense. After all, it is an enormous responsibility being in control of the nutritional well-being of another human. Good nutritional habits before conception give the baby an even healthier start. Good nutrition can improve infant birth weight and reduce infant mortality. This is not a time to diet! Weight gain and some increased fat deposition is necessary and quite healthy. Be sure to increase calcium, iron, and protein. Your physician may recommend a vitamin supplement, since many vitamin needs are increased. Eat nutritionally-dense foods. Twinkies, chocolate chip cookies, and potato chips offer few nutrients to that growing baby.

Aging

Many factors may interfere with good nutrition in older adults—economics, isolation, dentures, chronic health disorders, and medications. The widower whose wife always prepared the meals may be eating fast foods or frozen dinners. The depressed and lonely widow may eat very little at all. Proper nutrition throughout life and into later life can minimize degenerative changes and help you maintain productivity and wellness. However, your 65-year-old body will not be the same one you fed at 25. If you decrease activity and your body composition changes (increase in fat; decrease in lean), then caloric intake should be decreased. Maintaining an active lifestyle can keep energy requirements from decreasing drastically. Even though energy needs may drop as you age, nutrient needs do not diminish significantly. You must make your calories count! Be sure to eat adequate fiber and calcium, and fewer fats and refined sugars. Most of all, do not fall prey to nutritional quackery (special pills and elixirs of youth).

Nutrition for Sports and Fitness

Do you play competitive football? Are you training for a marathon? Is lap swimming every morning your fitness routine? Nutrition complements physical activity as you pursue a wellness lifestyle. However, the nutritional needs of an active person vary little from those more sedentary. If you are physically active, you burn more calories and have less chance of gaining weight (while eating more). Nevertheless, you do not need a special diet. There have been many myths and propaganda surrounding athletic performance and nutrition. Let us set you straight on the facts. An athlete does not benefit from consuming more protein (not even a body builder). Protein supplements are a waste of money. The main fuel for exercising muscles, glycogen, comes from carbohydrates. The best are complex (breads, pastas, potatoes, rice, fruit), which provide plenty of vitamins and minerals. Athletes participating in intense workouts twice a day need to consume a high complex carbohydrate diet (450–500 grams/day compared with approximately 350 grams/day in the average American diet).[28] High-sugar snacks consumed before exercising can actually decrease performance. Carbohydrate loading (that is, manipulating diet and training in order to increase glycogen stores in the muscles) has not been shown to be effective for athletes participating in events requiring less than 1 1/2 to 2 hours of continuous, noninterrupted effort.[29]

The benefits of vitamin and mineral supplementation is a current area of study in regard to nutrition for competitive athletes. Large doses of vitamins C, E, and beta-carotene have shown promise in minimizing muscle damage and soreness in hard-working athletes.[30] Nonetheless, the evidence in this area is spotty. Much more research is needed before athletes should begin consuming megadoses of vitamins with the idea of enhancing athletic performance.

Dehydration is a major contributor to poor athletic performance. Due to the loss of fluids from perspiring, some believe that special "energy" drinks are best at replacing this loss. Actually, the best liquid to drink is cool water. It is absorbed more quickly than anything else. Athletes, like everyone else, should drink 8–10 glasses of water every day. They should also drink a cup or more of water immediately before exercise, and another 1/2 to 1 cup every 15 minutes during exercise. Do not wait until you are thirsty. Thirst is not a reliable indicator of dehydration because it usually does not occur until after 2–4 pints of body water are lost. Also, there is no need for salt tablets. A 2-pound water loss results in an average sodium loss of 1 gram (easily replaced by the salt in our foods). We eat more than enough sodium. What is important is drinking enough water to keep sodium distributed throughout the body. In regard to nutrition, the key to sports and fitness performance is the same key to general wellness and vitality—a balanced diet.

Summary

Even though diet is not singled out as a specific risk factor for coronary heart disease, dietary factors are often interrelated with patterns of physical activity as major contributors to heart disease, stroke, obesity, atherosclerosis, osteoporosis, and some types of cancer. While many dietary components are involved in diet and health relationships, a primary factor is our high consumption of fats (especially saturated fats). These are often consumed at the expense of fruits, vegetables, and complex carbohydrates that may be more conducive to health.

Like many, you may admit to having some poor nutritional habits. You may rationalize this by saying:

- I'll do better after I get out of school and have more time. (Frankly, you will probably be busier after graduation!)
- But I feel fine! (Like smoking, poor eating habits may not noticeably affect your health for years.)
- I don't have any control over what the cafeteria serves. (However, you do have *choices* in the cafeteria and between meals.)
- I don't have enough money to buy the right foods. (On the contrary, milk is cheaper than soft drinks; a bunch of bananas costs less than a bag of potato chips.)
- I'm going to die anyway, so I might as well eat what I like. (Yes, we are all going to die. However, lifetime dietary habits significantly affect the *quality* of the last 10 to 20 years of your life.)

Wellness involves making informed choices, rather than rationalizing! Improved eating habits can positively affect your health—both now and later in life. The heart of good nutrition is *seven dietary principles* and *three simple words*. A diet that emphasizes variety, moderation, and balance is a big step toward achieving high-level wellness. A variety of foods is available to you, and it is up to you to make responsible choices—complex carbohydrates high in fiber and foods low in fat, cholesterol, sodium, and refined sugars.

References

1. "ADA Survey of Dietary Habits." *Nutrition Today* 26 (December 1991): 5.

2. Farthing, Maryann C. "Current Eating Patterns of Adolescents in the United States." *Nutrition Today* 26 (March/April 1991): 35–39.

3. Signorielli, Nancy. "Television and Health: Images and Impact." *Mass Communication and Public Health.* Edited by Charles Atkin and Lawrence Wallack, 96–113. Newbury Park, CA: SAGE Publications, Inc., 1990.

4. *The Surgeon General's Report on Nutrition and Health.* Washington D.C.: U.S. Department of Health and Human Services, DHHS (PHS) publication 88–50210, 1988.

5. "Improving America's Diet and Health: From Recommendations to Action." *Nutrition Today* 27 (January/February 1992): 34–36.

6. Williams, Melvin H. *Nutrition for Fitness and Sport.* Dubuque, IA: Wm. C. Brown Publishers, 1992.

7. Williams, Melvin H. *Nutrition for Fitness and Sport.*

8. "The Importance of Fiber." *University of California at Berkeley Wellness Letter* 8 (April 1992): 4–5.

9. Kantor, Mark A. "Nutrition, Cholesterol, and Heart Disease, Part IV: The Role of Dietary Fiber." *Nutrition Forum* 6 (July/August 1989): 25–29.

10. "The Importance of Fiber."

11. Williams, Melvin H. *Nutrition for Fitness and Sport.*

12. "Eat Right America." *Journal of the American Dietetic Association* 92 (March 1992): supplement.

13. U.S. Department of Agriculture, U.S. Department of Health and Human Services. *Nutrition and Your Health: Dietary Guidelines for Americans,* 3rd edition. Home and Garden Bulletin No. 232, 1990.

14. *The Surgeon General's Report on Nutrition and Health.*

15. Kantor, Mark A. "Nutrition, Cholesterol, and Heart Disease, Part III: How Diet Affects Blood Cholesterol Levels." *Nutrition Forum* 6 (May/June 1989): 17–20.

16. *Nutrition and Your Health: Dietary Guidelines for Americans.*

17. Williams, Melvin H. *Nutrition for Fitness and Sport.*

18. Clark, Nancy. "Dairy Tales." *Runner's World* 24 (June 1989): 44–50.

19. Finday, Steven. "Latest Dispatch from the Vitamin Front." *U.S. News and World Report* 107 (November 6, 1989): 100–101.

20. Clark, Nancy. "Dairy Tales."

21. *Recommended Dietary Allowances,* 10th ed. National Academy of Sciences—National Research Council, 1989.

22. *The Surgeon General's Report on Nutrition and Health.*

23. Smith-Schneider, Lisa M., Madeleine J. Sigman-Grant, and P. M. Kris-Etherton. "Dietary Fat Reduction Strategies." *Journal of the American Dietetic Association* 92 (January 1992): 34–38.

24. "The New Food Label." *Nutrition Today* 27 (January/February 1992): 37–38.

25. U.S. Department of Agriculture, Human Nutrition Information Service. *Eating Better When Eating Out.* Home and Garden Bulletin No. 232–11, 1991.

26. *Eating Better When Eating Out.*

27. Wardlaw, Gordon. "Eating Vegetarian." *Healthline* 10 (July 1991): 2, 4.

28. McBean, Lois D., editor." Eating for Top Performance. "*Nutrition Reports.* Dairy Council of Michigan, Okemos, MI, Winter 1991.

29. Williams, Melvin H. *Nutrition for Fitness and Sport.*

30. Williams, Melvin H. *Nutrition for Fitness and Sport.*

Suggested Readings

Amato, Paul R., and Sonia A. Partridge. 1989. *The New Vegetarians.* New York: Plenum Press.

"Are You Eating Right." *Consumer Report.* 57 (October 1992). 644–51.

Bailey, Covert. 1984. *The Fit-or-Fat Target Diet.* Boston: Houghton Mifflin Co.

Benefits of Nutritional Supplements. 1987. Washington, DC: Council for Responsible Nutrition.

Berning, Jacqueline, and Suzanne Nelson Steen. (eds.) *Sports Nutrition for the 90s.* Gaithersburg, MD: Aspen Publishers, Inc.

Brown, Judith E. 1991. *Everywoman's Guide to Nutrition.* Minneapolis, MN: University of Minnesota.

Clark, Nancy. 1990. *Nancy Clark's Sports Nutrition Guidebook.* Champaign, IL: Human Kinetics Publishers.

Diet and Health: Implications for Reducing Chronic Disease Risk. 1989. Washington DC: National Academy of Sciences.

Earl, Robert, Donna V. Porter, and Nancy S. Wellman. "Nutrition Labeling: Issues and Directions for the 1990's." *Journal of the American Dietetic Association* 90 (November 1990): 1599–1601.

Jones, Jeanne. 1992. *Eating Smart.* New York: Macmillan Publishing Co.

Li, Virginia C. "On Diet and Dieting: Reaching High Level Wellness." *Wellness Perspectives* 7 (Winter 1990): 61–75.

Meyer, Jean and Jeanne P. Goldberg. 1990. *Dr. Jean Meyer's Diet and Nutrition Guide.* New York: Pharos Books.

Munnings, Frances. "Osteoporosis: What is the Role of Exercise?" *The Physician and Sportsmedicine* 20 (June 1992): 127–38.

Peterkin, Betty B. "Dietary Guidelines for Americans, 1990 edition." *Journal of the American Dietetic Association* 90 (December 1990): 1725–1727.

Piscatella, Joseph C. 1991. *Controlling Your Fat Tooth.* New York: Workman Publishing Co.

Rolfes, Sharon Rady, and Linda Kelly DeBruyne. 1990. *Lifespan Nutrition: Conception Through Life.* St. Paul, MN: West Publishing Co.

"The New Food Label." *Nutrition Today* 27 (January/February 1992): 37–38.

The Surgeon General's Report on Nutrition and Health. 1988. Washington DC: U.S. Department of Health and Human Services, DHHS (PHS) publication 88–50210.

Tribole, Evelyn. 1992. *Eating on the Run.* Champaign, IL: Human Kinetics Publishers.

Williams, Melvin H. 1992. *Nutrition for Fitness and Sport,* 3rd edition. Dubuque, IA: Wm. C. Brown Publishers.

For More Nutrition Information Contact:

National Center for Nutrition and Dietetics
216 West Jackson Blvd., Suite 800
Chicago, IL 60606–6995

Human Nutrition Information Service
United States Department of Agriculture
6505 Belcrest Road
Hyattsville, MD 20782
(301) 436–7725

NUTRITION HOTLINE: 1–800–366–1655
- a registered dietitian will answer your questions Monday-Friday, 10:00 am-5:00 pm (EST)
- prerecorded messages 24 hours a day

10
Weight Management

Chapter Objectives

After reading this chapter, you will be able to:

1. Differentiate between overweight and obesity.
2. Explain the purpose of the Body Mass Index (BMI), and identify a BMI associated with health problems.
3. List seven health conditions associated with obesity.
4. Identify how the location of fat on the body is linked to health risks.
5. Describe how each of the following factors contribute to obesity: energy balance, fat cells, set point, heredity, metabolism, and nutrient composition of food.
6. Define basal metabolic rate (BMR), and identify five factors that affect it.
7. List four reasons why crash/fad dieting does not work for permanent weight loss.
8. Define and explain the "yo-yo syndrome" (weight cycling).
9. List five guidelines to follow in evaluating any weight loss plan.
10. Identify and explain the three major components of effective lifetime weight management.
11. Give five examples of behavior modification techniques.
12. List five ways exercise helps in weight management.
13. Identify weight loss myths, fads, and gimmicks.
14. Compare and contrast the eating disorders: bulimia and anorexia nervosa.

Terms

- Anorexia nervosa
- Basal Metabolic Rate (BMR)
- Behavior modification
- Body fat
- Body image
- Body Mass Index (BMI)
- Bulimia
- Calorie (kcal)
- Cellulite
- Eating disorder
- Essential fat
- Fat cell (adipose cell)
- Fat-free mass
- Glycogen
- Lean-body mass (muscle mass)
- Liposuction
- Obesity
- Overweight
- Set point
- Storage fat
- Yo-yo syndrome (weight cycling)

Americans are obsessed about weight. It is likely that you know your weight within 5 pounds. Every birth announcement gives the baby's weight to the exact ounce. Weight scales are commonplace in American bathrooms and even on street corners. This preoccupation has made weight control a multibillion dollar business. Americans spent approximately $8.3 billion in 1991 on weight loss products and services (not including diet soft drinks, artificial sweeteners, or exercise club memberships).[1] It is estimated that this amount will top $12.4 billion in 1996.

The craze to lose weight (whether needed or not) is reflected by the more than 65 million Americans who report that they are dieting.[2] Bookstore shelves and magazine racks are crammed with diet plans guaranteed to help you lose those extra inches. Television, radio, and newspapers further advertise a multitude of weight loss options. With all of this attention, one would predict that the American population is very lean. Actually, obesity is a major health problem in our country. We are getting fatter—not thinner! Few dieters attain their weight loss goals, and most are unable to keep weight off over a period of time. Estimates vary, but approximately 26 percent of the total population in this country is considered obese (i.e., a body mass index for women greater than 27.3, and for men greater than 27.8).[3] Many health professionals feel that obesity is THE most common and serious health problem facing America today. On the other extreme, the incidence of anorexia nervosa and bulimia nervosa is at epidemic proportions. The paradox of these facts reveals how complex America's weight problem is.

Maintaining a reasonable body weight is a definite wellness issue. Your body is the vehicle by which you function in society. Being overfat can affect you physically, emotionally, socially, and even occupationally. Since the purpose of wellness is to strive toward full potential, maintaining a reasonable body composition is one step toward achieving wellness. Knowledge gives you the tools to plan your lifetime weight management scheme. It is important that you understand body composition facts, effective weight loss principles, weight management guidelines, and the influence of heredity and environment on weight control.

The Impact of Culture

Why people diet and how they go about dieting is heavily bound in culture. In the 1880s, full-figured actress Lillian Russell was the epitome of beauty and voluptuousness. During these times, a surplus of fat was equated with wealth and success. The twentieth century brought about a decline of fatness as a social asset. Insurance companies began observing the increased death rate among those extremely overweight. The socially elite began diminishing the enormity of banquet menus. President William Howard Taft, weighing in at 355 pounds in 1909, began facing ridicule for his size. Corsets gave way to exercise, massage, raised hemlines, and penny scales. Hollywood stars, such as Jean Harlow and Gloria Swanson, gave diet and beauty advice that focused on reducing food intake. Thinness became equated with glamour, success, and desirability. After the Depression, the knowledge that excessive fat was linked to heart disease became a publicized issue. Weight reduction became a national pastime—a craze. Mail order companies began making large profits with their weight loss

The pursuit of a model-like body is an unhealthy pressure

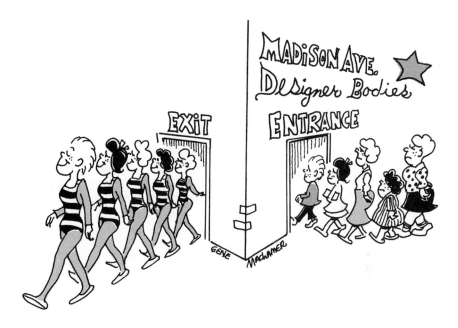

gimmicks. The market eventually gave way to new low-calorie foods and drugs designed to fool the body's hunger sensations. At the same time, labor-saving machines reduced the energy output necessary in daily life. The message that emerged by the 1960s was "Thin is in." The desire for an unrealistic slimness, particularly among women, has caused many to be preoccupied with their bodies and with dieting. This standard is perpetuated in all channels of social influence—families, peers, and the media. The message is pounded home over and over: "You can never be thin enough." This notion was documented in a 1980 study by David Garner[4] and colleagues. His study of data from *Playboy* centerfolds and Miss America Pageant contestants from 1959 to 1978 indicated a shift toward a thinner ideal shape for women in our culture. The same study showed a significant increase in diet articles in popular women's magazines over the same period. They further demonstrated that American women during this time period were actually *increasing* in weight based on actuarial tables. A recent follow-up study[5] shows that the cultural ideal for women's body size has remained thin, and perhaps even thinner. The body size of recent Miss America contestants has decreased even more, and *Playboy* centerfolds' measurements have plateaued at a very low level. This "cultural index of the ideal woman's body" is now 13 percent to 19 percent below the expected weight for age and height, as determined by actuarial tables. Since a body weight below 15 percent of expected weight is one of the criteria for diagnosing anorexia nervosa, what does this say about our cultural "ideals"?

With extreme slimness as a cultural norm, it becomes clear why fear of fat, fad dieting, surgical fat removal, and eating disorders abound. When the overweight and obese evaluate themselves in society's mirror, they define themselves as unattractive and as failures. Such harsh evaluations are a result of an acceptance of society's distorted concept of the "ideal" body. Everyday advertisements suggest that we invest money, time, and hope into trying to reach this ideal. Unfortunately, the results are often feelings of guilt, despair, and inferiority.

Weight management begins with an acceptance of your personal body type, and a healthy perception of your body image. Your basic body build and frame size are genetically determined. That is why 140 pounds may look different on you than on someone else. Once you accept this, you can proceed with being the best you can be. Making wishful statements like . . . "If only I looked like that, life would be better" . . . takes away the energy that could be used to take charge of your life and improve *all* dimensions of wellness! The media and fashion industry need to take responsibility for using models who depict fitness and health, rather than emaciation. Some already have. With the popularity of fitness and wellness programs in our country, we hope the image is changing. The "one size fits all" standard must change.

Understanding Body Composition

Your body is composed of body fat and fat-free mass. **Fat-free mass** includes muscle, bone, body fluids, and organs. Muscles, which are part of your fat-free mass, are often specifically referred to as **lean-body mass** or **muscle mass. Body fat** is classified as either essential fat or storage fat. **Essential fat,** required for normal body functioning, is stored in major body organs and tissues such as the heart, muscles, intestines, bones, lungs, liver, spleen, kidneys, and throughout the central nervous system. Females have additional essential fat in the breasts and pelvic region for child-bearing and other hormone-related functions. **Storage fat** is the extra fat that accumulates in adipose cells (or fat cells) around internal organs and beneath the skin surface to insulate, pad, and protect the body from trauma and extreme cold. As you learned in chapter 4, there are different ways of assessing body composition. Knowing your body composition (especially your percentage of body fat) can help you set realistic weight goals.

Overweight versus Obesity

Too often the terms *overweight* and *obesity* are used interchangeably. **Overweight** refers to body weight greater than that which is normal.[6] "Normal" is most often thought of as an average weight for a specific height. The Metropolitan Life Insurance Company began publishing height-weight charts in the 1940s, listing desirable weight ranges for specific heights based on three classes of frame size. These charts, based on mortality rates of persons who purchased life insurance policies, have been widely distributed. Metropolitan regularly updates these charts. You have probably seen one of these charts in a physician's office or magazine, and looked to see where you rank. There has been considerable controversy and criticism over the appropriateness of these height-weight charts, since they do not take into account different shapes, skeletal sizes, or variances in muscle development. The frame sizes give too much latitude of choice, and non-Caucasians are underreported in these tables. Also, the mortality data for life insurance purposes does not necessarily correlate to a desirable weight for wellness, vitality, and quality of life.

A more suitable measure for assessing the relationship between weight and health risk is the **Body Mass Index (BMI),** as illustrated in figure 10.1. This nomogram helps you calculate your BMI, which is a ratio between weight and height. BMI is computed from the equation:

$$BMI = \frac{\textbf{weight in kilograms}}{\textbf{(height in meters)}^2}$$

Take a few seconds and determine your BMI. A reasonable weight goal is indicated with a ① on the center scale. A BMI of 20–25 is associated with the lowest risk of health problems for most people. Your health risk increases as your BMI

Figure 10.1

Nomogram for body mass index.

1983 Metropolitan Life Insurance Company Tables Courtesy, Statistical Bulletin, Metropolitan Life Insurance Company.

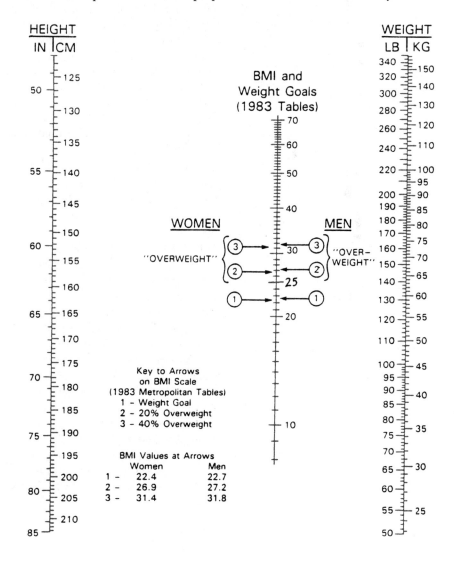

increases. A BMI of 25–27 may be associated with health problems for some people. This is the caution zone. A BMI over 27 is associated with increased risk of health problems such as heart disease, high blood pressure, and diabetes. A BMI *below* 20 may also be associated with health problems in some people. A disadvantage of using the BMI is that it remains a measure of weight and height, not fatness (i.e., it doesn't distinguish between body fat and muscle). The BMI should be used with caution as an *absolute* indicator of obesity. Nevertheless, it is regarded by the scientific community as a means to correlate health risks and body size, especially when more scientific measures are unavailable (see chapter 4).[7]

Understanding the difference between being overweight and obese is important. A weight scale can only measure how much you weigh, not how much fat you have. Standard height-weight tables do not assess your "fatness." An athlete may be considered overweight according to a height-weight chart but is actually very low in fat, due to muscular development. Overweight can also be a result of increased bone density or fluid. On the other extreme, a normal-weight, sedentary person may actually have too much fat. **Obesity** means an excessive accumulation of body fat.[8] We consider a woman to be obese if she is over 30 percent body fat. A man over 25 percent body fat is obese. A BMI above 27 is normally classified as obesity. At this level, the excess body fat becomes a chronic health threat. Since several medical problems are associated with being obese, rather than being overweight, it is important that you have an idea of your body fat percentage and your BMI, rather than just your weight.

Risks Associated with Obesity

Being a few pounds overweight poses no serious threat to long-term health. However, this is not true for obesity. Although women generally face more cultural pressure to be thin than men, obesity poses significant health threats for both men and women. In *Healthy People 2000*, obesity is identified as a risk factor in five of the 10 leading causes of death.[9] These major killers associated with obesity are: heart disease, some types of cancer, stroke, diabetes, and atherosclerosis. Obesity can aggravate high blood pressure, cardiovascular problems, liver disorders, and arthritis. Obesity is often found in conjunction with diabetes and gallbladder disease. Obesity complicates surgery and pregnancy. Pulmonary problems, heat intolerance, and reduced fertility are more prevalent in the obese. Among obese women there is an increased risk of endometrial and breast cancers. Obese men face an increased chance of colon, rectum, and prostate cancer. Obesity restricts mobility, increases fatigue, and decreases overall body efficiency.

Recent investigations even point to the location of excess fat as a risk factor. Fat distributed primarily in the abdominal area, (called "apple-shape" obesity) is characteristic of many men (but also present in some women). Apple-shape obesity increases the risk for hypertension, high cholesterol, diabetes, and breast cancer. Fat distributed in the lower extremities, around the hips, buttocks, and thighs (called "pear-shape" obesity), does not present as great a risk.[10] Pear-shape obesity is more common in women. The two types of fat have biochemical differences. Abdominal fat experiences much more enzyme activity, dumping more fatty acids into the bloodstream. Hip-thigh fat activity is more stagnant. Unfortunately, this hip-thigh fat is more difficult to lose than abdominal fat. Some obesity experts feel that one's waist-to-hip ratio is as important as the BMI in predictng potential weight-related health problems. Waist-to-hip ratio can be calculated by dividing the number of inches around the waistline by the circumference of the hips. For example, someone who has a 30-inch waist and 40-inch hips would have a ratio of .75. A woman whose ratio is .8 or higher is at risk, as is a man whose ratio is .95 or above. Whereas the distribution of fat has a strong genetic link, a comprehensive program of a low-fat, reduced-calorie diet and regular exercise can help reduce body fat stores, regardless of where they are located.

While obesity is known to decrease life expectancy, the psychological and social consequences of obesity are often overlooked. Obese people face a tremendous amount of prejudice and discrimination in our society. Their educational and professional opportunites often suffer. The stigma of obesity commonly results in anxiety, depression, and poor self-esteem.

What Causes Obesity?

For years the popular explanation for obesity was that people became obese simply because they ate too much. They were gluttons! Obesity was viewed as a condition resulting from a lack of self-control around food. Today, research points to obesity as a complex puzzle of metabolic, genetic, psychological, and environmental factors—not solely a lack of individual willpower. It is evident that no single factor results in obesity. In fact, obesity research is in its infancy. In an attempt to explain the causes of obesity, several factors have to be examined to understand the complexities of weight control. These include energy balance, fat cells, set point, heredity, metabolism, and the nutrient composition of food.

The Energy Balance Equation

The energy balance equation states that energy input (calories consumed) must be equal to energy output (calories expended) for body weight to remain constant. Any imbalance in energy input or energy output will result in a change in body weight. If you eat more calories daily than your body expends in activity, you will store the excesses as fat. If you eat fewer calories than you burn, you will lose weight. It is unrealistic to assume that the equation must be exactly equal everyday to maintain your weight. Some days you eat more; some days less. Some days you are more active than others. Obviously, several days of imbalance in one direction will produce a change in body weight.

This explanation assumes that "a calorie is a calorie." A **calorie** (actually a **kcal**) is a measure of energy. One pound of body fat equals 3,500 calories of stored energy. Therefore, consuming an extra 3,500 calories will cause you to gain one pound of fat. If you burn an extra 3,500 calories with activity, you will lose one pound. To cause a reduction in body weight you simply (1) reduce calorie intake below the energy requirement; (2) increase the calorie output through additional physical activity above energy requirements; or (3) combine the two methods by reducing calorie intake and increasing calorie output. So, how do you lose 10 pounds? By creating a calorie deficit of 500 calories daily (by either increasing exercise or decreasing food intake) for 7 days, you will lose 1 pound (3,500 calories). By maintaining this deficit, you will be 10 pounds lighter in 10 weeks.

However, weight loss is not necessarily this simple. For some, dieting causes feelings of fatigue, resulting in a decrease of energy expenditure. As body weight is reduced, the energy costs of movement go down proportionately, thus reducing caloric output. Also, individual differences in resting metabolic rates, cellular makeup, and lean tissue need to be considered. That is why knowledge about other factors is necessary to fully understand the complexities of weight loss.

Regardless of the problem of relying solely on the energy balance equation as the only way to understand weight loss and weight gain, it is the best way of explaining why, in this age of modernization and decreased physical demands, so many Americans are too fat. Most are not active enough to utilize the calories consumed! How many calories do you need to maintain a desirable body weight? Table 10.1 helps you estimate your daily caloric need based on your activity level. Remember, this is only an approximation and may vary between individuals. To lose or gain weight, the calorie intake must be adjusted upward or downward.

Table 10.1

Determining Your Daily Caloric Needs

Desirable weight × Activity level = Calories needed daily

Activity Level	Calories Needed per Pound per Day
Sedentary (most Americans, office job, light work)	13
Moderate Activity (weekend recreation)	15
Very Active (vigorous exercise 3 times per week)	16
Competitive Athlete	17+

Example: 140 lbs. (desirable weight) × 15 (moderate activity) = 2,100 calories

Fat Cells

The size and number of fat cells in the body determine degrees of fatness. **Fat cells** (also known as **adipose cells**) are storage sites for energy. The body increases fat storage in two ways: by increasing the number of fat cells, and by increasing the size of the fat cells. As expected, the body increases its number of fat cells during childhood and teenage growth spurts. Fat cells also expand and contract as energy is stored or burned. In fact, they can expand 2 to 3 times their normal size but cannot enlarge endlessly. At some point, new fat cells are created in response to the body's need to store more excess energy. Contrary to earlier theories, it is now well-accepted that increases in fat cell *number* can occur throughout adult life.[11] This capacity to increase cell numbers when a maximum cell size is reached depends on the age and sex of the person, as well as the site of the fat tissue.[12] Unfortunately, once a fat cell has been created, it exists for life. Fat cells do not seem to be destructible.

Therefore, the fat cell theory proposes that weight reduction in adults is a result of decreasing the size of the fat cells, shrinking them by using the energy stored in them, or not filling them at all. This theory also explains why people who grow a large number of fat cells during childhood have a predisposition to obesity as adults. They can reduce the amount of fat stored in the cells, but the excess number of fat cells is still there, waiting to be filled again.

Fat cells are with you forever.

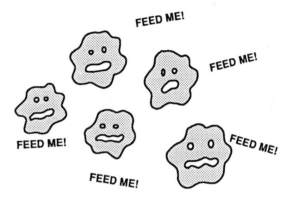

Knowing that obese children often become obese adults, it is easy to see one way to prevent obesity. Control the development of new fat cells during childhood and teenage years with regular exercise and sensible eating. This makes more sense than letting children become obese in the first place. This fact makes us question why daily physical education is being cut from most school programs. In this day and age, children need more daily exercise, not less!

When going on a low calorie diet, the adult with an excessive number of fat cells gets caught in a trap. A large number of empty fat cells is a biologically abnormal state. The body's natural tendency is to defend its fat cell size. As a result, the appetite control center in the brain is stimulated, causing the dieter to eat more calories. This condition of "starved fat cells" is the reason why most all dieters (especially in the obese category) eventually regain their lost weight. This is also the reason why obese people on treatment programs tend to stop losing weight when their fat cells shrink to "normal size".[13] In this way, obesity can become a lifelong condition. *Prevention* is the key!

Set Point Theory

The set point theory maintains that every individual is programmed to be a certain weight, and that the body regulates itself to maintain that "set" weight. Studies of people in alternating states of semi-starvation and gorging have shown that, once intervention ceases, they return to their former weights.[14] What determines your **set point**? The hypothalamus in the brain may act as a body weight thermostat, lowering body metabolism and increasing hunger if fat levels fall below the set point. Here is where the set point theory and fat cell theory merge. The set point mechanism is thought to respond to signals sent out by the fat cells as to the amount of fat in storage. The weight at which this occurs may depend on the number of fat cells. Consider two 200-pound women. Sara has a normal number of fat cells, which are enlarged. Mary has an excessive number of fat cells of normal size. Sara has a greater chance of weight loss, because she can reduce her cell size, and still sustain adequate fat volume. Mary faces a harder battle, because her body will work to maintain her cell size. This is another reason for not getting too many fat cells to begin with. This theory also helps explain why attempts at permanent weight loss by crash dieting are not successful. The body naturally fights against this starvation state.

The set point theory is based on survival. How else could populations endure famine, or our ancestors survive periods of food shortages? Heredity influences the set point, too. Some people have naturally higher set points, causing maintenance of higher levels of body fat. Some individuals have naturally low set points.

Can you change your set point? Some studies show that exposure to high-fat diets (a typical American diet?) actually raises the set point, and that regular, vigorous exercise can lower the set point.[15] Exercise stimulates changes in metabolism, thus causing the body to use fat, rather than protect against its losses.

Heredity

"I can't lose weight; it's in my genes!" Many would view this exclamation made by many obese persons as an excuse for their physical state. New research about genetic influences of obesity lends some (but not *total*) credibility to this exclamation. Children with obese parents do have a greater tendency to become obese adults.[16] Is this an inherited tendency or a result of inappropriate behaviors learned and reinforced at home? Studies of families (especially twins) have provided insights to this question. A classic study[17] conducted by Claude Bouchard showed that adult identical twins were similar in *total* fat gain and *distribution* of fat gain when consistently overfed for 100 days. There were huge differences between pairs of twins as to body weight gains, body composition changes, and waist/hip circumference changes. Within twins, however, there were striking similarities. Similar research[18] shows that adult twins tend to be similar in body weight and body mass index regardless of whether they were raised together in the same home or separated in early childhood and raised in different environments. These and other findings seem to validate the important role heredity has in obesity. Nevertheless, heredity is only a *tendency* or predisposing factor that can be influenced by environmental components and behaviors, unlike a genetic trait (like eye color) that cannot be changed.[19] Those people who are predisposed to be overweight or obese will have more difficulty controlling their weight, but it is certainly not impossible for them to attain and maintain a healthy weight.

Metabolism

Every individual expends a certain amount of energy, even at rest, to sustain the vital functions of the body. This energy requirement is called the **Basal Metabolic Rate (BMR)** and accounts for approximately 70 percent of calories burned in one day.[20] A true measure of basal (resting) metabolism is taken when you have been lying quietly, but awake, and without food for 12 to 15 hours. Most men have a BMR requirement of 1,600–1,800 calories daily; most women need 1,200–1,450 calories daily. Since BMR is such a large component of your daily energy expediture, it can significantly affect body weight over time. It is an important, yet highly individual factor in the development of obesity.

Your BMR is a result of several interrelated factors, including age, gender, body size, nutritional status, musculature, activity level, and genetics. Table 10.2 depicts how BMR is affected by each of these factors.

Table 10.2

Factors That Affect Basal Metabolic Rate

Age	BMR declines with age, attributed partially to physical inactivity, which results in less muscle mass and more fat.
Gender	Women generally have lower BMRs than men (about 5%–10% lower) due to smaller size, greater body fat, and less muscle mass.
Body size	Smaller body surface area results in lower BMR.
Nutritional status	Fasting, very low calorie diets, or long-term undernutrition lowers BMR.
Musculature	Increased muscle mass or tone increases BMR. Muscle tissue is more metabolically active than fat. As muscles atrophy from inactivity, BMR declines.
Activity level	BMR increases during exercise and may remain elevated somewhat after exercising.
Genetics	We all inherit physiological tendencies, and, as a result, BMR is inherently higher in some people and lower in others.

Some theorize that the obese have "sluggish" metabolisms. That is, they need fewer calories for normal body functions than the average person, and they turn food into energy very slowly.[21] While some of the obese may have some of the factors that cause a lower-than-normal metabolism, the crucial question remains: Are they fat because their metabolism is low, or is their metabolism low because they are fat? Fat, being storage tissue, is inactive and has a low metabolism, whereas muscle tissue is active and has a high metabolic rate.

Nutrient Composition

The energy balance equation approach to weight loss/gain is based on the premise that all calories are "created equal." That is, for weight loss, the *source* of calories is not important as long as the total calorie deficit is greater than the caloric intake. Recent findings report that total caloric intake is not correlated to obesity as much as dietary fat is![22] The premise is that "a calorie *is not* a calorie"! Some researchers have even narrowed the association between dietary fat and body fat specifically to saturated fat intake.[23] Why does this occur? Saturated fat is converted into body fat with greater ease than are carbohydrates. For every 100 carbohydrate calories consumed, 23 calories are burned up metabolizing it (i.e., converting it to a storable form), and about 77 calories are actually stored. In contrast, for every 100 fat calories consumed, only about 3 calories are used to convert it to storable form, leaving a whopping 97 calories available for body fat![24] (There *is* one predominently-carbohydrate substance that has been found to convert to body fat quite easily—alcohol![25] Alas—beer bellies!) Studies show that normal-weight and overweight persons may consume approximately the same number of calories, whereas the overweight persons derive a greater proportion of their calories from fat.[26] When fat intake is reduced and carbohydrate intake is not restricted, people can still lose weight—even when the total daily intake of calories is increased. Knowing this, isn't it absurd that most people's first attempt at losing weight is to go on a radical, restrictive diet?

What about Dieting?

Most people who want to lose weight think immediately of going on a diet. This notion is reinforced by the number of new fad diets advertised each year. These popular diets are viewed by the user as a temporary inconvenience that will be discontinued as soon as the weight goal has been reached. "Going on a diet" implies "going off" it. Dieters assume that weight will be lost quickly and immediately. Chances are, however, that the excess pounds have accumulated gradually over a period of years. These pounds are maintained by ingrained habits. Most fad diets rely on rigid food choices. Food becomes the enemy, and mealtime a battle to be fought. Practicing restraint can result in food cravings, binges, guilt, and feelings of self-deprecation. Most popular diets do not emphasize physical exercise. In fact, more than half of the overweight adults trying to lose weight are doing so by eating fewer calories. Less than one-third are increasing physical activity.[27] This is a reflection of our sedentary lifestyle, and the emphasis on "dieting" as a means to control weight. Diets have special appeal and sound so easy. Most of them, however, are nutritionally inadequate, too low in calories, and can be dangerous.

When you go on a very-low-calorie diet, up to 70 percent of the weight loss during the first three days is water.[28] This is predictable since your body prefers carbohydrates for energy. Being starved of carbohydrates, it uses **glycogen** (stored carbohydrates) for energy. As you use this glycogen, you lose water, since each gram of carbohydrate is stored with 3 grams of water. Your body also uses protein for energy, resulting in a loss of muscle tissue. Crash dieting can cause headaches, ketosis, and loss of bone mineralization. If you go on a very-low-calorie diet (less

The multitude of diet books can be confusing to the consumer

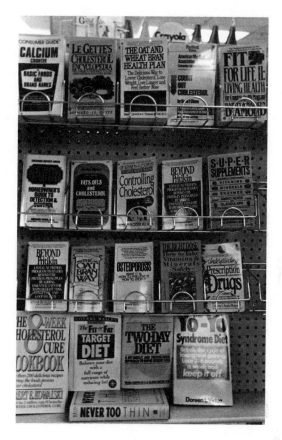

than 800 calories per day), your body slows its metabolism (BMR) significantly.[29] After all, your body doesn't know that there is a grocery store just a block away. It thinks you are dying from starvation! Therefore, your body saves energy by burning fewer calories. This conservation of energy causes the diet to be even less effective. Depression, irritability, fatigue, and feelings of deprivation often follow. The survival urge to eat eventually wins out and weight is regained. When this happens, the crash dieter may become fatter for five reasons:

1. If old eating habits are resumed, the regained weight is fat; some of the weight loss was most likely lean tissue.

2. Metabolism could remain slowed for months.

3. Overeating (especially a preference for dietary fat) may occur in response to the past deprivation.

4. More fat cells could develop as the existing cells fill to capacity and divide.

5. Metabolic alterations can occur (i.e., fat is stored more efficiently; the body conserves fat stores as a protective phenomenon against future losses).

Liquid Diets

In recent years, liquid diets and diet powders have become popular with millions of dieters. These diet drinks are used as replacements for several meals each day. Some physician- or hospital-supervised plans require that the entire diet be comprised of liquid replacements. Such a diet may provide all of the nutrients you need in a day (even fiber). However, a few problems can occur that may contribute to diet failure and weight regain:

1. It eliminates the need to make meal-planning decisions and choices. Diet re-education is fundamental to making weight management skills a permanent behavior.

2. It eliminates chewing, which is important for healthy teeth and gums.

3. It limits the real fiber (from fruit skins, vegetables, and grains) that your digestive system needs.

4. Unless a hospital or doctor supervises such a diet, side effects can occur: fatigue, nausea, dizziness, hair loss, constipation, dry skin, heart beat irregularities, and even death, if abused.

5. Do they work? About 95 percent of those who lose weight by such restrictive dieting regain it.

There is nothing in a liquid meal replacement that causes weight loss. It simply provides a measured amount of calories, plus some vitamins and minerals in an easy-to-fix form. Only for those morbidly obese people (with a BMI over 30), whose lives are in jeopardy because of their weight, may a strict hospital-monitored liquid diet program be justified.

Yo-Yo Syndrome

Fad dieting does not produce lasting results, and repeated bouts of dieting result in improved efficiency in the body's adaptive response to semistarvation. Since the body interprets drastic dieting as a mortal threat, basal metabolic rate slows as in an effort to maintain life. This metabolic response causes greater difficulty in losing weight and greater efficiency in gaining weight.[30] As a result, many obese people have repetitive cycles of weight loss and weight gain. This cycle is known as the "**yo-yo**" **syndrome** (also called **weight cycling**). In this cycle, fat is often lost slower and regained faster with each repeated dieting bout. Therefore, yo-yo dieting affords the body repeated opportunities to enhance its efficiency at storing energy—a function of fat cells. Yo-yo dieters also tend to regain their weight in the more risky abdominal location. Incessant dieting may actually be the reason why many Americans are fatter today than ever!

Weight cycling not only alters metabolic processes, it can be dangerous. A report based on a 32-year analysis of weight fluctuations in 3,130 men and women in the Framingham Heart Study has found that this gain-lose-gain cycle may be as risky as staying obese.[31] That is, individuals with a high weight variability are more likely to be victims of heart disease or premature death than those whose weight remains stable! This is not to say that weight loss is contraindicated. Millions of overweight people stand to benefit from loss of fat. However, since dieting is a major factor in body weight fluctuation (and since most diets don't work on a long-term basis), the yo-yo syndrome is a serious public health issue. In fact, even though nearly 50 percent of women who diet are not overweight, the weight cycling risks are seen at all weight categories— whether thin or obese.[32] These facts accentuate even more dramatically the need to learn *skills* for maintaining weight loss and to *prevent* obesity from occurring altogether.

Reliable Diet Programs

Are there any reliable weight loss plans? Yes. There are some very good programs available. Weight Watchers International, which has been in operation since 1963, is one example of a plan that is considered safe and effective. It is especially important for the morbidly obese to seek professional help in losing weight. These persons would be wise to consult one of the excellent hospital-based programs available in many communities. Since new fad diets appear almost weekly, and disappear almost as quickly, it is unrealistic to assess every particular diet for strengths and weaknesses. Instead, use the following guidelines in evaluating any weight loss plan:

1. It should use real, regular food available in supermarkets.

2. It should provide an energy deficit to allow slow, safe weight loss of 1 to 2 pounds per week.

3. It should encourage the reduction of fat in the diet.

4. It should teach lifelong changes that allow freedom and flexibility for individual lifestyles.

5. It should make possible the enjoyment of social situations such as eating out, holidays, and special occasions.

6. It should allow for basic energy needs (never under 1,200 calories daily) and be nutritionally balanced (the basic food groups, U.S. dietary guidelines, etc.).

7. It should not be too costly.

8. It should require exercise.

A final question to ask yourself when considering a diet plan should be, "Can I live on this diet for the rest of my life?"

The goal of weight loss is fat loss, which takes time and long-term lifestyle change. Many diets are variations on the food restriction theme, are unpleasant, and fail to teach modification of eating behavior. Just about any type of food restriction will result in weight loss. The key is keeping the weight off by learning to live with food.

Effective Weight Management

The factors that contribute to obesity are so numerous and complex that it is impossible to pinpoint one cause. Having knowledge of the theories of obesity should help you understand some of these complexities. Fat cells, metabolism, set points, genetics, and energy expenditure all play a role. Behaviors that have developed over a period of time are also intricately involved. One unrefuted truth emerges in nearly all weight control studies—*permanent weight control involves a lifelong commitment to good eating habits and regular exercise.* There is evidence that young adults in their early twenties gain a disproportionate amount of weight by the time they are thirty, making them an important population segment for obesity prevention efforts.[33] If you are in this age group, this fact should help motivate you to commit to a lifetime weight management plan. Weight management is a lifestyle. Rather than isolated bouts of crash dieting or sporadic exercise, maintaining a reasonable body composition is a result of lifelong integration of three components: (1) nutritional knowledge; (2) eating management (behavior modification); and (3) exercise.

Nutritional Knowledge

Dieters are notorious for trying faddish diet plans. Thus, it is essential to have a good framework for making sensible, well-balanced food choices. Basic weight management principles are not different from general good nutritional recommendations (low fat, sugar, salt, high complex carbohydrates, fiber). Simply cutting the fat from your diet reduces a tremendous number of calories. "I lost weight without eating less!" is often the exclamation of persons who substitute fiber-rich grains, fruits, and vegetables for fat in their diets. Being aware of caloric values of foods, the food groups, vitamin needs, sources of "hidden" fats, and energy needs can help you make sensible food choices. Cooking technique alone can cut many calories. And don't forget to read labels while shopping.

Eating is one of life's pleasures. Traditional diets often feature a lot of "can" and "cannot have" foods. This "all or nothing" approach to food contributes to binging, overeating, and other abnormal eating behaviors. Sensibility in food choices does not mean that you will never again eat chocolate cake. There should never be "guilt" or "forbidden" foods. Instead, lifetime weight management means seeing how much or where chocolate cake fits into your total diet. Reduce, don't eliminate certain foods. Balance your food choices over time. Control portions. Gradual, rather than drastic, changes in dietary patterns lead to successful maintenance. Healthful eating does not happen by accident. It is essential to learn about the nutritive value of foods and devise strategies for making good choices over the course of the day.

Eating Management

Why do you eat? "Because I am hungry!" you answer. If everyone ate only when they were in the physiological state of hunger, very few would have a weight problem. We are surrounded with opportunites to eat more than we need to. Eating behavior is strongly influenced by psychological, social, and emotional factors. Controlling eating habits begins with having an understanding of why you eat and what antecedents trigger eating. Do you eat when you are bored? Lonely? Angry? Stressed? Do you eat when you turn on the television? Read? Do you eat when something smells good? When others are eating? When you want to please Aunt Margaret? As discussed in chapter 1, keeping records for a few days may help you identify the antecedents that trigger a behavior—in this case, eating. You will find at the end of this book a sample eating diary that you may want to use to understand your personal eating behavior.

Eating habits can be changed by behavior modification techniques. **Behavior modification** is based on the premise that all behaviors are learned responses to environmental cues or antecedents. In using these techniques, eating becomes a more conscious act, and healthier behavior patterns are integrated into the day-to-day routine. These include slowing the act of eating, altering susceptibility to the cues (e.g., separating eating from other activities, such as watching TV), and breaking behavior chains. Table 10.3 gives examples of some behavior modification techniques.

Table 10.3
Behavior Modification Techniques

1. Keep an eating diary to maximize awareness of eating.
2. Eat in one room only; sit at a table—don't stand.
3. Make eating a ritual.
4. Keep a weight graph.
5. Never read or watch TV while eating.
6. Use smaller plates.
7. Always leave some food on your plate.
8. Drink a lot of water throughout the day and during meals.
9. Prepare, serve, and eat one portion at a time.
10. Do not place serving dishes on the table.
11. Grocery shop from a list and never on an empty stomach.
12. Leave the table after eating and clear dishes directly into the garbage; brush teeth immediately or chew gum.
13. Keep problem food out of sight or not in the house at all.
14. Keep healthy food accessible and visible.
15. Eat slowly; chew each bite thoroughly; put utensils down between bites; eat with nondominant hand; cut food into smaller pieces.
16. Rehearse strategies in advance for eating out, special occasions, and high-risk situations.
17. Substitute alternative activities for eating (write a letter; go for a walk; jog; pay bills; sew; play tennis; etc.).

Changing eating behavior demands commitment and perseverence (unlike the "easy" and "simple" pitch delivered by many popular women's magazines). In order to continue with or maintain a weight loss, you must be able to identify your own high-risk situations where difficulties with feelings or social situations threaten a relapse. Developing and practicing coping strategies for dealing with these situations is an essential part of eating management. And, very importantly, behavior change in regard to eating management works best when you are reinforced by social support—family, friends, dietitians, community, and weight-loss groups.[34]

Exercise

Most obese individuals do not consume significantly greater amounts of food than nonobese individuals.[35] Some even say that we eat less food than Americans did in the 1900s. Are you surprised? Yet we have gotten fatter because calorie output has declined drastically. Our diet hasn't changed as much as our exercise habits! Television viewing, which substantially decreases activity levels and may influence diet, is a strong factor in obesity.[36] Computers, video games, and VCRs have further decreased overall activity levels. American technology has been ingenious in discovering ways for us to save energy, thus throwing off our energy balance. Electric garage door openers, riding lawn mowers, electric toothbrushes, and drive-in banks are just a few examples of "activity-robbing" conveniences.

The secret to lifelong weight management is exercise, not dieting! Exercise is one of the few factors positively correlated with long-term weight maintenance.[37] A year-long study[38] of overweight men and women compared body weight losses between 2 groups: those who dieted only; and those who combined diet with exercise (brisk walking/jogging three times per week for 25–45 minutes). The "diet-plus-exercise" group increased loss of body fat, especially in the dangerous abdominal fat area. Regular, aerobic exercise contributes to fat loss in several ways.

It Burns Calories   Table 10.4 shows how many calories you burn per minute in various activities. Note that the larger person burns more energy than the lighter person engaged in the same activity. Also notice how aerobic activities burn considerably more calories per minute than light, day-to-day tasks. Most people burn approximately 100 calories per mile whether walking or jogging. If this does not seem like a lot, look at it this way: You only burn about 1 calorie per minute while sitting. Remember that weight gain does not occur overnight; nor does weight loss. A pound of fat is lost by burning 3,500 calories. No one ever said it must all be done at once, and only by jogging. Find ways to weave increased energy expenditure into day-to-day living: walk to work, take stairs instead of elevators, ride a bike on errands, etc.

There is some controversy as to whether exercise increases postexercise basal metabolic rate.[39] If there is some slight increase in metabolism after exercise, the total effect on energy balance is minimal. The greatest benefits of exercise in weight control are in the calories burned in the actual exercise and the positive effects it has on maintaining lean body mass.

It Prevents Loss of Lean Body Mass (Muscle Mass)   Aerobic exercise enhances the burning of body fat. It also tend to build muscle tissue. Since muscle cells are metabolically active, they burn more calories in basal metabolism than fat cells.

It Is a Natural Appetite Suppressor   Moderate exercise has a tendency to decrease the appetite for a period of time after the workout because blood is diverted from digestive organs to skeletal muscles. You may feel thirsty, but not

Table 10.4

Caloric Expenditure Per Minute for Various Activities

Source: From Physiological Measurement of Metabolic Functions in Man. *C. Frank Consolazio, Robert E. Johnson, and Louis J. Pecora, pp. 331–332. Copyright 1963 McGraw-Hill Book Company. Reprinted by permission of the publisher.*

Body Weight	117	143	170	196
Sitting, quietly reading	.9	1.1	1.4	1.6
Driving a car	1.8	2.1	2.6	2.9
Household tasks (dusting, sweeping)	2.3	2.9	3.4	3.9
Showering	2.7	3.3	3.9	4.5
Basketball (moderate)	5.5	6.7	7.9	9.2
Bicycling (4.6-min./mile, 13 mph)	8.3	10.2	12.1	14.0
Dance (aerobic-medium)	6.2	7.0	7.8	9.0
Dance (waltz)	4.0	4.9	5.8	6.7
Golf (foursome)	3.2	3.9	4.6	5.3
Racquetball	7.6	9.3	11.0	12.7
Running (8.5-min./mile, 7 mph)	10.8	13.3	15.7	18.2
Swimming (crawl, 50-yds./min.)	8.3	10.1	12.0	13.9
Tennis (recreation)	5.4	6.6	7.8	9.0
Volleyball (moderate)	4.4	5.4	6.4	7.4
Walking (13.3-min./mile, 4.5 mph)	5.1	6.3	7.5	8.6
Weight training	6.2	7.5	8.9	10.3

usually hungry. This is why exercising during a lunch break helps you control weight. After exercising, you feel satisfied with a light lunch. Extremely intense exercise tends to lower blood sugar, which stimulates appetite. So, to burn fat, keep your exercise at a moderate intensity, and work to increase the duration. (Be sure not to view exercise as an excuse for eating more!)

It May Lower Your Set Point   The set point theorists believe that regular, vigorous exercise is the one sure way to lower your body's fat level. Maintaining an active lifestyle stabilizes the set point at this lower level.

It Promotes the Maintenance of Weight Loss   Most health professionals agree that losing weight is easy; keeping it off is much more difficult. To avoid the negative consequences of weight cycling, much more attention is being given to *maintenance* of weight loss. Exercise has been shown to be one of the few factors correlated with long-term weight maintenance.[40] A change in lifestyle that includes a consistent exercise regimen across the life span is the fundamental key to successful weight-loss maintenance.

Other Ways Exercise Helps with Weight Management   For overweight, sedentary individuals, exercise may not be a richly reinforcing experience at first. It may be difficult to get out and exercise in public. They may feel self-conscious about their bodies. They may have negative feelings about exercise because of past embarrassing experiences. As exercise becomes a satisfying habit, the individual begins to experience a new sense of well-being and power. Anxiety and depression are reduced. As weight comes off, self-image is enhanced. Self-esteem and self-confidence are improved. These psychological benefits received from regular participation in physical activity are often the additional impetus necessary for adhering to a weight loss/maintenance program. This positive self-concept helps reinforce all other areas of weight management, including food selection, reduced anxiety, and feelings of control.

Commonly Asked Questions about Weight Control

Q. I have seen a lot of advertisements from health salons promoting effortless exercise machines for weight loss. Do they work?

A. Because many people do not understand the basic principles of fat metabolism, they fall prey to the appeal of these ads. After all, they say you don't have to sweat or even change clothes! It takes only minutes! Roller machines, oscillating tables, electrical muscle stimulators, and power-driven vibrators are promoted as equipment that removes fat or breaks up fatty deposits. These devices are worthless gimmicks. They have no value in reducing fat because of the lack of effort on the part of the participant. Remember, fat loss is a result of burning more calories than you consume. Since these machines are doing the work, few calories are burned. Using active machines such as stationary bicycles, rowing machines, stair climbers, and cross country skiing machines are effective ways to burn calories, because *you* exert energy.

Q. What about body wraps, rubberized suits, and other special weight-reducing apparel? I've worn some of these and they seem to work.

A. Waist belts or body wraps do nothing more than squeeze water out of one tissue area into another. Think about the indentation that occurs on your wrist after wearing a rubber band there for several minutes. This circumference loss is only temporary until rehydration occurs. Rubberized or vinyl suits can be dangerous, especially if worn while exercising. These suits trap the heat and perspiration given off by the body, not allowing the natural process of evaporation—the body's normal cooling process. It is like a turkey basting in its own juices! Water, not fat, is lost by the body, and the danger of life-threatening overheating is possible. Again, as soon as the body is rehydrated, weight is regained.

Weight loss gimmicks reduce your wallet, not your waist

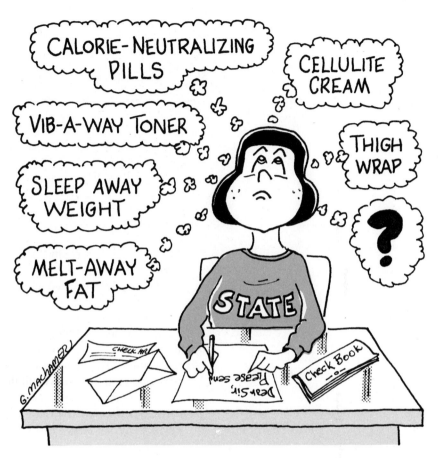

Q. *I see a lot of weight-loss pills and candies in the drug stores and available by mail-order. Are they effective?*

A. Over-the-counter products are promoted to do everything from curb the appetite to magically melt away fat. If you purchase these gimmicks, you are looking for the "quick fix," not a lifestyle change. Those desperate to lose weight are often easy prey for drugs and products that promise the metabolically impossible. The side effects (nervousness, sleeplessness, irritability) make such products a questionable lifetime weight management program. Many manufacturers of these products recommend adherence to a diet while taking their product. (Of course, this is usually in small print and is probably the real cause of any short-term weight loss that takes place!)

Q. *I have cellulite on my thighs. Is there any special way to remove it?*

A. There is no such thing as **cellulite.** It is a slang term used to describe the dimpled fat found primarily on the buttocks and thighs of women. Concentrated areas of fat tend to bulge in some women because with age their connective fibers are taut and their skin thin. This fat is like any other fat, in that only a comprehensive program of exercise and calorie reduction will remove it. No miracle creams, saunas, diets, or devices specifically break up cellulite. Buying a product that claims to do this only reduces your wallet!

Q. *The only place I feel I have too much fat is on my abdomen. Is there any way to just lose fat there?*

A. The concept of "spot reduction" (that is, selectively burning off fat from a particular body area) is a myth. No one can dictate where body fat will accumulate or be removed. Genetics determine your body build and preferred fat storage sites. Exercising a specific body area does not burn fat in just that area. Fat stores from throughout the body are mobilized during exercise. So, your abdomen will lose fat only after a combined program of total-body aerobic exercise and calorie management, not solely by doing 100 curl-ups a day. It is possible to "spot tone," however. Those 100 curl-ups create very strong abdominals!

Q. *I have read that eating grapefruit with other foods burns excess fat. Is this true?*

A. There is no magic food combination that specifically burns fat, just as there is no "negative-calorie" food (that is, food that burns more calories than it contains).

Q. *My friend had his stomach stapled and lost a considerable amount of weight. What about this and other surgical treatments of obesity?*

A. Surgery for obesity should not be taken lightly and should be considered only as a last resort for the morbidly obese (those at least 100 pounds above ideal weight). Even the nonsurgical means of jaw-wiring and inserting balloons in the stomach are drastic measures in tackling obesity. As with any major medical procedure, these methods have inherent risks and medical complications. Also, their long-term effectiveness is questionable, unless a drastic lifestyle change accompanies the procedure. **Liposuction** (suctioning fat from under the skin) has become popular as a method of removing body fat from selected body parts. This surgical procedure, performed by physicians who specialize in cosmetic surgery, is another questionable approach to weight loss.

Q. *I am heavily involved in competitive sports. As a result, I am very muscular. When I stop competing, how do I avoid having all of that muscle turn into fat?*

A. Your concern is fueled by a common misconception. Muscle can no more turn into fat than a cat can turn into a dog. The reverse is also true. Fat cannot become muscle. The cellular makeup of each is totally different. If you stop activity altogether, your muscles will atrophy and lose tone. Calories not needed to fuel your body will be stored as fat. To avoid this, continue some regular exercise and modify your calorie consumption, being sure your energy input and output are relatively equal.

Q. *Most of my friends talk about wanting to lose weight. But I want to gain some weight. How do I do it?*

A. First of all, realize that body build is genetic. Some people are built like greyhounds, some like German shepherds! Once you assess your body type and potential, engage in weight training and a general exercise program to increase your muscle density. You do not want to put on excess fat by indiscriminately eating more food. Protein drinks are not the answer; nor are high fat and sugar snacks. Do make sure you increase your calorie intake some to compensate for the energy burned while exercising, but make healthy food choices. Complex carbohydrates are best. Ways to healthfully increase your caloric intake include these:

- Replace sodas with fruit juices.
- Replace cookies, and doughnuts with nuts, raisins, bran muffins, yogurt, milk, and fruit.
- Replace hamburgers and fries with thick-crust vegetable-topped pizza.
- Prepare hot cereals with milk instead of water; add nuts, peanut butter, fruit, wheat germ.
- Top cold cereal with bananas, raisins, etc.
- Eat hearty soups.
- Add garbanzo beans, seeds, tuna, croutons, cottage cheese, lean meat to salads.

Q. *I am concerned because my sister is very much overweight. She doesn't act like it bothers her, but I think it does. What can I do to motivate her to lose weight?*

A. Often we have relatives or friends who have health-robbing habits (smoke, overweight, nonexerciser, etc.). Because we care about them, it is natural to want to help. In the case of your sister, do not nag or criticize her. Instead, set a good example, and talk about why you do the things you do (select certain foods, behavior modification tricks, etc.). Try to include her in your practices. Invite her to go on a walk, bike riding, or to an aerobics class. Grocery shop or eat out together. Share recipes and food preparation ideas. Show that you care. Make a pact with her (you will try to stop biting your fingernails, while she tries to lose weight). Be there for her. However, realize that she is ultimately responsible for herself. Nevertheless, be her friend, confidante, and number one cheerleader.

Q. *I have heard that I will burn more fat if I work out at the lower end of my target heart rate range rather than at a high intensity. Is this true?*

A. This low-intensity fat-burning idea is a misunderstanding based on an oversimplification. It is true that the higher the exercise intensity, the more the body prefers to use glycogen rather than fat for fuel. Some have interpreted this to mean that to burn fat, low-intensity exercise is best. However, the type of fuel used during exercise does not make a great deal of difference. The most important exercise variable is *total* caloric expediture. Because you don't fatigue as quickly when exercising at a low intensity, you may be able to work out for a longer period of time and feel more comfortable while doing it.

Eating Disorders

We live in a society obsessed with thinness. In our culture, thin signifies power, success, and control. This indoctrination begins early in life, and the hundreds of hours we spend in front of the television, at the movies, and looking through magazines drives home the message. The famous, the glamourous, and the models are thin. Every day we see flat stomachs, perfect breasts, flawless teeth, narrow waists, and unblemished complexions. Our culture especially socializes girls to be concerned about their physical appearance. Females have a tendency to define their worth in relation to what they perceive others think about them. For them, thinness equates with attractiveness and social approval. The message is "Work hard in school, but be popular and pretty." On the contrary, a male's self-concept is linked to physical dominance and sports competence. Most adolescent boys desire to be bigger and stronger. Studies have shown that females consistently desire to weigh less than their ideal body weight, whereas males do not.[41]

For adolescents, self-esteem is often determined by body image. **Body image** is the mental picture a person has of his or her body, and the associated attitudes and feelings toward it. This image is not necessarily consistent with actual physical appearance. The changes of puberty bring more fat stores to the average girl. As this new physical self meets the mental self, a negative body image may result. More fat is natural and normal to the adolescent female, but it opposes what she thinks everyone prefers! Feeling these pressures, women often compare themselves to a norm of unrealistic thinness. Since few measure up to the fashion industry's ideal, dieting is commonplace. At the same time obesity is dramatically rising among children in our country, thin 9-year-olds are dieting and fretting about their weight! The dilemma of preventing obesity, yet avoiding a fostering of "thin mania" presents a tremendous challenge.

The frequency of dieting among teenage girls is alarming. In some cases dieting is carried to such an extreme that the behavior becomes obsessive. Fear of fat, fad dieting, and a distorted body image can lead to a psychological eating disorder. An **eating disorder** is defined as "a disturbance in eating behavior that jeopardizes a person's physical or psychosocial health."[42] You should bear in mind that preoccupation with weight and dieting are not synonymous with an eating disorder. An eating disorder is an extremely serious psychopathological state. Eating disorders are now viewed as multidimensional in cause and nature: psychiatric, physiological, and social. Thus, the treatment must include all components. Certain populations are especially at risk for developing eating disorders. These include gymnasts, dancers (especially ballet), cheerleaders, pom-pom performers, distance runners, and models. Even though more women than men suffer from eating disorders, there is a higher than normal incidence of eating disorders in certain subgroups of males where slenderness is encouraged: models, dancers, wrestlers, and long distance runners.

High school and college-age students are vulnerable due to academic and social stresses, as well as peer pressure to conform. Rather than a strict addiction, eating disorders are a response to our societal influences, dieting culture, fat discrimination, over-achieving perfectionism, and media's images. Two of the most common eating disorders are bulimia and anorexia nervosa. They may occur separately or together.

Bulimia Nervosa

Bulimia is a Greek word meaning "ox" and "hunger." The disorder was so named because the sufferer eats like a hungry ox. That is, bulimia is characterized by a compulsive need to eat large quantities of food (binging) to the point of gorging, followed by purging through vomiting, use of laxatives, or fasting. Often the binge is a response to an intense emotional experience, such as stress, loneliness, or depression rather than the result of a strong appetite. Nevertheless, most bulimics are not aware of what precipitates these uncontrollable binges, nor are they able to stop them. The diagnostic criteria for bulimia is:[43]

1. Recurrent episodes of binge eating, i.e., rapid consumption of a large amount of food in a discrete period of time.

2. A feeling of lack of control over eating behavior during the eating binges.

3. Self-induced vomiting, use of laxatives or diuretics, strict dieting or fasting, or vigorous exercise in order to prevent a weight gain.

4. Persistent overconcern with body shape and weight.

5. Two binge episodes a week for at least 3 months.

Bulimia is the most common eating disorder. Some surveys suggest the prevalence of bulimia to be as high as 19 percent in college-age women and 5 percent in college-age men.[44]

Bulimia frequently starts as normal, voluntary dieting behavior, which later becomes compulsive, uncontrollable, and pathological. The bulimic's eating binge involves a rapid gulping down of enormous quantities of food. Preferred foods are high in calories, sweet tasting, and can be eaten rapidly without preparation—ice cream, cookies, candy, bread, cheese, chips, doughnuts. The consumption of this food is not a pleasurable pastime, but a compulsion. Up to 20,000 calories can be consumed in one sitting, followed by abdominal pain and discomfort. The binge generates guilt, depression, and anxiety. Purging follows, reducing the anxiety and fear. Then the cycle begins again.

The bulimic is aware of her abnormal behavior and has great fear of not being able to stop. She has feelings of guilt and shame about her behavior. Bulimia is a secret habit and can continue for many years undetected. The weight of most bulimics is normal, or fluctuates within 10 pounds, as a result of the binge-purge cycle.

The physical effects of bulimia include electrolyte imbalance (especially potassium), low blood sugar, esophageal lacerations, dehydration, and nerve and liver damage from low potassium. Tooth enamel is eroded by the stomach acid brought up with vomiting. Severe abdominal pain is common. In rare cases, actual rupture of the stomach has occurred. Bone density is lost if the disorder continues for many years.

People with bulimia need professional help and are often tearful and desperate when they finally seek help. Psychotherapy is necessary to understand the underlying cause of the disorder, as well as to help reshape the bulimic's feelings of self-worth and self-confidence. Bulimics tend to be extroverted perfectionists—high achievers—and are often academically or vocationally successful. Yet, bulimics have troubled interpersonal relationships, low self-esteem, poor impulse control, high levels of anxiety and depression, and are self-critical and sensitive to rejection. It is not uncommon to see other impulsive behaviors among bulimics, including kleptomania, alcohol and drug use, and sexual promiscuity.[45] The treatment goal is to get the bulimic to cope with her stresses and body image insecurities through less destructive ways, and to feel more comfortable with herself in today's world. Bulimia is difficult to cure, and some struggle with this disorder for life.

Anorexia Nervosa

Far less common than bulimia, **anorexia nervosa** is a psychological disorder in which self-inflicted starvation leads to a drastic loss of weight. Whereas the bulimic has a general dissatisfaction with her body weight, the anorexic is obsessed with achieving thinness. Individuals with anorexia nervosa have an iron determination to become thin and an intense, irrational fear of becoming fat. They vehemently deny their impulse to eat, their appetite, and their enjoyment of food. The term "anorexia" is actually a misnomer, because loss of appetite is usually rare until late in the illness. While bulimics feel shameful about their abnormal behavior, anorexics justify their weight loss efforts.

Found primarily in early and middle adolescent females, anorexia may result in physical deterioration to the point of hospitalization, or even death. Anorexia carries a 19:1 female-to-male ratio with a prevalence estimated at 1 percent among adolescent girls.[46] The diagnostic criteria for anorexia is:[47]

1. Refusal to maintain body weight over a minimal normal weight for age and height, e.g., weight loss leading to body weight 15 percent below that expected.

2. Intense fear of weight gain or becoming fat even though underweight.

3. A disturbance in the way in which one's shape and weight is experienced.

4. In females, amenorrhea for at least 3 consecutive cycles.

Anorexia often starts as innocent dieting that turns into irrational behavior characterized by severe caloric restriction, fasting, relentless exercising, diuretic and laxative use, and, in some cases, self-induced vomiting. The anorexic pursues and maintains thinness despite an emaciated appearance that is so apparent to others.

Anorexics display an extraordinary amount of energy directed to exercise and school work in spite of the starvation state. However, they avoid social relationships, have a low self-esteem, and are fearful of change. Despite an aversion for eating, the anorexic is preoccupied with food. She may prepare elaborate meals for others, collect recipes, carry or hide snacks, and memorize the caloric content of various foods. Bizarre eating habits are commonplace. One anorexic cut a raisin in two and chewed each half for five minutes. In many situations they may pretend to be eating but are actually putting food into their napkin or feeding the dog under the table.

Family stress and social pressure contribute to this disorder. Most anorexics come from middle to upper class families that place a high premium on achievement, perfection, and physical appearance. Their families are often overcontrolling and overprotective. Anorexics exhibit extreme perfectionism accompanied by a profound sense of ineffectiveness. Only by restricting food intake do they feel a sense of control and a means of coping with life's stresses.

Anorexia causes the physiological complications that accompany any malnutritive state: chronic fatigue, skin becomes dry and scaly, hair falls out, menstruation ceases, blood pressure drops, and cardiac complications occur. Constipation is commonplace. Bone growth is retarded, increasing the risk of fractures and osteoporosis. Anorexics have an unusual sensitivity to cold due to their low body-fat percentage.

Treatment for anorexia nervosa involves medical, psychological, and nutritional help. The major obstacle to treatment is the patient's denial that any problem exists. The entire family must be involved, since the anorexic's behavior has deep psychological origin—low self-esteem, struggle for control and independence, and fear of physical sexual development.

What Can Be Done?

The risk factors for bulimia and anorexia nervosa are similar in many ways, that is, female gender, ambiguity in sex roles for women, and sociocultural emphasis on thinness. Since both eating disorders appear to be increasing in incidence, implementation of prevention programs is desperately needed. The most obvious and effective site for prevention is in the schools. However, all segments of society need to absorb some of the responsibility, including parents, coaches, advertising executives, the media, and the entertainment business. Society needs to send the message of healthy acceptance of self and body. Not everyone is meant to be a size 6!

If you suspect a friend, roommate, or relative of having an eating disorder, you probably wonder what you can do to help. Eating disorders are not solely about food and eating but are manifestations of emotional distress. Therefore, just begging someone to "start eating" or "put on some weight" is futile. Also, ignoring the situation, or "waiting to see what happens" will not solve the problem.

The first step to recovery is indisputable—locate professional help as soon as possible! Congress has mandated that every state establish a system of community mental health centers to assist people with a variety of psychological problems. These centers are a good source for providing treatment or helping you locate professionals who specialize in treating eating disorders. Even though psychotherapy has become more prevalent and accepted in the last 25 years, some still avoid it. For whatever reason, psychotherapy still carries a stigma with some people.

Since your anorexic or bulimic acquaintance may deny her condition or balk at your suggestion for help, it may be very difficult to pursuade her to seek help. However, both physical and psychological evaluation are crucial at the onset of treatment. You cannot force someone to get help. It is important, however, to be direct and honest with them while showing sincere concern and support. You may have to be tough, even make the appointment, and insist on accompanying them to see the specialist.

Other Sources of Help:

American Anorexia/Bulimia Association
418 East 76th Street
New York, NY 10021
(212) 734–1114

Anorexia Nervosa and Related Eating Disorders
P.O. Box 5102
Eugene, OR 97405
(503) 344–1144

National Association of Anorexia Nervosa and Associated Disorders
P.O. Box 2771
Highland Park, IL 60035
(708) 831–3438

The National Anorectic Aid Society
1925 East Dublin-Granville Road
Columbus, OH 43229
(614) 436–1112

Summary

Obesity is a complex disorder. No longer is it considered just a problem of overeating or lack of willpower. It is caused by a multiple number of factors—some within your control and some beyond. Genetics, environment, and culture combine to complicate the simple act of nourishing our bodies. It is important to understand body composition and be able to differentiate between overweight and obesity. Since many health problems are associated with obesity, concern with weight control should begin sufficiently early in life to reduce the risk of developing obesity. Prevention is the "treatment" of choice. The factors affecting obesity give insight into the complexities of losing excess body fat.

"Monday I start my diet" is far too often the cry as the way to lose weight. This "diet mentality" has actually contributed to the obesity problem. Dieting and concerns about appearance have also contributed to the increasing incidence of eating disorders. Effective weight management involves nutritional knowledge, behavior management, and exercise. Whereas dieting is temporary, restrictive, and negative, lifestyle weight management is a positive, flexible means of dealing with food for life and health. It is a lifestyle of healthy eating and regular exercise, amidst established cultural patterns and social and economic forces. No gimmick or gadget can replace this lifestyle approach.

Regular exercise is the key ingredient in maintaining a healthy body composition. Technological advances have increased the quality of our lives in many ways but have eliminated much daily physical exertion. It is a challenge to find ways to fit activity into your life. However, lifelong weight management and total wellness depend on it. Only when we start considering food as fuel and accepting a range of healthy body weights will obesity begin to be eradicated.

References

1. "Recession Hits Weight Loss Industry." *Obesity & Health* 6 (January/February 1992): 8.

2. "Issues in Weight Control." *Journal of the American Dietetic Association* (supplement) 92 (January 1992): 17–22.

3. "Issues in Weight Control."

4. Garner, David, Paul Garfinkel, Donald Schwartz, and Michael Thompson. "Cultural Expectations of Thinness in Women." *Psychological Reports* 47 (October 1980): 483–91.

5. Wiseman, Claire V., James J. Gray, James E. Mosimann, and Anthony H. Ahrens. "Cultural Expectations of Thinness in Women: An Update." *International Journal of Eating Disorders* 11 (January 1992): 85–89.

6. Williams, Melvin H. *Nutrition for Fitness and Sport*, 3rd ed. Dubuque, IA: Wm. C. Brown Publishers, 1992.

7. "Body Mass Index Makes Comparisons Easier." *Obesity & Health* 5 (January/February 1991): 8.

8. Williams. *Nutrition for Fitness and Sport*.

9. Department of Health and Human Services, Public Health Service. *Healthy People 2000: National Health Promotion and Disease Prevention Objectives*. Washington DC: Department of Health and Human Services, 1990.

10. Stamford, Bryant. "Apples and Pears: Where You 'Wear' Your Fat Can Affect Your Health." *The Physician and Sportsmedicine* 19 (January 1991): 123–24.

11. "'Unhappy' Fat Cell Seeks Balance." *Obesity & Health* 6 (March/April 1992): 25.

12. "'Unhappy' Fat Cell Seeks Balance."

13. "'Unhappy' Fat Cell Seeks Balance."

14. Keesey, Richard E. "A Set-Point Theory of Obesity." *Handbook of Eating Disorders*. Edited by Kelly D. Brownell and John P. Foreyt, 63–87. New York: Basic Books, 1986.

15. Keesey. "A Set-Point Theory of Obesity."

16. "What Causes Obesity." *Reebok Instructor News* 5 (Winter 1992): 4–5.

17. Bouchard, Claude et al. "The Response to Long-Term Overfeeding in Identical Twins." *The New England Journal of Medicine* 322 (May 24, 1990): 1477–82.

18. Stunkard, Albert J., Jennifer R. Harris, Nancy L. Pedersen, and Gerald E. McClearn. "The Body-Mass Index of Twins Who Have Been Reared Apart." *The New England Journal of Medicine* 322 (May 24, 1990): 1483–87.

19. "Issues in Weight Control."

20. "What Causes Obesity."

21. National Dairy Council. *Weight Management.* Rosemont, IL, 1988.

22. Dattilo, Anne M. "Dietary Fat and Its Relationship to Body Weight." *Nutrition Today* 27 (January/February 1992): 13–19.

23. Dattilo. "Dietary Fat and Its Relationship to Body Weight."

24. Hands, Elizabeth S. *Food Finder*, 3rd ed. Salem, OR: ESHA Research, 1990.

25. Suter, Paolo M., Yves Schutz, and Eric Jequier. "The Effect of Ethanol on Fat Storage in Healthy Subjects." *The New England Journal of Medicine* 326 (April 9, 1992): 983–87.

26. "Issues in Weight Control."

27. "Weight-Loss Regimens Among Overweight Adults." *The Journal of the American Medical Association* 262 (September 1, 1989): 1163, 1167.

28. Williams. *Nutrition for Fitness and Sport.*

29. Williams. *Nutrition for Fitness and Sport.*

30. Goodrick, G. Kenneth, and John P. Foreyt. "Why Treatments for Obesity Don't Last." *Journal of the American Dietetic Association* 91 (October 1991): 1243–47.

31. Lissner, Lauren, Patricia M. Odell, Ralph B. D'Agnostino, Joseph Stokes III, Bernard E. Kreger, Albert J. Belanger, and Kelly D. Brownell. "Validity of Body Weight and Health Outcomes in the Framingham Population." *The New England Journal of Medicine* 324 (June 27, 1991): 1839–44.

32. Berg, Frances. "Yo-Yo Dieting Threatens Heart." *Obesity & Health* 5 (November/December 1991): 93–94.

33. King, Abby C., and Diane L. Tribble. "The Role of Exercise in Weight Regulation in Nonathletes." *Sports Medicine* 11 (May 1991): 331–49.

34. "Why Treatments for Obesity Don't Last."

35. King, and Tribble. "The Role of Exercise in Weight Regulation in Nonathletes."

36. Gortmaker, Steven L., William H. Dietz Jr., and Lilian W. Y. Cheung. "Inactivity, Diet, and the Fattening of America." *Journal of the American Dietetic Association* 90 (September 1990): 1247–55.

37. King, and Tribble. "The Role of Exercise in Weight Regulation in Nonathletes."

38. Wood, Peter D., Marcia L. Stefanick, Paul T. Williams, and William L. Haskell. "The Effects on Plasma Lipoproteins of a Prudent Weight-Reducing Diet, With or Without Exercise, In Overweight Men and Women." *The New England Journal of Medicine* 325 (August 15, 1991): 461–66.

39. Poehlman, Eric T., Christopher L. Melby, and Michael I. Goran. "The Impact of Exercise and Diet Restriction on Daily Energy Expenditure." *Sports Medicine* 11 (February 1991): 78–101.

40. King and Tribble. "The Role of Exercise in Weight Regulation in Nonathletes."

41. "Body-Weight Perceptions and Selected Weight-Management Goals and Practices of High School Students—United States, 1990." *The Journal of the American Medical Association* 266 (November 27, 1991): 2811–12.

42. Harris, Robert T. "Anorexia Nervosa and Bulimia Nervosa in Female Adolescents." *Nutrition Today* 26 (March/April 1991): 30–34.

43. *Diagnostic and Statistical Manual of Mental Disorders*, 3rd ed. (revised). Washington, DC: American Psychiatric Association, 1987.

44. Harris. "Anorexia Nervosa and Bulimia Nervosa in Female Adolescents."

45. Harris. "Anorexia Nervosa and Bulimia Nervosa in Female Adolescents."

46. Harris. "Anorexia Nervosa and Bulimia Nervosa in Female Adolescents."

47. *Diagnostic and Statistical Manual of Mental Disorders*, III-R.

Suggested Readings

Anderson, Arnold E. 1990. *Males With Eating Disorders.* New York: Brunner/Mazel, Publishers.

Bailey, Covert. 1991. *The New Fit or Fat.* Boston: Houghton Mifflin Co.

Bennion, Lynn J., Edwin L. Bierman, and James M. Ferguson. 1991. *Straight Talk About Weight Control.* New York: Consumers Union.

Berg, Frances M., ed., 1993. *Health Risks of Obesity.* Hettinger, ND: Obesity and Health.

Brehm, Barbara A., and Betsy A. Keller. "Diet and Exercise Factors That Influence Weight and Fat Loss." *IDEA Today* (October 1990): 33–46.

Brownell, Kelly D., and John P. Foreyt, eds. 1986. *Handbook of Eating Disorders.* New York: Basic Books, Inc.

Brownell, Kelly D., Judith Rodin, and Jack H. Wilmore. 1992. *Eating, Body Weight and Performance in Athletes: Disorders of Modern Society.* Philadelphia, PA: Lea and Febiger.

Brownell, Kelly D., and Suzanne Nelson Steen. "Modern Methods for Weight Control: The Physiology and Psychology of Dieting." *The Physician and Sportsmedicine* 15 (December 1987):122–37.

Edwards, Ted L., Jr., and Barbara Lau. 1988. *Weight Loss to Super Wellness*, 2nd ed. Champaign, IL: Human Kinetics Publishers, Inc.

Ferguson, James M. 1988. *Habits Not Diets: The Secret to Lifetime Weight Control.* Palo Alto, CA: Bull Publishing Co.

Field, Howard L., and Barbara B. Domangue, eds. 1987. *Eating Disorders Throughout the Life Span.* New York: Praeger Publishers.

Frankle, Reva T., and Mei-Uih Yang, eds. 1988. *Obesity and Weight Control.* Rockville, MD: Aspen Publishers.

Gilbert, Sara. 1989. *The Psychology of Dieting.* London and New York: Routledge.

Gortmaker, Steven L., William H. Dietz, and Lilian W. Y. Cheung. "Inactivity, Diet, and the Fattening of America." *Journal of the American Dietetic Association.* 90 (September 1990): 1247–55.

Harris, Robert T. "Anorexia Nervosa and Bulimia Nervosa in Female Adolescents." *Nutrition Today* 26 (March/April 1991): 30–34.

Hsu, Lee Keung George. 1990. *Eating Disorders.* New York, NY: Guilford Press.

"Issues in Weight Control." *Journal of the American Dietetic Association* (supplement) 92 (January 1992): 17–22.

Jablow, Martha M. 1992. *A Parent's Guide to Eating Disorders and Obesity.* New York: Delta Publishing.

Kane, June Kozak. 1990. *Coping With Diet Fads.* New York: The Rosen Publishing Group.

Kano, Susan. 1989. *Making Peace With Food: Freeing Yourself From the Diet/Weight Obsession.* New York: Harper & Row.

Katch, Frank I., and William D. McArdle. 1993. *Nutrition, Weight Control and Exercise,* 4th ed. Philadelphia, PA: Lea and Febiger.

King, Abby C., and Diane L. Tribble. "The Role of Exercise in Weight Regulation in Nonathletes." *Sports Medicine* 11 (May 1991): 331–49.

LeBow, Michael D. 1988. *The Thin Plan.* Champaign, IL: Human Kinetics Publishers, Inc.

Leon, Gloria R. "Eating Disorders in Female Athletes." *Sports Medicine* 12 (October 1991): 219–27.

Li, Virginia C. "On Diet and Dieting: Reaching High Level Wellness." *Wellness Perspectives* 7 (Winter 1990): 61–75.

Logue, Alexandra Woods. 1991. *The Psychology of Eating and Drinking,* 2nd ed. New York: W. H. Freeman and Co.

"Losing Weight: What Works, What Doesn't." *Consumer Reports* 58 (June 1993): 347–57.

Miller, Wayne C. 1992. *The Non-Diet Diet: A Simple 100-Point Scoring System for Weight Loss Without Counting Calories.* Englewood, CO: Morton Publishing Co.

Palmer, R. L. 1988. *Anorexia Nervosa.* New York: Penguin Books.

Papazian, Ruth. "Never Say Diet?" *Healthline* 11 (October 1992): 4–7.

Scanlon, Deralee. 1991. *Diets That Work.* Los Angeles, CA: Lowell House.

Schlundt, David G., and William G. Johnson. 1990. *Eating Disorders: Assessment and Treatment.* Boston: Allyn and Bacon.

Schwartz, Hillel. 1986. *Never Satisfied: A Cultural History of Diets, Fantasies, and Fat.* New York: The Free Press.

Seid, Roberta Pollack. 1989. *Never Too Thin.* New York: Prentice-Hall Press.

Sherman, Roberta Trattner, and Ron A. Thompson. 1990. *Bulimia: A Guide for Family and Friends.* Lexington, MA: D.C. Heath and Co.

Shisslak, Catherine, Marjorie Crago, and Mary E. Neal. "Prevention of Eating Disorders Among Adolescents." *American Journal of Health Promotion* 5 (November/December 1990): 100–106.

"The Business of Weight Loss." *Journal of the American Dietetic Association* 91 (October 1991): 1243–60.

"Treatment of Obesity in Adults." *The Journal of the American Medical Association* 260 (November 4, 1988): 2547–2551.

Williams, Melvin H. 1992. *Nutrition for Fitness and Sport,* 3rd ed. Dubuque, IA: Wm. C. Brown Publishers.

Wolf, Naomi. 1991. *The Beauty Myth: How Images of Beauty Are Used Against Women.* New York: W. Morrow.

11

Cancer Prevention and Personal Safety

Chapter Objectives

After reading this chapter, you will be able to:

1. Define *benign, malignant, metastasis,* and *carcinogen.*
2. Identify the proportion of Americans who will eventually have cancer, according to present rates of incidence, and how many of these cancers are related to lifestyle and environmental factors.
3. Identify how cancer deaths rank in overall death statistics.
4. Identify cancer's seven warning signals.
5. List five primary prevention factors for reducing cancer risk and the three major controllable risk factors included in that list.
6. Recognize what age groups are most vulnerable to skin damage from sun overexposure.
7. Choose the recommended sunscreen SPF rating for skin protection.
8. Recognize the hours of the day that are particularly bad for sun exposure.
9. Choose foods that reduce cancer risk from a list of foods.
10. List three secondary prevention factors for cancer.
11. Recognize the proper procedure and schedule for conducting a breast self-exam and testicular self-exam.
12. Recognize the most common cancer in young men, ages 15–34.
13. Identify the leading cause of death among people under the age of 40.
14. List five guidelines for wearing a seat belt properly.
15. Identify the statistical profile of a low-risk and a high-risk driver.
16. List two responsible precautions that you can take to minimize your risk of injury/trouble in each of the following situations:
    a. Airplane travel
    b. Apartment or home fire
    c. To prevent falls in the home
    d. Around a lake while swimming or boating

e. During a lightning storm

f. While staying in a hotel

17. List six responsible precautions you can take to minimize your risk of being attacked, assaulted, or robbed.

Terms

- Benign
- Beta-carotene
- Cancer
- Carcinogen
- Cruciferous

- Free radicals
- Human papilloma virus (HPV)
- Malignant
- Melanoma
- Metastasis

- Precancerous
- Primary prevention
- Secondary prevention
- Tumor

A wellness lifestyle implies taking responsibility for your own health and making wise choices. The purpose of this chapter is to discuss two wellness concerns that are strongly affected by personal lifestyle choices. They are cancer risk and personal safety. Some of these choices are simple, such as buckling your seat belt every time you get into the car. Others, such as decreasing the risk of cancer, require a more complex series of decisions involving food selection, practicing self-exams, and avoiding carcinogens such as tobacco products. You will learn which behaviors increase health risks and how to decrease these risks to enhance your own state of wellness.

Cancer

Cancer is not a single disease, but a group of over one hundred different diseases, all characterized by abnormal cell growth and replication. Normally, cells grow and are replaced in an orderly manner. Enough new cells grow to replace those that are worn out and injured. Cancer cells lack controls to stop the growth process and continue to grow and multiply without restraint. This loss of control of cell growth may be due to a variety of factors. Ultraviolet radiation from sunlight, tobacco smoke, viral infections, diet, and chemicals in food and in the environment all have been implicated.

It is possible that all of us at some time experience potentially cancerous changes in our cells. These **precancerous** cells usually die or are destroyed by the immune system. Few live long enough to cause harm. If one abnormal cell survives, it can replicate into billions of cells, forming a lump or **tumor.** Tumors may be **benign** or **malignant.** Benign tumors are usually nonthreatening. Although they can grow large enough to interfere with organs and bodily functions, they seldom cause death. They usually resemble surrounding tissue, remain localized, and spread by expansion, like a wart or mole. They do not spread to other parts of the body. They can be removed completely by surgery and are not likely to recur. Malignant tumors are cancerous. They differ from surrounding tissue and tend to spread through **metastasis.** In metastasis, cells break away from the primary tumor and migrate to other tissues through the lymph or blood systems where they continue to grow. They have lethal potential because they invade and destroy normal tissues and spread to other parts of the body.

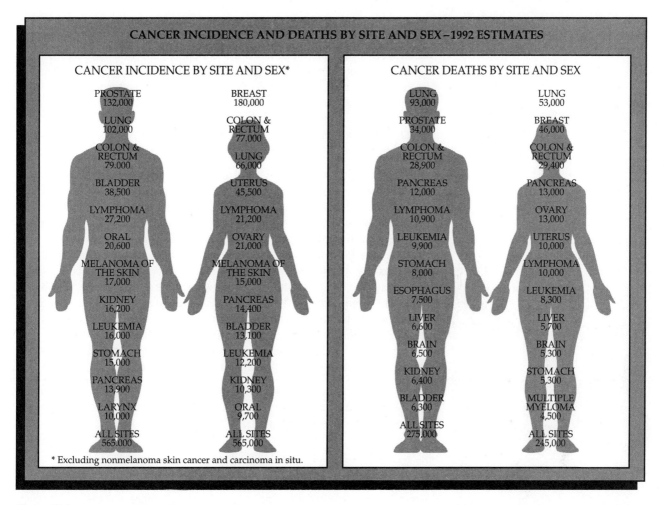

CANCER INCIDENCE AND DEATHS BY SITE AND SEX–1992 ESTIMATES

CANCER INCIDENCE BY SITE AND SEX*

PROSTATE 132,000	BREAST 180,000
LUNG 102,000	COLON & RECTUM 77,000
COLON & RECTUM 79,000	LUNG 66,000
BLADDER 38,500	UTERUS 45,500
LYMPHOMA 27,200	LYMPHOMA 21,200
ORAL 20,600	OVARY 21,000
MELANOMA OF THE SKIN 17,000	MELANOMA OF THE SKIN 15,000
KIDNEY 16,200	PANCREAS 14,400
LEUKEMIA 16,000	BLADDER 13,100
STOMACH 15,000	LEUKEMIA 12,200
PANCREAS 13,900	KIDNEY 10,300
LARYNX 10,000	ORAL 9,700
ALL SITES 565,000	ALL SITES 565,000

* Excluding nonmelanoma skin cancer and carcinoma in situ.

CANCER DEATHS BY SITE AND SEX

LUNG 93,000	LUNG 53,000
PROSTATE 34,000	BREAST 46,000
COLON & RECTUM 28,900	COLON & RECTUM 29,400
PANCREAS 12,000	PANCREAS 13,000
LYMPHOMA 10,900	OVARY 13,000
LEUKEMIA 9,900	UTERUS 10,000
STOMACH 8,000	LYMPHOMA 10,000
ESOPHAGUS 7,500	LEUKEMIA 8,300
LIVER 6,600	LIVER 5,700
BRAIN 6,500	BRAIN 5,300
KIDNEY 6,400	STOMACH 5,300
BLADDER 6,300	MULTIPLE MYELOMA 4,500
ALL SITES 275,000	ALL SITES 245,000

Figure 11.1

Cancer incidence and deaths by site and sex–1992 estimates.

Source: Cancer Facts and Figures-1992. *American Cancer Society.*

Cancer Incidence

Cancer is the second leading cause of death overall in the United States.[1] According to present rates, about one in three Americans will eventually have cancer. Even though gains have been made in cancer treatment and survival, the total number of cancer deaths has increased. While cancer is most common in people over 55, it can strike at any age. The earlier a cancer is detected, the simpler the treatment and the higher the survival rate. For this reason, it is important to understand cancer risk factors, warning signals, and to practice self-exams. See figure 11.1 for an overview of cancer incidence.

How to Cut Your Risk of Cancer (Primary Prevention)

People hear so much about cancer, they often get the feeling that everything causes cancer. If everything causes cancer, then there seems to be no use in trying to avoid it. They feel that there is little they can do to make a difference in their cancer risk, or that it is not worth the effort. They are wrong. Cancer, like heart disease, is largely preventable. Approximately 85 percent of cancers may be related to lifestyle and environmental factors over which you have control.[2] These cancers occur as a result of cumulative exposure to **carcinogens,** substances that cause cancer, over a period of time. The avoidance of factors that might lead to the development of cancer is termed **primary prevention.** The major primary prevention factors are controllable: tobacco usage; sun overexposure; and diet. Other primary prevention factors include: reducing alcohol consumption; avoiding hazards in the workplace; and minimizing exposure to radiation and environmental contamination. Choices you make daily can greatly cut your cancer risk. It is a matter of education and habit change. Here is what you can do.

Avoid Tobacco in Any Form   This includes cigarettes, pipes, cigars, snuff, and chewing tobacco. Tobacco contains many carcinogens that increase risk of developing several types of cancers. (See chapter 12 for additional information on the effects of tobacco.) In addition, when a smoker is exposed to other carcinogens, there seems to be a synergistic effect that multiplies cancer rates beyond what would be expected from the effect of each alone. For example, smoking, combined with the use of alcohol, greatly increases the risk of cancer. The number of smokers is decreasing in the United States. However, the use of smokeless tobacco, especially "dipping snuff," has increased.[3] Whereas lung cancer is most often implicated with tobacco use, tobacco products can produce a variety of oral cancers, including the lip, tongue, mouth, and throat.

The good news is that cancers caused by smoking are 100 percent preventable. If you are a nonsmoker, don't start. If you are a smoker, quit.

Reduce Sun Exposure   Overexposure to the sun is the main cause of skin cancer. It is estimated to strike one of every six Americans, making it the most common cancer.[4] We have been a nation of sun worshipers, and are paying dearly for our folly. How ironic that the price of a "healthy" tan can be not only premature skin aging and wrinkling, but skin cancer. You can protect yourself by following the guidelines in table 11.1.

Eat Healthfully and Manage Weight   Certain foods seem to be related to an increase or decrease in some kinds of cancers; for instance, a high-fat diet seems to play a role in the development of breast, colon, and prostate cancers. Studies show that by eating high-fiber foods, fruits, and vegetables and by avoiding high-fat red meat, bacon, and processed meats, we could reduce our overall cancer risk. However, a lot of Americans are not making these simple dietary adjustments. A 24-hour diet survey of 12,000 Americans by the National Cancer Institute indicated that 40 percent had eaten no fruit and 80 percent had consumed no whole grain breads or cereals.

Concerns have been voiced about pesticide and chemical residues in fruits and vegetables, as well as irradiation of fresh produce and poultry. There is no doubt that the production, processing, and transportation of food in our mass-markets world raises some serious concerns that necessitate further research.

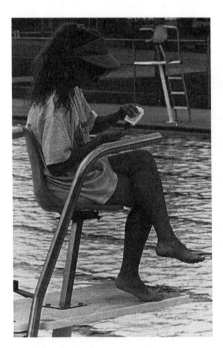

If you have an outdoor job, be aware of sun overexposure

Table 11.1

How to Reduce Sun Exposure

1. Avoid prolonged exposure to the sun when ultraviolet (UV) radiation is strongest, between 10:00 A.M. and 3:00 P.M., even on overcast days.
2. Plan activities for early morning or late evening.
3. When you will be working or playing outside for even 15–20 minutes, *apply a sunscreen rated SPF 15 or higher*. Reapply after swimming or perspiring.
4. Avoid tanning, even in tanning parlors or with sunlamps. There is no such thing as a safe tan. Tanned skin is damaged skin. The UVA light emitted by tanning booths still can cause sunburn, premature skin aging, and increased risk of skin cancer.
5. Protect children from too much sun. Skin damage occurs with each unprotected sun exposure and accumulates over a lifetime. Perhaps most of the damage is done in childhood and adolescence. Even one bad burn in childhood can double the risk of skin cancer.
6. Know what skin cancer looks like, and examine your skin at least once a month. If you find unusual moles or skin spots, have them examined by your physician.

Nevertheless, we do know that sun exposure, a fatty diet, and tobacco products are three highly controllable areas where your behavior has a major impact. Taking positive steps in these three areas makes more sense than worrying about food products over which you have little control.

Obesity is also linked to cancer. Obese individuals increase their risk of cancer of the breast, colon, and the male and female reproductive organs. The more overweight a person is, the greater the risk. People who carry extra weight in the abdomen are at higher risk for breast and endometrial cancer.[5, 6] The good news is that those who are "apple"-shaped (as opposed to "pears," who have bigger thighs and hips) can reduce their risk by losing weight.[7] It appears to be fairly easy for apple-shaped people to lose weight where it counts since fat leaves the abdomen first. While the explanation for the reduced risk is uncertain, researchers believe that weight loss reduces the amount of sex hormones available to stimulate possible precancerous cell growth in the reproductive organs.

Table 11.2

Ways to Increase Fiber Intake

Instead of	*Eat*
White bread	Whole grain bread
White rice	Brown rice
Mashed potatoes	Baked potato in the skin
Orange juice	Orange
Applesauce	Unpeeled apple
Processed cereals	Whole grain cereals
Potato chips	Popcorn, plain or lightly seasoned

By making positive choices in your daily diet and following the guidelines listed here, you can promote good health now and can reduce your cancer risk in the future.

1. Decrease fat intake.

2. Eat more high-fiber foods such as whole grain breads and cereals, fruits, and vegetables (table 11.2). Fiber, the nondigestible part of plant cells, seems to protect against colon cancer by speeding potentially harmful substances through the digestive tract and reducing contact time between carcinogens and the intestines.

3. Eat **cruciferous** vegetables. Broccoli, cauliflower, brussel sprouts, turnips, cabbage, and other members of the mustard family help prevent certain cancers from developing. They contain chemicals that activate an enzyme in the intestine that breaks down carcinogens and helps prevent colon cancer.

4. Include foods rich in vitamins A, C, and E each day. Citrus fruits, tomatoes, green peppers, baked potatoes, broccoli, and strawberries are high in vitamin C. Dark green and deep yellow fresh vegetables and fruits such as carrots, corn, spinach, peaches, and apricots contain a form of vitamin A called **beta-carotene.** Green and leafy vegetables, whole grains, egg yolks, nuts and wheat germ contain vitamin E. These three vitamins neutralize **free radicals,** potentially dangerous substances that produce precancerous cellular damage.[8]

5. Charcoal-grilled, salted and nitrite-cured, smoked, and pickled foods should be consumed in moderation. Charring and cooking meats at high temperatures for long periods of time produces carcinogens. The preservative nitrate in processed meats such as hot dogs, luncheon meats, bacon, beef sticks, and beef jerky forms cancer-causing substances when broken down by the body.

6. Drink lowfat milk daily. Calcium appears to neutralize potentially carcinogenic substances in the digestive tract, reducing risk of colorectal cancer. Also, processed cheese contains a cancer inhibitor, a form of linoleic acid, which may be incorporated into body cells of people who consume it, locking in a defense against cancer.[9]

Reduce Alcohol Consumption   Avoid alcohol or limit alcohol intake to two drinks a day or less. Excessive alcohol consumption increases risk of several cancers. Oral cancer is 15 times higher in drinkers who also smoke. Liver cancer occurs more frequently among heavy drinkers of alcohol especially when accompanied by cigarette smoking or chewing tobacco.

Other Ways to Reduce Cancer Risk   Make regular exercise a habit. There is evidence that the body's immune system may help in preventing cancer. Research has shown that exercise enhances overall health and well-being and strengthens the immune system. Researchers also speculate that exercise decreases the production of some reproductive hormones in both men and women, decreasing risk of cancers that depend on these hormones to develop.[10]

The results of the Harvard Alumni study should convince sedentary Americans to become more physically active in order to improve health and reduce their cancer risk. Researchers reported that males who burned at least 1,000 calories a week in physical activity had half the risk for colon cancer of inactive men.[11] Researchers speculate this is true for women, as well. (One thousand calories is the approximate equivalent of walking ten miles.) Other studies show the more you exercise the more protection you get. Exercise appears to prevent colon cancer by helping to speed food through the digestive system, leaving less time for carcinogens to remain in contact with the colon. And, as you already know, exercise is the key to weight management.

Avoid excessive exposure to radiation. While most medical X rays are low-dose, it is still wise to use protective shields to cover body areas not being X-rayed. There is also a potential problem of radioactive radon gas in the home in certain areas of the country.

Be aware of hazards in the workplace. Exposure to asbestos and other industrial materials increases risk, especially when combined with smoking. Minimize exposure to these products by wearing protective clothing and equipment and by following standard safety procedures.

Limit environmental contamination from PCBs and the insecticide DDT. PCBs were once used in a wide variety of products including: paint, pesticides, plastics, adhesives, ink, fire retardants, and electrical insulation. Both PCBs and DDT were banned by the U.S. Environmental Protection Agency in the 1970s, but because contamination of the environment was so widespread, they are still found in the food chain. These chemicals have been found in large amounts in the fat samples of some women who have breast cancer. PCBs and DDT are thought to be promoters or inducers, rather than direct carcinogens.

Early Detection (Secondary Prevention)

Secondary prevention is taking action to diagnose cancer as early as possible. This includes knowing cancer's warning signals (table 11.3), practicing self-exams, and getting regular cancer-related checkups by a physician. If cancer is detected in its early localized stages, it is easier to treat. Once metastases spread from the primary site, it becomes much more difficult to cure. Although not all cancers can be detected through self-exams, these, along with awareness of cancer's seven warning signals, can alert a person to the need to consult a physician.

Table 11.3

Cancer's Seven Warning Signals

Source: Courtesy of American Cancer Society

1. Change in bowel or bladder habits
2. A sore that does not heal
3. Unusual bleeding or discharge
4. Thickening or lump in breast or elsewhere
5. Indigestion or difficulty in swallowing
6. Obvious change in wart or mole
7. Nagging cough or hoarseness

If you have a warning signal, see your doctor!

See your physician for cancer-related checkups. Even if you have no symptoms, it is important for early detection of cancer to have periodic cancer-related checkups (see table 11.4). Until all cancers can be prevented, it is important to protect yourself with the knowledge of cancer signs, self-exams, early detection, regular checkups, and prompt treatment.

For most people without symptoms, cancer-related checkups are recommended every three years from age 20–39 and annually for those over age 40. People who are high risk for certain cancers may need tests more often.

Common Cancers

While many types of cancers exist, some are much more common than others. The most common cancers in order of occurrence for men are prostate, lung, colon/rectum and, in the 15- to 34-year old age group, testicular. For women, they are breast, colon/rectal, lung, and uterine.[12] Although they are the most frequently occurring cancers of all (over 600,000 cases next year), skin cancers are not usually included in cancer statistics since almost all nonmelanoma skin cancers are easily cured **if detected early.**[13] Even so, this year there will be an estimated 8,800 skin cancer deaths, 6,700 from malignant melanoma and 2,100 due to other skin cancers.[14]

Skin Cancer   Skin cancer accounts for 40 percent of all cancers, and fair-skinned people who don't tan easily are most susceptible.[15] The problem is particularly severe for young men, who have a higher rate of skin cancer than do women.[16] Another recent concern is that in the upper atmosphere, the thinning ozone layer now allows more of the sun's damaging ultraviolet radiation to reach the skin, which may cause even higher skin cancer rates. Approximately 90 percent of all skin cancers can be prevented by protecting the skin from the sun's rays.[17]

Table 11.4
Cancer Check-ups

Breast Cancer	Do a monthly self-exam; clinical examination of the breast every three years from ages 20–40 and then every year; a screening mammography by age 40; age 40–49 every 1–2 years, age 50+, yearly.
Colorectal Cancer	Have a digital rectal examination by a physician during an office visit yearly after age 40; the stool blood test every year after age 50; the proctosigmoidoscopy examination every 3–5 years after age 50.
Uterus/Cervic Cancer	Get an annual Pap test and pelvic exam for women who are or have been sexually active or are age 18+. After three or more consecutive satisfactory annual exams, the Pap test may be performed less frequently at the physician's discretion.
Testicular Cancer	Do a monthly self-exam.
Skin Cancer	Perform a monthly self-exam.
Prostate Cancer	Men over age 40 should have an annual rectal/prostate examination as part of his regular annual checkup.

Malignant **melanoma,** a dark wartlike or molelike lesion, has a deadly tendency to metastasize and may be fatal. Its incidence is increasing faster than any other cancer. Thirty percent of all melanomas occur in people under age 45. It is important to know what skin cancer looks like and to examine your skin at least once a year. If you find unusual moles or skin spots, the American Academy of Dermatology suggests using this ABCD test for early detection of malignant melanoma (see fig. 11.2). If detected early, skin cancer has an 85 percent to 99 percent cure rate.

Lung Cancer   Lung cancer is a rare disease except among smokers. As you know, exposure to sidestream cigarette smoke increases the risk for nonsmokers. Lung tissue damage and cellular changes that precede lung cancer have been observed in 93 percent of active smokers, but in only 6 percent of exsmokers and 1 percent of nonsmokers.[18] If a smoker quits, these early precancerous cellular changes are reversible, and the damaged bronchial lining often returns to normal. If the smoker continues, the abnormal cell growth may progress to cancer.

Figure 11.2

ABCD test for malignant melanoma

A—Asymmetry: Is one half unlike the other?

B—Border irregularity: Does it have an uneven, scalloped edge rather than a clearly defined border?

C—Color variation: Is the color uniform, or does it vary from one area to another—from tan to brown to black, or from white to red to blue?

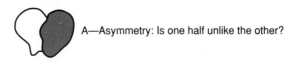

D—Diameter larger than one-fourth inch: At its widest point, is the growth as large as or larger than a pencil eraser?

Lung cancer, the leading cancer killer for both men and women, has a low survival rate because it is seldom discovered in its earliest stages. By the time it has grown large enough to produce noticeable symptoms or to be visible on X ray, it is already well advanced. It metastasizes readily through the bloodstream to the brain and other organs and is difficult to treat. The five-year rate for lung cancer survival is 13 percent, and has not changed, despite advances in cancer treatment, in 40 years.[19]

Colon and Rectal Cancer   A genetic tendency to develop noncancerous polyps in the colon, combined with a diet high in animal fat and low in fiber, may cause half, perhaps all colon cancer. One study found that adults whose childhood diets were low in salads and cruciferous vegetables or high in processed meats were more likely to get colon cancer as compared to adults who ate healthier diets. This does not mean that you are doomed by poor childhood eating habits, but that eating vegetables and cancer-preventative foods is good insurance at any age. Dietary habits and preferences are formed young and practiced over a lifetime. Chronic exposure to carcinogens in high-fat and highly refined and processed foods can eventually stimulate precancerous changes in cells.

Breast Cancer   Breast cancer is the most common cancer in women and the second leading cancer killer. It is estimated that one out of every nine women will eventually develop breast cancer.[20] This fact has frightened many women. Nobody is doomed, but everyone should understand that the "one-in-nine" statistic is a *lifetime risk.* Getting older is the most important risk factor for breast cancer. Look at the risk at specific ages, according to the American Cancer Society:[21]

by age 50:	1 in 50
by age 60:	1 in 23
by age 70:	1 in 13
by age 80:	1 in 10
by age 85:	1 in 9

Young women should not feel complacent because breast cancer can occur at any age. Although rare, about 2 percent of breast cancers are in men. Other risk factors for breast cancer include: a sister or mother who has had breast cancer, especially if it occurred before menopause; early onset of menstruation (before age 12), and experiencing menopause after age 50 (both situations increase the lifelong exposure to high estrogen levels); obesity; and never having given birth. These factors together account for only 25 percent of all breast cancer. White women have a somewhat higher risk than black or Hispanic women or those of Asian origin.

The incidence of breast cancer is slowly rising, but no one knows why. It could be partly because more women are being diagnosed at earlier ages, thanks to mammography. It might be partly attributed to some as-yet-unidentified dietary or environmental factor (i.e., PCBs or DDT). High fat intake is currently a suspect.

Breast Self-Examination

1. In the shower:
Examine your breasts during bath or shower; hands glide easier over wet skin. Fingers flat, move gently over every part of each breast. Use the right hand to examine the left breast, left hand for the right breast. Check for any lump, hard knot, or thickening.

2. Before a mirror:
Inspect your breasts with arms at your sides. Next, raise your arms high overhead. Look for any changes in the contour of each breast: a swelling, dimpling of skin, or changes in the nipple.

   Then rest palms on hips and press down firmly to flex your chest muscles. Left and right breast will not exactly match; few women's breasts do.

   Regular inspection shows what is normal for you and will give you confidence in your examination.

3. Lying down:
To examine your right breast, put a pillow or folded towel under your right shoulder. Place right hand behind your head—this distributes breast tissue more evenly on the chest. With left hand, fingers flat, press gently in small circular motions around an imaginary clock face. Begin at outermost top of your right breast for 12 o'clock, then move to 1 o'clock, and so on around the circle back to 12. A ridge of firm tissue in the lower curve of each breast is normal. Then move in an inch, toward the nipple, keep circling to examine *every part of your breast,* including nipple. This requires at least three more circles. Now slowly repeat procedure on your left breast with a pillow under your left shoulder and left hand behind head. Notice how your breast structure feels.

   Finally, squeeze the nipple of each breast gently between thumb and index finger. Any discharge, clear or bloody, should be reported to your doctor immediately.

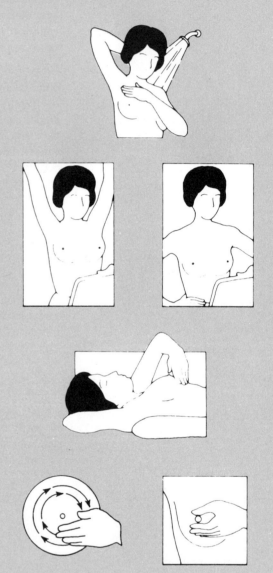

Source: Reprinted by permission of the American Cancer Society.

Figure 11.3
Breast self-examination

Since early detection is important, all women need to learn and perform breast self-examination once a month. With regular self-exams, women become more familiar with their breasts, making detection of any changes more likely. Figure 11.3 shows how to perform a breast self-examination.

Prostate Cancer   This is the most common cancer (excluding skin cancer) and the second leading cause of cancer deaths in men.[22] The warning signs of prostate cancer are: weak or interrupted urine flow; inability to urinate or difficulty starting and stopping urine flow; the need to urinate frequently, especially at night; blood in the urine; pain or burning on urination; continuing pain in the lower back, pelvis, or upper thighs. Most of these symptoms are nonspecific and may be similar to benign conditions such as infection or prostate enlargement.

Prostate cancer generally occurs in men over 50; risk increases with age. Studies indicate that dietary fat may increase the risk of this cancer.[23]

Testicular Cancer   Most people think that cancer is a disease old people get. Cancer of the testicle is different. It is not one of the most common types of cancer in this country, but it is the most common cancer in young men between the ages of 15 and 34.[24] Warning signs include a swelling or hard lump in the testicle, a dull ache in the lower abdomen and groin, a sensation of heaviness, or pain in the testes. Your risk of getting testicular cancer is 40 times higher if you have a testicle that never descended into the scrotum or descended after age 6.

Lives could be saved if more testicular cancers were detected and treated early. The 5-year survival rate of testicular cancer is 91 percent.[25] Treatment does not mean losing your "manhood" or your ability to have normal sex, and it doesn't mean you can't have children.

Men themselves discover most testicular cancers by learning how to examine their testicles. In doing this once a month, you can greatly increase the chances of finding a testicular cancer early if it does occur. All young men should learn and practice the monthly testicular self-examination shown in figure 11.4, from adolescence on. The technique is simple:

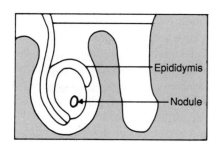

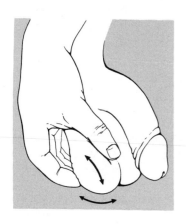

Figure 11.4
Testicular self-examination

1. Perform the examination once a month, after a warm bath or shower, when the scrotal skin is most relaxed.

2. Examine each testicle gently with the fingers of both hands by rolling the testicle between the thumb and fingers.

3. Feel for a small lump, about the size of a pea, generally on the front part of the testicle. There is a natural structure at the back of each testicle called the *epididymis.* Learn what it feels like so you will not confuse it with an abnormal lump.

4. If you do find a lump, tell your physician about it **right away.** Remember, not all lumps are cancerous. Don't let fear keep you from getting the medical attention that could save your life. Cancer will not go away if you ignore it.

Uterine Cancer   With the widespread use of Pap smears for early detection, the death rate from uterine cancer has declined. Cervical cancer, often seen in young women, has been linked to the **human papilloma virus (HPV)** which can be spread through sexual contact. Risk factors for cervical cancer include a history of viral genital infections such as herpes and genital warts, becoming sexually active at an early age, or having had several different sex partners.

A Pap test, in which cells from the cervix and uterine lining are examined under a microscope, is a simple procedure that can be done at intervals by physicians as a part of each pelvic examination. If cervical cancer is detected at an early stage, it can easily be removed.

Personal Safety

Throughout this book we have tried to increase your awareness of risks and personal choices that affect your wellness. Injuries and illnesses stemming from accidents and environmental hazards sometimes seem to be beyond the average person's control. Especially accidents—which are the fourth overall cause of death in the United States (and the number one cause of death among teens and young adults)—often appear to be a matter of "chance."[26] In fact, the risks you are exposed to while driving a car, traveling on a vacation, getting around campus, and working around an apartment or house can be substantially reduced by heeding basic safety precautions. Some of these precautions seem like common sense to most. Yet, for whatever reason, many fail to follow even "common sense" precautions. Federal, state, and local regulations have been established to help protect us from a variety of traffic, fire, water, and air travel tragedies. But laws and regulations cannot *make* people act. When you strive for high-level wellness, *all* lifestyle choices are taken seriously. Since the wellness concept is centered on an ongoing personal commitment to positive choices, safety awareness and responsibility cannot be excluded.

We tend to focus solely on the impact an accident has on our physical dimension of wellness. The truth is, such a trauma can equally affect our emotional, social, occupational, and even spiritual dimensions! Consider the following: one American in 6 sustains an accident-related injury that results in measurable economic loss.[27] Of these:

- one-fourth occur on the job or during commutes
- one-fourth involve people who work at home
- thirty percent occur during leisure time
- about 20 percent involve motor vehicles

The remainder of this chapter focuses on choices that can help you control risks in your immediate environment.

Automobile Seat Belts

Motor vehicle crashes are the leading cause of death among people age 40 and younger. In talking about motor vehicle collisions, we deliberately chose not to use the word "accident," which is sort of a luck/fate approach. Instead, we use "crash" because it is well understood what specific things can be done to reduce risks. Drunken-driving laws, child car-restraint regulations, mandatory seat belts, availability of air bags, and designated driver programs have done a lot to curtail traffic fatalities. Still, approximately 48,000 Americans die annually in car crashes, costing the U.S. $40 billion.[28] Of these casualties, half of the people could have been saved if they had used their seat belts, *and* fully half of the serious injuries incurred in collisions could have been prevented by the use of seat belts.[29] Although drivers initially resisted seat belt use, 39 states and the District of Columbia have enacted seat belt laws, and compliance is growing. The importance of using seat belts cannot really be overstated. For, even if all the other advice in this book is practiced (exercise regularly, eat a nutritious diet, don't smoke, etc.), *one* accident without a seat

Table 11.5

Why I Don't Buckle Up

> 1. **Seat belts are uncomfortable.**
>   Unlike the original floor-anchored belts, new belts are designed to let you move freely until a collision occurs. Plus, they are a lot more comfortable than a body cast or traction!
> 2. **I'm only going to the store down the street.**
>   Seventy percent of crashes occur within 25 miles of home, and 80 percent occur at speeds less than 40 mph.[30] People not wearing seat belts have been killed at speeds less than 12 mph!
> 3. **The belt will prevent me from being thrown clear of the accident.**
>   Exactly! Your chances of being killed are 25 times greater if you're thrown out of the car.[31]
> 4. **The seat belt will trap me in a burning or submerged car.**
>   Only one-half of one percent of all crashes result in fire or submergence.[32] Unfortunately, television action shows capitalize on such scenes. If you do find yourself in this terrifying predicament, wouldn't it be better to have been restrained and thus conscious enough to get out of the vehicle, rather than have had your head smashed into the windshield, leaving you unconscious and incapable of escaping?

belt could immediately and irrevocably end any wellness program. It does not make sense, if we care about health and wellness, to not buckle up. Table 11.5 lists the most common excuses people give for choosing not to use their seat belts. Hopefully you do not use the same flimsy excuses.

To prevent injury, seat belts must not only be worn, but worn properly every time. You are most likely to survive an automobile crash without injury if you follow these recommendations:

1. Wear the seat belt low across the pelvis, not the abdomen. In a crash, a force of 20 to 50 times your body weight is exerted against the belt. The bony pelvis can withstand this load, whereas internal organs would be injured if the belt is higher, across the abdomen.

2. Keep the belt snug. A loose belt offers little protection, and may compound injuries if you are thrown against it. You can also slide forward under a loose belt and suffer head or neck injuries from the shoulder strap.

3. Never wear the shoulder strap under your arm or around behind your back. When properly worn, this strap rests on the middle of the collarbone and the upper chest.

4. Never share a belt. In a crash, a parent sharing a belt with a child can crush the child. Each passenger must have his own belt. Also, know that it is impossible to hold a child in your arms in the event of a collision. In a crash, a twenty-pound baby is propelled forward with the force equivalent to four hundred pounds.[33]

5. Pregnant women should wear the seat belt under the abdomen—across the upper thighs and as low on the hips as possible. The shoulder strap should go across the shoulder and chest. The fetus is at *much greater* risk when the mother does not wear a seat belt! The leading cause of fetal death in a crash is death of the mother.[34]

Many new automobile models are including inflatable airbags as standard equipment. These bags will be valuable in preventing thousands of deaths and injuries. But remember, airbags protect only in head-on collisions, not side-impact crashes. Your seat belt is still your first line of defense in all crashes.

Driving Safety

Driving is on average approximately 10 times more dangerous than traveling by airplane or train.[35] However, if you are a low-risk driver, you are far less likely to die in a car crash than a high-risk driver. Statistics define a low-risk driver to be a 40-year-old who is sober when driving and wears a seat belt; a high-risk

What is your excuse for not wearing a seatbelt?

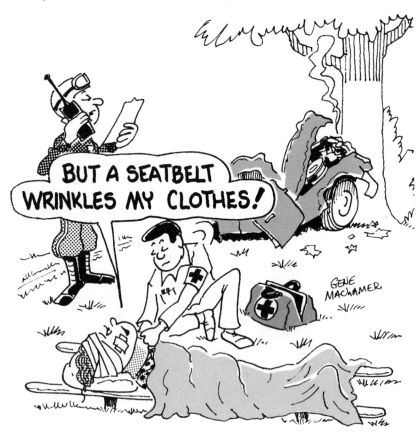

driver is an 18-year-old, intoxicated male traveling in a light-weight car without wearing a seat belt.[36] The best driver is also a defensive driver—one who can anticipate potential danger and respond appropriately. Attitude is a key ingredient in defensive driving. Speeding, following too closely, and improper lane changing are the most common traffic infractions leading to crashes.[37] Driver inattention is also a major contributor to crashes.

Airplane Safety

Unfortunately, many people take a fatalistic attitude toward airplane crashes. Despite sensational headlines, deaths due to airplane crashes are quite low when compared to other modes of transportation. According to statistics collected by the National Transportation Safety Board, passengers who think systematically in advance about their own safety are more likely to survive an airplane accident.[38] How often have we observed airplane travelers settle into their seats, bury their heads in a newspaper, and ignore the safety instructions given by the flight attendants? Taking the first few minutes on a plane to review all safety instructions, observe safety features on the plane, and make an escape plan is a responsible wellness behavior. The following steps will help prepare you for an emergency:

- Locate the nearest exit and count the number of rows to the exit, so you could find it if the lights were out.
- Keep your seat belt fastened throughout the flight.
- Study the seat-pocket safety card.
- If possible, wear comfortable clothes and shoes.

Contrary to popular belief, where you sit in the plane has not been found to be a significant survival factor; however, sitting in an aisle seat may quicken an escape.

Personal Safety Awareness

. . . falls, drownings, fires, tornadoes, floods, rape, lightning, thefts, chokings, bicycle accidents, assaults, vandalism. . . .

These predicaments don't just happen to *other* people. You may find yourself facing any of the above situations at some time. Though chance is one factor, you do have some control over your own fate. You have the capacity to handle a variety of emergencies, possibly minimizing any ill effects. Advanced planning and preparation is the key. Look carefully at table 11.6 and think seriously about each item as it relates to you. Do you adhere to these common-sense safety precautions?

Crime Prevention As much as we hate to admit, crime and violence are a very real part of contemporary American life. Whether you are at school, traveling, at work, or going about daily living routines, anyone can become a victim. Even on the assumed "idyllic settings" of college campuses, assaults, sexual attacks, and

Table 11.6

Nine Wellness Tips to Avoid Trouble

1. Fall-proof your home/apartment.

    Falls are the second leading cause of accidental death in the United States.[39] Stairs, loose carpeting, icy sidewalks, improper lighting, wet tile, etc., help contribute to these statistics. Take charge of your environment to make it safe!

2. Install smoke detectors throughout your home/apartment.

    Test them periodically, and replace batteries at least once a year. Plan and rehearse evacuation procedures in preparation for a fire. The heat build-up and toxic gases from a fire can be even more threatening than the flames themselves. In most cases, you only have a few minutes after the smoke detector goes off to safely escape a building.

3. When checking into a hotel, locate the nearest fire exits to your room. Count and memorize the number of doorways between your room and these fire exits.

4. Always wear a helmet when riding a motorcycle or bicycle.

5. Learn to swim. Never swim alone or dive into shallow water (or water of unknown depth).

6. Always wear a life preserver when boating.

7. Find shelter immediately during a lightning storm. Once inside, stay away from telephones, metal objects, and open doors and windows.

8. Never use electrical appliances near a sink or tub filled with water.

9. When walking, jogging, or cycling at night, always wear light clothing or reflective apparel.

thefts occur. You can help protect yourself from being a victim with some basic precautions. There is nothing extraordinary about the following personal safety tips. They are simply examples of assuming self-responsibility for your own wellness.

1. Always lock your house, apartment, residence hall room, and car—even when you are there.

2. At night, park in well-lit spots and walk in brightly lit areas.

3. Never walk alone at night or in unpopulated areas. Use a campus escort service if available.

4. Be aware of suspicious persons in buildings, hallways, parking areas, elevators, stairwells, and around restrooms. Note their description and contact the police or security.

5. Don't let strangers know when you are home alone.

6. Glance into your car, checking the seats and floor before getting in.

7. Never hitchhike or pick up hitchhikers.

8. If you are being harassed, turn and proceed toward lights and people.

9. Watch your alcohol consumption. Drinking puts you at risk and vulnerable to assault, robbery, and rape.

10. Secure all valuables and don't flaunt expensive possessions.

11. When you are walking alone, walk with your shoulders back and your head held high. Keep a strong and steady pace. Remain alert and be aware of your surroundings. Muggers and rapists rarely attack those who appear assured and confident. Also, walk facing traffic, even if you're on a sidewalk. This prevents an assailant in a car from sneaking up on you from the rear.

12. Have a defensive plan in mind should you encounter trouble.

We know that not all accidents and injuries are preventable. Some just happen. However, many accidents and personal traumas *are* preventable with some basic precautions. Too often after an accident or tragic event we have heard someone say: "I wish I would have . . ." Being careful may seem boring to some, but it *is* the wellness way!

Summary

You can significantly increase your chances of living a healthy, active life, free of disabling disease, by daily personal choices. Your risk of cancer can be greatly decreased by emphasizing primary prevention awareness. This involves reducing dietary fat, increasing consumption of complex carbohydrates and foods rich in vitamins A, C, and E, reducing consumption of alcohol, and avoiding overexposure to sunlight and carcinogens. Secondary prevention is also important. It includes awareness of cancer's seven warning signals, medical checkups, and regular self-exams. Any tobacco product is deadly. Smokers have an increased chance of heart disease, cancer, respiratory disease, and premature death as compared to nonsmokers. Smokeless tobacco causes oral cancer, gum disease, and tooth loss. Smoking is quickly losing its appeal and has fallen to an all-time low as nonsmokers begin to assert their right to breathe clean air.

Accidents are the fourth most common cause of death in the United States behind heart disease, cancer, and stroke. However, accidents (especially automobile crashes) are the number one cause of death among young people. All accidents and crime are not just a matter of "chance." You can substantially reduce your risks of being a victim by heeding basic precautions. Acting to control risks in your immediate environment is a powerful way to enhance your total wellness.

References

1. American Cancer Society. *Cancer Facts and Figures*—1993. American Cancer Society, 1599 Clifton Road, N.E., Atlanta, GA 30329–4251.

2. The United Cancer Council. *Cancer Prevention: Fact and Fiction.* Washington, DC: U.S. Government Printing Office.

3. *Cancer Facts and Figures*—1993.

4. The Skin Cancer Foundation, 1992. New York.

5. Shapira, D.V., N.B. Kumar, G. H. Lyman, et al. "Upper Body Fat Distribution and Endometrial Cancer Risk." *JAMA.* 1991; 266(13) 1808–1811.

6. Shapira, D.V., N.B. Kumar, G. H. Lyman, et al. "Abdominal Obesity and Breast Cancer Risk." *Annals of Internal Medicine,* 1990; 112(3): 182–186.

7. Shapira, D.V., N.B. Kumar, G. H. Lyman, "Estimate of Breast Cancer Risk Reduction with Weight Loss." *Cancer.* 1991; 67(10): 2622–2625.

8. "Free Radicals and Antioxidants: Finding the Key to Heart Disease, Cancer, and the Aging Process." *University of California at Berkeley Wellness Letter.* Oct. 1991.

9. Eichner, Edward R. "Exercise, Lymphokines, Calories, and Cancer." *The Physician and Sportsmedicine.* Vol. 15. June, 1987: 109–116.

10. "Fitness and Cancer." *The Physician and Sportsmedicine.* Vol. 19, No. 12, Dec. 1991.

11. Lee, I. M., R. S. Paffenbarger, C. Hsieh. "Physical Activity and Risk of Developing Colorectal Cancer Among College Alumni." *Journal of National Cancer Inst.* 1991; 83(18): 1324–1329.

12. *Cancer Facts and Figures—1993.*

13. *Cancer Facts and Figures—1993.*

14. *Cancer Facts and Figures—1993.*

15. Laszlo, J. *Understanding Cancer.* New York: Harper and Row, 1987.

16. *Cancer Facts and Figures—1993.*

17. *Cancer Facts and Figures—1993.*

18. U.S. Department of Health and Human Services. *Cancer of the Lung. Research Report.* Washington, DC: U.S. Government Printing Office, 1987.

19. *Cancer Facts and Figures—1993.*

20. *Cancer Facts and Figures—1993.*

21. "One in Nine American Women will . . ." *University of California at Berkeley Wellness Letter.* July 1992.

22. *Cancer Facts and Figures—1993.*

23. *Cancer Facts and Figures—1993.*

24. U.S. Department of Health and Human Services. *Testicular Cancer. Research Report.* Washington, DC: U.S. Government Printing Office, 1987.

25. *Cancer Facts and Figures—1993.*

26. University of California, Berkeley. *The Wellness Encyclopedia.* Boston: Houghton Mifflin Co., 1991.

27. Castelli, Jim. "Study Reveals Causes, Costs of Accidents." *Safety & Health* 144 (August 1991): 61–64.

28. Rothman, Howard. *The Employee Handbook for Building a Healthier Lifestyle.* Brookfield, WI: International Foundation of Employee Benefit Plans, 1991.

29. Campbell, Sharon Lynn. "Six Reasons Why People Don't Buckle Up." *Safety & Health* 143 (February 1991): 78–80.

30. Campbell. "Six Reasons Why People Don't Buckle Up."

31. Campbell. "Six Reasons Why People Don't Buckle Up."

32. Campbell. "Six Reasons Why People Don't Buckle Up."

33. *The Wellness Encyclopedia.*

34. *The Wellness Encyclopedia.*

35. *The Wellness Encyclopedia.*

36. *The Wellness Encyclopedia.*

37. Sandler, Roberta. "Safe Driving: It's Up to You." *Safety & Health* 143 (April 1991): 74–75.

38. *The Wellness Encyclopedia.*

39. "Fall-Proof Your Home." *Safety & Health* 144 (October 1991): 46–48.

Suggested Readings

American Cancer Society, *Cancer Facts and Figures—1993*, 1599 Clifton Road, N.E., Atlanta, GA 30329–4251.

Bromley, Max L. and Leonard Territo. 1990. *College Crime Prevention and Personal Safety Awareness.* Springfield, IL: Charles C. Thomas, Publisher.

"Extinguish Fire-Safety Myths." *Safety & Health* 144 (September 1991): 76–77.

Laszlo, John. 1987. *Understanding Cancer.* New York: Harper and Row.

Morra, Marion. 1990. *Triumph: Getting Back to Normal When You Have Cancer.* New York, NY: Avon.

Schoemaker, Joyce M. and Charity Y. Vitale. 1991. *Healthy Homes, Healthy Kids.* Washington, DC: Island Press.

Smith, Michael Clay and Margaret D. Smith. 1990. *Wide Awake: A Guide to Safe Campus Living in the 90's.* Princeton, NJ: Peterson's Guides, Inc.

Tkac, Debora (ed.). 1990. *Lifespan-Plus: 900 Natural Techniques to Live Longer.* Emmaus, PA: Rodale Press.

University of California, Berkeley. 1991. *The Wellness Encyclopedia.* Boston: Houghton Mifflin Co.

Whittemore, Gerard. 1986. *Street Wisdom for Women.* Boston: Quinlan Press.

Resources

American Cancer Society, Inc.
National Headquarters
3340 Peachtree Road NE
Atlanta, GA 30326

Sexually Transmitted Disease Hot Line   1–800–227–8922

Y-Me Breast Cancer Support Program   1–800–221–2141

Living With Cancer, Inc.
P.O. Box 3060
Long Island City, NY 11101

1–800–ACS–2345

Cancer Information Clearinghouse,
National Cancer Institute
Building 31, Room 10A18
9000 Rockville Pike
Bethesda, MD 20225
(800) 4-CANCER for all areas except:
Alaska: (800) 638–6070
Hawaii: (800) 524–1234

12
Substance Abuse

After reading this chapter, you will be able to:

1. Give three out of five reasons why alcohol/drug dependence is considered a disease.
2. Define the following terms: drug, addiction, alcoholism, tolerance, passive smoking, 'roid rage, and synergy.
3. List five factors that affect alcohol absorption.
4. Describe the effects of alcohol on the central nervous system and personal behavior.
5. Differentiate between alcohol use, abuse, and alcoholism.
6. Identify family behaviors that reduce one's risk of alcohol related problems.
7. Identify the blood alcohol concentration (BAC) regarded as legally drunk.
8. Describe the "Zero . . . One . . . Three Rule for Responsible Drinking."
9. Explain why a person may not feel intoxicated but have a BAC of .10 percent or more.
10. List the harmful effects of alcohol on the body.
11. Choose a correct guideline to follow if you overindulge in alcohol.
12. Choose a correct guideline to follow if a friend passes out from alcohol overindulgence.
13. List five tips/strategies for drinking less or not at all.
14. Evaluate your personal alcohol use.
15. Identify the birth defects caused by a mother's alcohol consumption while pregnant.
16. Differentiate between fetal alcohol syndrome (FAS) and fetal alcohol effect (FAE).
17. Identify the health hazards related to passive smoking.
18. Identify two most common illegal drugs used in the United States today.
19. Identify side effects of marijuana, cocaine, anabolic steroids, and caffeine abuse.
20. Describe the relationships between cocaine and crack and between crank and ice.
21. List four drugs that affect physical performance and describe how they do so.

22. List three of four common kinds of nonprescription drugs that can lead to physical dependance if overused.
23. Describe how prescribed drugs can be abused.
24. Give three examples of drugs that act synergistically to produce harmful effects.

Terms

- Addiction
- Alcohol (ethyl alcohol/ethanol)
- Alcoholism
- Amotivational syndrome
- Amphetamines
- Anabolic steroids
- Blackout
- Blood alcohol concentration (BAC)
- Caffeine

- Cocaine
- Crack
- Crank
- Delta-9-tetrahydrocannabinol (THC)
- Diuretics
- Drug
- Fetal alcohol effect (FAE)
- Fetal alcohol syndrome (FAS)
- Ice

- Marijuana
- Narcolepsy
- Nitrosamine
- Passive smoking
- 'Roid rage
- Synergy
- Testosterone
- Tolerance

We all live in a drug saturated environment. We have drugs for everything—anxiety, depression, infection, and pain. A **drug** is a chemical that alters a person's physical or mental condition. The question is not whether to use drugs, since most people do; but rather, when, where, why, and how much they are to be used. Most of us use over-the-counter drugs, such as aspirin. Others use prescribed drugs for a medical condition. Still others misuse and abuse legal and illegal drugs at the cost of their bankbooks, relationships, and even their lives (see table 12.1). We first address alcohol because it is the most abused legal drug in our society. This chapter includes alcohol use assessments, responsible drinking guidelines, and strategies for drinking less to help you make decisions about your alcohol use. Other drugs addressed include tobacco, illegal recreational drugs, drugs affecting physical performance, and over-the-counter and prescription drugs. Before we discuss specific drugs, let's examine addiction in general.

Addiction

Addiction is a pathological or abnormal relationship with an object or event.[1] It is an illness that progresses from a definite, though often unclear, beginning toward an end point. Beginning as a voluntary, pleasurable act, it then becomes reflexive and compulsive. The most insidious of all addictions is alcoholism, which has been recognized as a disease by the American Medical Association since 1956. This recognition eliminates notions that the alcoholic is a weak-willed person, who could quit drinking if he/she wanted. Recognizing alcoholism and other drug dependence as a disease implies five things:

- *The disease can be described.* The compulsion to drink (or to use other drugs) is manifested in habits that are inappropriate, unpredictable, excessive, and constant.

- *The course of the disease is predictable and progressive.* It will get worse; it is as simple as that. Sometimes there will be plateaus when the drinking and/or drug behavior seems to

Table 12.1

It's Not Just a College Problem

Source: National Institute on Drug Abuse, 1987

Drugs used today are more potent, more dangerous, and more addictive than ever. Initial drug use occurs at an increasingly early age. It erodes the self-discipline and motivation necessary for learning and is closely tied to dropping out of school. Fifty-seven percent of all high school seniors in the United States have used an illicit drug at least once before they finish high school. Thirty-six percent have used an illicit drug other than marijuana.

In the average class of 30 high school seniors:

- 15 or more have tried marijuana at least once
- at least one uses marijuana daily
- 23 have reported being around people who were smoking marijuana
- 27 have tried alcohol
- at least one uses it almost daily
- 17 report that they are often around people who are using alcohol to get high
- 10 say most or all of their friends use enough to get drunk at least once each week
- 5 have tried cocaine
- 7 have tried nonprescription sedatives and tranquilizers
- 6 have tried inhalants
- 4 have tried hallucinogens
- 7 have tried amphetamines
- 6 use cigarettes daily

remain constant for months or even years. But over time the course of the disease is inevitably toward greater and more serious deterioration. This deterioration can be physical, mental, and spiritual.

- *The disease is primary.* Alcoholism/drug dependency is a primary disease. Other problems the victim may have cannot be treated until the dependency is treated first.
- *The disease is permanent.* Once you have it, you have it. Trying to learn to use drugs/drink moderately will not work. The chances for successful treatment are much better in the earlier stages of the disease.
- *The disease is terminal.* If you have a chemical addiction and do not successfully arrest it, you will die from it. Whether the chemical complicates a heart condition, high blood pressure, liver problems, bleeding ulcer, or precipitates a stroke or suicide, it is still the agent that causes the death.

A useful assessment for recognizing any chemical dependency is to ask, "Is the alcohol or other drug causing *any* continuing disruption in my life—or the lives of those close to me?" (i.e., physical, mental, emotional, social, or economic). If the answer is "yes" and you do not stop drug use, then this constitutes harmful dependence.

Addictive Relationships Other Than Alcohol or Drugs

In past years, the focus of the term addiction has been centered exclusively around the use of alcohol and other drugs. Recently, a more neutral term, "dependence," has been substituted for addiction. *Dependencies* or *addiction-like* behaviors may include other objects or events such as food, gambling, sex, shoplifting, work, spending, exercise, and television. Even though these addictive objects or events are different, they all produce the desired and pleasurable mood change the addict seeks. For example:

- The gambler feels excited when studying a racing form.
- The alcoholic feels relaxed and happy when drinking at the neighborhood bar.
- The food addict feels rewarded and comforted when eating or shopping for food.
- The shoplifter senses a thrill when stealing a magazine from the drug store.
- The sex addict gets aroused when browsing in a pornographic bookstore or when searching for a new sex partner.
- The addictive spender feels exhilarated during a shopping spree.
- The workaholic feels an extreme sense of accomplishment while working all day on Sunday.

All of these objects and events have a normal, socially acceptable function. Food is to nourish, gambling is for fun and excitement, sex is for intimacy, and drugs are to help overcome illness. Most people have a normal, healthy relationship with these things, but dependent behavior results in an abnormal relationship. Dependent individuals seek a pleasurable mood change to fulfill personal needs. The addict turns to the addiction just as someone else may turn to a spouse or best friend for support, nurturing, and intimacy. As the addiction progresses, the addict becomes more and more preoccupied, withdrawn, and isolated. Table 12.2 illustrates how this type of behavior affects all the dimensions of wellness.

We know that chemical addictions produce physiological dependence resulting in withdrawal symptoms when the substance is denied. When the object of other dependencies (i.e., food or gambling) is withdrawn, withdrawal symptoms also result (i.e., anxiety or irritability).

A person can switch an addictive relationship from object to object and event to event. For example, former alcoholics can become chain smokers. Switching from object to object helps create the illusion that the "problem has been taken care of," when in reality one dangerous relationship has replaced another.

Table 12.2

How Addictions Affect the Wellness Dimensions

Physical	Addicts don't take very good care of their bodies. Addictions over time affect various parts of the body—an alcoholic's liver; a bulimic's throat. Added stress of addiction takes its toll on the heart and every other organ of the body; malnourishment is common; the body's immune system breaks down. A body is more accident prone. Considerations and even attempts at suicide become real.
Social	Addicts become withdrawn and isolated from others, become loners, interact only with the object or event of addiction; responsibility to family, school, job, etc., diminishes.
Emotional	Feelings of guilt and shame increase; depression is common; unresolved issues increase; mood swings increase; anxiety increases; fits of rage for no reason occur; paranoia develops (addict starts to question everyone and everything).
Intellectual	Logic breaks down; the addict's behavior doesn't make sense to him/her; school work falters; he/she loses touch with world events; judgment is impaired.
Spiritual	Addicts are not "connected" in a meaningful way to the world around them; they lose feelings of belonging and being an important part of the world; lose sense of knowing oneself; importance of self drifts farther and farther away; values and priorities shift; they begin to rationalize.
Occupational	Quality of job/school performance decreases as the addict becomes more and more preoccupied; absenteeism increases; relationships at work/school deteriorate; promotions and recognition are passed by.

Individuals with addictions or who exhibit addictive-like behaviors to substances, objects, or events need professional help. A partial listing of organizations, agencies, or resource centers that give information and assistance with addictions can be found at the end of this chapter.

Addictive Personality

Is there such a thing as an "addictive personality"? Do some individuals possess such a personality? This controversial topic continues to produce heated debate among psychologists. Although the addictive personality type has not been confirmed by research, some feel that this personality type does exist. They believe the addictive personality may be found in persons who don't know how to have healthy relationships, have been taught not to trust people, and have never learned to "connect" with others, community, one's emotions, and spiritual powers greater than oneself.[2]

These experts believe that early life experiences determine whether or not a person will live in a state of dependency. They would argue that the family environment is the most important component because the family is where we learn about relationships. For example, in abusive families, the children are often treated as objects, thus developing low self-esteem and mistrust in people. Also, in neglectful families, children may learn to be passive, to feel dead inside, and will seek out someone or something that makes them feel alive. This theory reflects the idea that people often form addictions because of the positive feelings (mood change) they experience when using a particular substance or repeating a behavior.

Experts claim there is no single characteristic or constellation of traits that is inevitably associated with addiction. So who is vulnerable? Possibly the individual who:

- Has a low sense of self-esteem
- Has a sense of alienation
- Is unable to turn to others for comfort
- Possesses a need for instant gratification
- Is impulsive
- Displays antisocial behavior (Is willing to go outside the boundaries of what is normally accepted)
- Cannot control strong feelings

- Rebels against authority
- Likes to try exciting and dangerous things
- Lies easily
- Is a perfectionist—a high achiever
- Seeks approval from others
- Fears personal criticism
- Is overly concerned with how others perceive him/her
- Tends to be submissive and dependent

However, many people display these characteristics without becoming addicts. This leads some to believe the personality disorders and antisocial behavior that accompany chemical abuse are the result of this abuse, not the cause of it. They claim there is no way to predict who will become an addict.[3]

Alcohol

Alcohol is the most misunderstood drug in America. Some say alcohol is a beverage, or a drug, or a central nervous system depressant. They say it is a mood-altering chemical in liquid form, or that it is sinful and dangerous. Others say it is a rite of adulthood and is safe. What a conflicting set of statements! What is alcohol, and what does it do? **Alcohol** (technically known as **ethyl alcohol** or **ethanol**) is a central nervous system depressant. The central nervous system (CNS) is composed of the brain and the spinal cord. A CNS depressant is a chemical that slows brain functions. Alcohol slows reaction time, dulls alertness, and

There are many consequences of abusive drinking.

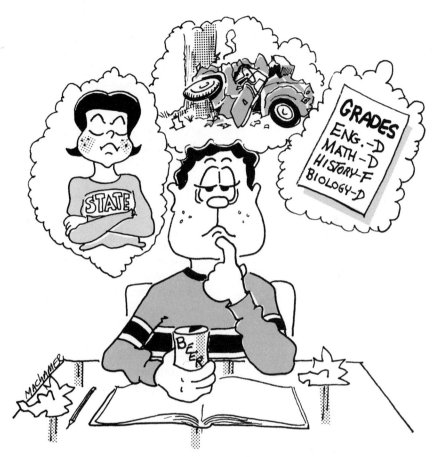

impairs body coordination. It intensifies emotions, lowers inhibitions, and increases risk-taking behaviors. It also disrupts judgment and reasoning power. On the positive side, alcohol is a good social-lubricant; on the negative, it can be unhealthy and unsafe if abused.

Alcohol Absorption

Most healthy bodies process alcohol in the same manner. Alcohol is water soluble and is transported throughout the body by the blood, which is mostly water. The amount of alcohol in the blood is expressed as a percentage, for example 0.10 percent **blood alcohol concentration (BAC)** or blood alcohol level (BAL). With the first sip, alcohol briefly irritates tissues of the mouth and esophagus. Alcohol rapidly enters the bloodstream through the small intestine and, to a small degree, through the stomach. A fraction exits in breath, sweat, and urine. Alcohol is chiefly metabolized (i.e., chemically broken down) in the liver, through which the entire blood supply circulates every four minutes. Enzymes in the liver metabolize alcohol into acetaldehyde, a highly toxic chemical. This is converted into acetate, and finally into carbon dioxide and water. The process is slow, roughly three hours for each ounce of pure alcohol. Despite vigorous folklore, virtually nothing will speed up liver function or sober up the intoxicated. A person who is drunk and drinks coffee does not become sober, only a wide awake drunk.

The mind-bending effects of alcohol begin soon after it hits the blood stream. Within minutes, alcohol enters the brain, numbing nerve cells and slowing their messages to the body. In the heart, cardiac muscles strain to cope with alcohol's depressive action, and the pulse quickens. If drinking continues, alcohol builds in the blood stream and disrupts the centers in the brain that govern speech, vision, balance, and judgment. As more alcohol is ingested, the drinker may lose consciousness. Alcohol is a hazardous anesthetic, with a narrow range between deadness and dead. At a BAC of 0.4 to 0.6 percent, the drinker is comatose and in danger of dying from respiratory failure.[4]

Speed of Alcohol Absorption

How quickly alcohol is absorbed into your bloodstream depends on five factors: body weight, gender, speed of consumption, food intake, and beverage preference. How is alcohol absorption affected by body weight and gender? It is not a myth that a man can drink the same amount of alcohol as a woman of equal weight and have a lower (BAC). This means a woman can get drunk faster than a man does. There are several explanations for this. First, women generally weigh less than men do, so the same amount of alcohol is concentrated in a smaller body mass. Second, even at the same weight, women typically have a higher percentage of body fat and less body water than men do. Since alcohol dissolves much more readily in water than in fat, the difference in body composition means that when alcohol enters a woman's body, it becomes more concentrated and therefore has a more potent effect than the same amount of alcohol would in a man's body. Third, there is an enzyme in the gastric system (small intestine and stomach) that metabolizes alcohol before it is absorbed into the bloodstream. This enzyme is found in greater amounts and is more active in men than in women. So even if a man and a woman weigh the same, have the same proportion of body fat, and drink the same amounts, more alcohol is likely to reach a women's blood, brain, and liver than a man's. This phenomenon leaves women more susceptible to liver disease. It is known that alcoholics, especially women, have virtually no gastric alcohol metabolism.[5]

Speed of consumption and food intake also affect the rate of alcohol absorption. A 12-ounce can of beer sipped over an hour's time is not absorbed into the blood stream as fast as a beer that is gulped down quickly. Food in the stomach inhibits alcohol absorption. Without inhibitors in the stomach, alcohol is absorbed extremely fast through the stomach walls and small intestines. Carbonated drinks, such as champagne, rum and coke, and whisky and soda, are absorbed even faster than water-diluted drinks.

The alcohol content of liquor (whiskey, gin, rum, etc.) is higher than that of beer or wine. Because of this, liquor causes intoxication sooner than an equal volume of beer or wine (fig. 12.1). A standard drink is defined as supplying half an ounce of absolute alcohol. This is the approximate amount found in each of the following: 12 oz. of regular beer (4% alcohol); 4 oz. of American wine (12.5% alcohol); 3 oz. of

Figure 12.1

Percentage of alcohol in beer, wine and liquor by volume.

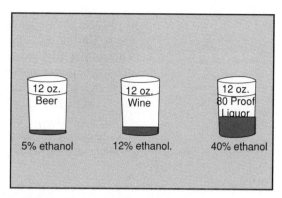

sherry (16.5% alcohol); 1 1/4 oz. of 80-proof distilled spirits ("hard liquor"); brandy, cognac, liqueurs, cordials—40% alcohol; or 1 oz. of 100-proof distilled spirits. One person's wine glass is another person's beer mug, so always measure your drinks.

Your alcohol history determines how quickly you feel the effects of this drug. It is based on your lifetime alcohol consumption, the frequency of your drinking, and the tolerance you have acquired. The number of drinks it takes for you to feel a "buzz" increases as your tolerance to alcohol increases. **Tolerance** is the body's physical adjustment to the habitual use of a chemical. An experienced drinker with a BAC of .10 percent may not feel drunk due to alcohol tolerance. An inexperienced drinker may feel intoxicated at that BAC because a tolerance has not developed (table 12.3).

Table 12.3

Percentage of Blood Alcohol Concentration

Source: Mothers Against Drunk Driving and PRIDE

		Body Weight (pounds)				
		120	140	160	180	200
Number of Drinks*	2	.06	.05	.05	.04	.04
	4	.12	.11	.09	.08	.08
	6	.19	.16	.14	.13	.11
	8	.25	.21	.19	.17	.15
	10	.31	.27	.23	.21	.19

Effects Related to Blood Alcohol Concentration (BAC)

BAC	EFFECT
.04	Reduced visual acuity, as much as wearing dark glasses, slight euphoria, and loss of shyness
.05	Relaxed state; judgment impaired, caution reduced
.08	Inhibitions lowered, may do the unexpected
.10	Movements and speech impaired; legally intoxicated
.20	Very drunk; loud and difficult to understand, emotions unstable, staggers, muscular coordination reduced; has the appearance of a "sloppy" drunk
.30	Loss of consciousness
.40+	Onset of coma; possible death due to respiratory arrest

*One drink equals 1 1/2 ounces 80-proof of alcohol, 12 oz. beer, or 5 oz. wine

If you are in a "chugging" contest, many of the above factors come into consideration. Chugging is not proof of maturity or a route to social acceptance. Chugging will only make you drunk, incoherent, and accident prone. It is dangerous and may cause convulsions, blackouts (loss of memory during a period of drinking), passouts (unconsciousness), vomiting, nausea, and even death. There are between 200–400 alcohol poisoning deaths annually in the United States.[6] Nearly all are due to "chugging" contests.

Considering all the factors that affect alcohol absorption rate, is your level of alcohol use a low- or high-risk behavior?

Impact of Alcohol

Alcohol is by far the most devastating drug—wrecking families and friendships, impairing health, wrecking careers, filling jails, hospitals, and morgues. In 1990, it cost American society an estimated 136 billion dollars and more than 100,000 lives.[7] Alcohol accounts for 50 percent of all deaths from motor vehicle crashes, one-third of all drownings, and about half of all deaths caused by fire.[8] Alcohol is linked to half of all homicides, a third of all suicides, and two-thirds of all assaults. Social workers report that alcohol is a factor in nearly 50 percent of their child-abuse cases. Over 36 percent of the male population in prison report that they were under the influence of alcohol at the time of their crimes.[9] The greatest tragedy of all is the fact that the *number-one* killer of teenagers is *drinking and driving.*[10] The majority of these drinkers started early, before they had even turned 13.[11] As you can see in table 12.4, more than 80 percent of college students

Table 12.4

Drinking Quantity/Frequency of College Students

Source: Hickenbottom, Bissonette and O'Shea (1987). "Preventive Medicine and College Alcohol Abuse." Journal of American College Health.

Percent	Category	Description
13	1	Nondrinkers
23	2	Occasional drinkers
25	3	Light drinkers (1–2 drinks once or twice a week and 3–4 drinks less than once a week)
21	4	Light-to-moderate drinkers (1–2 drinks more than twice a week, 3–4 drinks once or twice a week, and 5–6 drinks less than once a week)
11	5	Moderately heavy drinkers (3–4 drinks more than twice a week and 5–6 drinks once or twice a week and 7 or more drinks less than once a week)
5	6	Moderately heavy drinkers (5–6 drinks more than twice a week and 7 or more once or twice a week)
2	7	Heavy drinkers (7 or more drinks more than twice a week)

Over 80 percent report some drinking ranging from occasional to heavy.

report some drinking, ranging from occasional to heavy. Alcohol consumption is one of the major reasons for absenteeism among college students. It is involved in 90 percent of campus rapes, 25 percent of student deaths, is a factor in 40 percent of academic problems, and is a major contributor to campus violence. Thousands of college students will drop out because of drinking.

Long-Term Effects of Alcohol

Alcohol is a toxin, and its harmful effects on the body are great. A few drinks may make you drowsy and can interrupt patterns of sleep. Over time, heavy drinking can cause brain damage (speeds death of brain cells), damage nerve endings, and increase the risk of heart disease and cancer (mouth, throat, stomach, intestines, pancreas, and liver). It can depress the immune system and cause gastritis, pancreatitis, anxiety, delirium tremens (DTs) and malnutrition. Alcohol is a primary cause of liver failure. When alcohol is present in the liver, it preempts the breakdown of fats, which then accumulate within the liver cells. As fatty cells enlarge, they can rupture or grow into cysts that replace normal cells. After years of heavy drinking, fibrous scar tissue, or cirrhosis, impedes the normal flow of arterial and venous blood through the organ, resulting in liver failure and death.

Use and Abuse

About two-thirds of Americans use alcohol.[12] These individuals enjoy an occasional alcoholic beverage (no more than one to two drinks per week). Others, however, drink in moderation or abuse alcohol. Moderate drinking means no more than two drinks a day for most men and no more than one drink a day for most women. Who is the alcohol abuser? It is the individual who drinks more than *three per day* or more than *five drinks per week*.[13] It is the drinker who considers alcohol to be something other than a beverage to be consumed with meals or to celebrate special occasions. Alcohol abusers "use" alcohol as a medication to kill pain, to alter emotions (i.e., when mad or depressed), to help them sleep, or to cope with life. If you drink when pregnant or drink and drive, you are an alcohol abuser.

The morning after a night of abusive drinking, you may experience the following conditions: oversensitivity to light and sound; a hangover; dehydration; nausea; bloodshot eyes; "bags" under the eyes; and **blackout** (cannot remember all or parts of the night before). To avoid abusing alcohol follow the Zero . . . One . . . Three Rule for Responsible Drinking in table 12.5.

Table 12.5

The Zero . . . One . . . Three Rule for Responsible Drinking

Source: Concept partially developed by "Enjoy Michigan Safety Coalition." Funded by Michigan Office of Highway Safety Planning.

0 = No level of drinking is recommended. Never drink and drive—even one block
1 = Drink only one alcoholic beverage per hour if you do drink
3 = Never drink more than three alcoholic beverages per day (or more than five per week)

Alcoholism

No one plans on becoming an alcoholic, yet alcoholism is on the rise (see table 12.6). Even newborn infants may become addicted if the mother abuses alcohol during pregnancy. Most alcoholism is a result of abusive drinking. The difference between the alcoholic and the alcohol abuser is control over drinking. The abusive drinker can stop. The addict cannot. Ask yourself: Do you *want* it, or do you *need* it?

Table 12.6

Profile of Alcoholism in the United States

Source: National Center for Health Statistics, 1988

Alcoholism is one of America's most serious public health problems. A look at percentages of Americans who have been exposed to alcoholism:

- 42.8% of adults have lived with, been married to, or have had a blood relative who was an alcoholic or problem drinker.
- 18.1% of adults have lived with an alcoholic or a problem drinker at some time during their first 18 years of life.
- Far more women have been married to alcoholics or problem drinkers.
- Half of all traffic deaths can be traced to drunk driving; 54% to 74% of those convicted of drunk driving are alcoholics.
- Health care costs for untreated alcoholics are at least 100% higher than for nonalcoholics.
- 20% to 40% of all U.S. hospital beds are occupied by persons being treated for alcoholism or complications of alcohol abuse.
- Evidence shows that exposure to alcoholism predisposes people to become alcoholics themselves.

Alcoholism is a drug (chemical) dependence. It involves progressive preoccupation with drinking, leading to physical, mental, or social dysfunction. Approximately one of ten Americans is an alcoholic. The point where heavy drinking merges into alcohol dependence is blurry. The behaviors may appear to be the same. For example, both the addict and abuser may suffer from blackouts, passouts, arrests, hangovers, absenteeism, accidents, violence, poor job or school performance, and poor relationships.

Heredity explains some alcoholism because a history of alcoholism in the family puts you at higher risk. What you inherit is not the disease but a predisposition to the disease. Scientists are looking for biological markers (i.e., variations in neurotransmitters, certain blood enzymes and brain waves) hoping to eventually identify influential genes. One researcher reports that there are different types of alcoholics, just as there are different types of diabetics and schizophrenics.[14] He claims that a cluster of symptoms is needed in order to lead to dependence. Abusive drinking and craving are pivotal.

The answers to these questions about your drinking can help you decide if you need professional help.

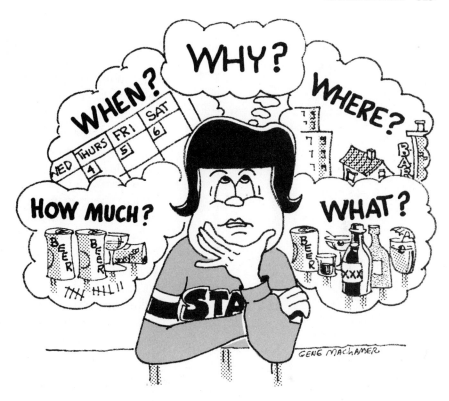

The way in which you were introduced to alcohol as a child strongly influences your attitudes and drinking behavior as an adult. Table 12.7 lists factors indicative of those who would experience the fewest problems with alcohol in adulthood. How do you stack up with these factors?

The alcohol abuser needs to change his drinking behavior by quitting or following the Zero . . . One . . . Three Rule for Responsible Drinking. The alcoholic must quit! No alcoholic should ever quit "cold turkey" (abruptly) without proper supervision, however, as the body has become dependent upon alcohol. When you abruptly stop using alcohol, you will probably experience some withdrawal symptoms, which can be dangerous. Some of these symptoms are profuse sweating, coldness, tremors or shakes, nausea, headaches, and hallucinations (auditory or visual).

It is imperative to identify early the 20 percent of drinkers whose lives can potentially be shattered by addiction to alcohol. For about 8 percent of the population, alcohol is relatively innocuous.[15] Most people have few difficulties with alcohol—many others cross the line into alcoholism—and those who do deny it furiously. That is the paradox of alcohol.

Table 12.7

Social Self-Assessment

Source: National Institute on Alcohol Abuse and Alcoholism.

You are least likely to have problems with alcohol if:

1. You were exposed to alcohol in relatively small quantities early in life by your family or within the context of a religious or cultural group.
2. Your family members viewed alcohol as a food and consumed small quantities, primarily at mealtime.
3. Your parents set a good example by practicing responsible drinking behaviors.
4. Your family did not view drinking alcoholic beverages as a means of demonstrating maturity, adulthood, or masculinity/femininity.
5. Abstinence was accepted as a legitimate choice with respect to the consumption of alcoholic beverages.
6. Drunkenness was not an acceptable form of behavior.
7. Alcohol was viewed as a beverage and not as the central focus of a group activity.
8. Rules and rituals associated with drinking were known and understood by all group members; they were both reasonable and agreeable to those members.

Anyone who drinks should ask the following questions. Does anyone in my family (even one member) have a history of alcoholism or drug abuse? Am I drinking too much? When am I drinking? Where am I drinking? What am I drinking? Why am I drinking? Are most of my friends heavy drinkers? Do I seek out events at which alcohol will be served? Do you "have to have a drink?" Do you make up excuses to drink? Do you intend to control your alcohol intake but never do?

If you are not satisfied with your answers, consider getting a professional assessment. Take the quiz in table 12.8 to find out if you have a drinking problem.

For those with an alcohol problem, help is available. There is hope. Many people have gone to treatment centers, hospitals, clinics, and self-help groups for assistance in dealing with drinking problems.

One popular group that offers assistance to alcoholics of all ages is Alcoholics Anonymous (AA). AA was founded in 1935 by two desperate alcoholics—a stockbroker and a surgeon. The group had only 100 members during the first four years. It now has a world-wide membership of over two million. AA is a fellowship of mutual and spiritual support that has endured in simplicity. No dues, no minutes, the only condition for membership is *a desire to stop drinking.*

Table 12.8

Drinking Habits Quiz

Source: National Institute on Alcohol Abuse and Alcoholism.

1. Do you think about drinking often?
2. Do you drink more now than you used to?
3. Do you avoid situations where it would be impossible to get a drink if you wanted one?
4. Do you sometimes gulp your drinks?
5. Do you often take a drink to help you relax?
6. Do you drink often when you are alone?
7. Do you sometimes forget what happened while you were drinking?
8. Has your drinking ever created problems between you and friends, you and your parents, or with the law?
9. Have you ever injured yourself or another person after drinking?
10. Do you need a drink to have fun?
11. Do you ever just start drinking without really thinking about it?
12. Do you drink in the morning to relieve a hangover?

(If you answered "yes" to four or more questions, you may be a problem drinker.)

Strategies for Dealing with Alcohol

Alcohol is an accepted drug in today's society, but you don't have to go along with the crowd. Who controls and makes decisions about your life—you or others? Take charge. Here are some helpful strategies for you and ways you can help others who have abused alcohol.

Strategies for drinking less or not at all include:

1. It is increasingly more acceptable to say "no thanks" to alcohol.
2. Let your waistline be your incentive. Alcoholic beverages are loaded with "empty" calories (high in calories, low in nutrients). There is some evidence that alcohol not only adds calories to the diet but also keeps the body from burning dietary fat properly. Alcohol in the blood stream slows down fat metabolism more than 30 percent while speeding up the burning of carbohydrates. This unused fat gets deposited on the thighs, hips, and stomach.[16]
3. If you do drink, follow the Responsible Drinking Guidelines found in table 12.5. Switch to juice or soft drinks after the three-drink maximum.
4. At restaurants, order food first, not an alcoholic beverage. That way you will have less time to drink.

5. After exercise, or when extra thirsty, avoid carbonated alcoholic drinks. They are absorbed too fast, and you may be tempted to gulp them down. Drink a glass of cold water first.

6. Don't hold the drink in your hand. Put it down somewhere—this will help slow down consumption.

7. Try cocktails without the alcohol (i.e., a Bloody Mary without the vodka) or nonalcoholic beer.

8. Dilute your drinks with water, ice, or extra fruit juice.

9. Make sure your drinks are accurately measured.

10. Volunteer to be the designated driver (you may even get free soft drinks).

If a friend has passed out from drinking alcohol:

1. Put him on his stomach. If you put him on his side or back, he may vomit, inhale his vomit, and suffocate.

2. Do not give him anything to eat or drink. He is unconscious. You could cause him to choke.

3. Be sure he is breathing okay—not shallow, but deep breathing. Shallow breathing means his brain is shutting down, and his involuntary functions are ceasing. Call for help!

4. Cover him with a sheet, not a blanket. If your friend has overdosed on alcohol, his internal body temperature has fallen. The shivering of his body stimulates him and helps to keep him alive. Too much external warmth will stop that important stimulation.

5. If he is shivering, call for help!

6. Gently shake your friend, and call him by his first name. He will probably respond in some manner. If he doesn't respond at all, call for help!

Alcohol and the Law

Society has responded to the alcohol problem with legislation. All 50 states now have a drinking age of 21 years. You are breaking the law if you are under the age of 21 and are using, possessing, or transporting alcohol. These laws partly discourage some students from drinking, which lowers the potential for accidents. Drinking to *any* extent reduces the ability of *any* driver (see table 12.3). Fifty percent of all fatal auto accidents in this country are alcohol-related.[17]

Most states have defined driving under the influence of alcohol as having a blood alcohol content (BAC) of .10 percent. Whether or not a person feels intoxicated is not the point, but whether he registers .10 on a breathalyzer (see table 12.3). The rationale for the law is that it may act as a deterrent to drinking and driving. Some states have dropped the figure to .08 percent; at least two states are considering .05 percent as presumption of intoxication. There is no safe drinking BAC! Look at table 12.9 for some sobering statistics.

Here is the message: You could be one of the persons who dies in the next 20 minutes due to alcohol-related accidents. Or you could be crippled or permanently injured for life. Do not let it be you. Most think it won't happen to them.

Irresponsible drinking complicates your life.

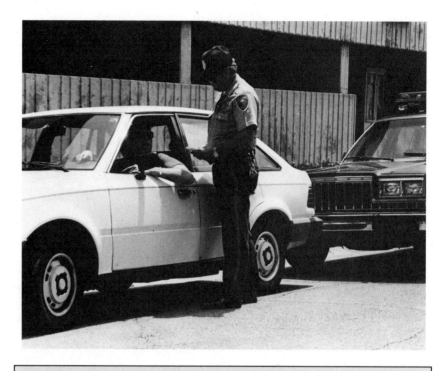

Table 12.9

Sobering Facts on
Drinking and Driving

*Source: National Highway Transportation Safety
Administration*

1. Drunk drivers are 25 times more likely than sober drivers to have accidents.

2. About 23,000 persons are killed each year in alcohol-related accidents. About 450 persons die each week, and every 20 minutes another life is lost in an alcohol-related accident.

3. More than 36 percent of the persons who die in alcohol-related accidents are passengers, drivers of the other vehicle, and pedestrians.

4. About one of every two Americans will be involved in an alcohol-related accident in their lifetime.

5. The social drinkers are a greater menace than commonly believed, as their critical judgment is impaired with a low BAC and they outnumber the obviously intoxicated drivers.

6. More are arrested for drunken driving—1.8 million a year—than for other crime in the U.S. Yet, the average drunken driver drives hundreds of times, thousands of miles, before being caught.

7. The average BAC of those arrested is .17 percent—equivalent to a 160-pound man drinking nearly 10 beers in two hours.

8. Repeat offenders: 24 percent are convicted for a second time within seven years; 8.6 percent for a third time; and 4.3 percent for four or more times.

Fetal Alcohol Syndrome (FAS) and Fetal Alcohol Effect (FAE)

Fetal alcohol syndrome (FAS) is a condition acquired by the unborn fetus and caused by the mother drinking alcohol during pregnancy. The alcohol passes through the placenta (within minutes) and affects the unborn child. There is no other cause for the FAS. Women need to understand that the placenta does not keep unwanted chemicals away from the fetus. We now know that what a mother eats, drinks, or smokes passes to her unborn child. Humans are supposed to be the wisest of creatures, yet it is not uncommon to see pregnant women drinking alcoholic beverages, smoking, and taking drugs they would never consider giving to their children. Then they expect their babies to come into the world healthy and cuddly. Alcohol is one of the leading causes of mental retardation in the Western World.[18]

Alcohol damages the vulnerable developing brain and may impair placental function, as well. This damage is irreversible. Since we are unsure exactly which brain cells of the fetus are destroyed, the expectant mother who drinks is denying her child development of his/her full potential. The damage can range from severe physical deformity, clumsiness, behavioral problems, stunted growth, to mental retardation. No one is certain how much alcohol it takes to cause damage to the fetus. Some women drink very little and their babies are still affected.

A far greater number of babies have more subtle symptoms that are rarely attributed to drinking mothers. This condition is called **Fetal Alcohol Effect (FAE).** The mother of a child diagnosed with FAE did not necessarily drink less during pregnancy than the mother of a child with FAS, but, for some biological reason, the baby was not as damaged physically. The FAE child shows traits of impaired memory, poor judgment, and reduced capacity to learn from experience. Many FAE children go through life undetected and misjudged. They often drop out of school or wind up on the margins of society.[19] Drinking while pregnant is like playing Russian roulette with your baby's life. Why take chances with your baby's future? The message is: There is no known safe level of alcohol consumption during pregnancy. FAS and FAE are totally preventable, but abstinence is the only way to guarantee that a baby will suffer no ill effects from alcohol.

Tobacco

If you are a regular smoker, you may be losing about six minutes of life expectancy for every cigarette you smoke. For most smokers that means a life expectancy reduced by five to eight years. The U.S. Surgeon General has described cigarette smoking as ". . . the chief preventable cause of death in our society."[20] More people die from smoking-related diseases than from alcohol, cocaine, heroine, suicide, homicide, car accidents, and AIDS combined. Despite all the frightening statistics, the warnings, and the publicity given to the health risks of smoking, each year thousands of young people start smoking.

The Decline of Smoking

Little was known about the health consequences of smoking until 1964 when the first Surgeon General's report on smoking and health was published. At that time, nearly half of our population smoked.[21] In the years since, millions of people have quit, and now smokers are less than a quarter of the population. Once considered sophisticated, smoking now seems to be most prevalent in the lower socioeconomic and the least educated groups. Studies reveal that smoking is twice as high among those with less than a high school education compared to those with a college education.[22]

Before World War II, smoking was considered a masculine activity, and few women smoked. After World War II, with increasing emancipation, women began smoking in ever-increasing numbers. As a result, lung cancer deaths for women tripled. While proportions of adult men and women smokers have dropped since 1964, surveys indicate that men have given up smoking more often than women.[23]

Smoking may have been considered glamorous once, but today attitudes are changing. Smoking commercials have been banned from radio and television since 1971. Cigarette advertisements and packages carry health warnings. Over 75 percent of adult smokers have either tried to quit smoking or would like to try.[24] Nonsmokers are tired of passive smoking—breathing air polluted by tobacco smoke—and are gaining the right to breathe clean air in workplaces and public areas.

Why Do People Smoke?

The most important influences in starting to smoke are family and friends. In families where one or both parents smoke, a person is twice as likely to be a smoker than when the parents are nonsmokers.[25] Many teenagers start smoking because they think "everybody else does," and they want to be like their friends or appear more grown up. They don't think much about the costs or health risks of smoking.

Nicotine, a drug in cigarette smoke, is addicting, as anyone who has tried to quit smoking has quickly discovered. Nicotine is an alkaloid drug synthesized by the tobacco plant in the same fashion that the opium poppy (the source of heroin) and the coca plant (the source of cocaine) synthesize their addictive substances. Habituation to nicotine may occur after smoking only three packs of cigarettes. Once a person is hooked on nicotine, it can be difficult to quit. Indeed, experts say that addiction to nicotine can be just as strong as addiction to cocaine or heroine. Without a steady supply of nicotine, withdrawal symptoms may occur. A person may become irritable, anxious, hostile, and crave tobacco. Nicotine withdrawal may also produce headaches, nausea, and inability to concentrate. Although these symptoms subside, the failure rate for people who try to quit smoking on the first try is more than 80 percent. Smokers' family and friends should be more aware that smoking is not just a "nasty habit," but a form of drug dependence.

Health Risks of Smoking

Of the 41,000 potentially toxic chemicals in cigarette smoke, the three major toxic substances are nicotine, carbon monoxide, and tar. Nicotine stimulates the cardiovascular system. Increased heart rate and blood pressure place a burden on the heart muscle, which now needs more oxygen. Carbon monoxide, a toxic gas, immediately reduces the blood's ability to carry oxygen and ultimately damages the inner surface of coronary arteries, increasing the rate of atherosclerosis. When combined with vasoconstriction, a narrowing of the arteries, this can cause ischemia (lack of oxygen) and coronary tissue damage. Smoking also increases arrhythmias, increases stickiness and clotting of blood cells, and decreases levels of HDL.[26] This is why smokers die from heart attacks at double the rate of nonsmokers.

Tar contains potent carcinogens. It also contains chemicals that irritate lung tissue and may promote chronic bronchitis and emphysema. These substances can paralyze and destroy the cilia that line the bronchi, allowing tar and other particles to accumulate in the lungs. This causes *smoker's cough,* which is the body's attempt to rid itself of the buildup of particulate matter. Long-term contact between lung tissue and tar can cause cellular changes leading to the development of cancer.

The reduction in a person's life expectancy due to smoking parallels increasing cigarette usage. Mortality rises the younger a person started smoking, the longer a person has smoked, the deeper a smoker inhales, and the higher the tar and nicotine content of the tobacco used. If that smoker is overweight, has moderately elevated blood pressure, or has a high cholesterol level, the risk of having a heart attack skyrockets.[27]

If you've smoked for many years, does it do any good to quit? Yes! Heart attack risk declines by about half in the first year after quitting. Risk continues to decrease with each year of abstinence, until, after 10 to 15 years, an exsmoker has almost the same risk of dying as if he had never smoked (see table 12.10). People who quit smoking may gain weight, but it is less of a health risk than continuing to smoke. The average weight gain is 6 pounds for men and 8 pounds for women, which brings them to average weight levels of persons who have never smoked. Regardless of how long or how much a person has smoked, quitting is beneficial.

Smokeless Tobacco

Cigarette smoking is not the only form of tobacco that presents health risks. Smokeless tobacco—snuff and chewing tobacco—is surging in popularity among young adult males. Advertised by athletes, smokeless tobacco seems to be viewed as a safe alternative to cigarette smoking, which is forbidden by coaches on athletic teams. The tobacco industry wants you to believe that snuff and chewing tobacco provide all the pleasure of cigarettes, minus the risks. But the evidence shows otherwise. Highly carcinogenic tobacco **nitrosamines** are released in concentrations 1,000 times higher in smokeless tobacco-saliva mixtures than in cigarette smoke.[28] Snuff and chewing tobacco cause many problems ranging from bad breath to cancer. A decrease in the ability to taste and smell, stained teeth, gum damage, tooth loss, and wear on the chewing surfaces of the teeth caused by grit in the tobacco are commonly experienced. Use of smokeless tobacco also causes leukoplakia, a precancerous condition that produces thick, rough, white patches

Table 12.10
When Smokers Quit

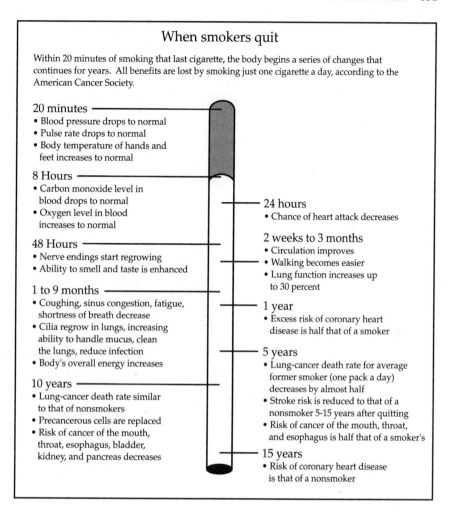

When smokers quit

Within 20 minutes of smoking that last cigarette, the body begins a series of changes that continues for years. All benefits are lost by smoking just one cigarette a day, according to the American Cancer Society.

20 minutes
- Blood pressure drops to normal
- Pulse rate drops to normal
- Body temperature of hands and feet increases to normal

8 Hours
- Carbon monoxide level in blood drops to normal
- Oxygen level in blood increases to normal

48 Hours
- Nerve endings start regrowing
- Ability to smell and taste is enhanced

1 to 9 months
- Coughing, sinus congestion, fatigue, shortness of breath decrease
- Cilia regrow in lungs, increasing ability to handle mucus, clean the lungs, reduce infection
- Body's overall energy increases

10 years
- Lung-cancer death rate similar to that of nonsmokers
- Precancerous cells are replaced
- Risk of cancer of the mouth, throat, esophagus, bladder, kidney, and pancreas decreases

24 hours
- Chance of heart attack decreases

2 weeks to 3 months
- Circulation improves
- Walking becomes easier
- Lung function increases up to 30 percent

1 year
- Excess risk of coronary heart disease is half that of a smoker

5 years
- Lung-cancer death rate for average former smoker (one pack a day) decreases by almost half
- Stroke risk is reduced to that of a nonsmoker 5-15 years after quitting
- Risk of cancer of the mouth, throat, and esophagus is half that of a smoker's

15 years
- Risk of coronary heart disease is that of a nonsmoker

on the gums, tongue, or inner cheek.[29] Experts predict an oral cancer epidemic beginning in two or three decades if the current trend continues.

In addition, smokeless tobacco is addictive. Nicotine from tobacco is absorbed into the bloodstream (one of the most efficient delivery systems known) and eventually produces dependency. Many people feel that the dependency produced by smokeless tobacco is harder to break than smoking.

Are You a Passive Smoker?

Nonsmokers, who outnumber smokers three to one, are growing tired of **passive smoking**—breathing air polluted by tobacco smoke. Especially when they read reports from the American Heart Association and the Environmental Protection Agency (EPA). The American Heart Association report states that secondhand smoking causes 53,000 deaths per year (37,000 of these from heart disease).[30] In 1993, the EPA officially declared secondhand smoke to be a human carcinogen that causes about 3,000 nonsmokers a year to die from lung cancer and about 12,000 deaths a year from other cancers. The EPA also reported that children exposed to secondhand smoke are at an increased risk of bronchitis, pneumonia, and asthma. Many states have passed laws restricting smoking in public places. Restaurants, airplanes, and trains have separate smoking and nonsmoking sections. Nearly all companies in America have restricted smoking in the workplace. Why has this occurred? How does smoke-filled air affect nonsmokers?

The passive smoker involuntarily inhales toxic fumes produced by the cigarette of the mainstream smoker. What nonsmokers may not realize is that these highly toxic substances are found in higher concentrations in sidestream than in mainstream smoke. Even though smoke is mixed with environmental air, it still

Smoking is everybody's business.

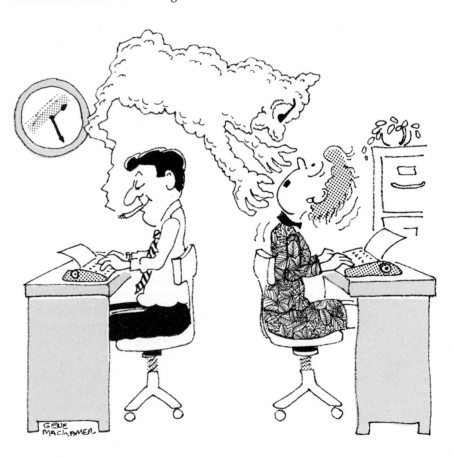

causes eye and nasal irritations, sore throats, coughing, and headaches in non-smokers. It may also be harmful to people with asthma, respiratory illness, cardiovascular disease, or an allergy to smoke. Families of smokers have more respiratory problems and more days of absence from work or school due to illness than families of nonsmokers. Children of smokers have more colds, ear infections, reduced lung function, and a greater chance of being hospitalized for acute respiratory infections than nonsmokers' children.[31] Studies have indicated that nonsmoking wives of heavy smokers have double the risk of lung cancer compared to other nonsmokers. The same thing may be true for their risk of emphysema, bronchitis, and other respiratory diseases.

Why Should I Quit?

The simple act of quitting smoking can add years to a person's life (table 12.10). Even more important, it increases the chance that those years will be healthy and active, drastically decreasing the chances of suffering painful, incapacitating, and costly illnesses. Overall quality of life will improve. You will save money, since cigarettes are expensive. A pack-a-day habit sends nearly $700 a year up in smoke. You can say goodbye to tobacco stains on your teeth and fingers. Your breath, hair, clothes, and surroundings will smell fresher. Your smoke will no longer annoy or harm other people, and this will particularly benefit your own family. No longer will cigarette burns or messy ashes ruin furniture, carpet, and countertops. Your risk of setting an accidental fire will be reduced. Your ability to taste and smell will return. As the effects of smoking are reversed, you will eliminate smoker's cough and increase your endurance so that you have more energy all day long. Besides reducing the health risks, you will overcome a potential drug addiction that may have taken control of your life.

How to Quit Smoking

In the past few years, millions of Americans have quit smoking. Of smokers who quit, most have done it on their own. There are many ways to quit. Some people try to gradually reduce the number of cigarettes they smoke. Others quit cold turkey. A new product is helping many quit by weaning them away from nicotine. The product is a small patch worn on the skin that minimizes the usual withdrawal symptoms. It is available by prescription only. It works by painlessly releasing decreasing doses of nicotine through tiny blood vessels near the surface of the skin. An even more successful cessation program is an approach combining nicotine chewing gum, nicotine patches, and behavior modification counseling.[32] The number one determinant of success, however, is simply the smoker's own desire to quit, based on some strong motivational goal, like saving money or improving health. If you are a nonsmoker wishing to help a smoker who is trying to quit, you should know that the support of family and friends is the second most important factor in successfully breaking the grip of the nicotine habit.

Giving up smoking can be a long-term process, and some people must try several times before they quit for good. About 20 percent succeed in quitting on the first try, which is about the same success rate as breaking an alcohol or heroin addiction. This doesn't mean that a person can't quit, because every year thousands of people do. But it takes effort, desire, support, and a firm commitment. If a person quits smoking, then starts again, she should not be considered weak-willed. Some former smokers say they still crave cigarettes long after they quit smoking. The smoker who does not succeed in quitting on the first try should try, try again. Mark Twain said it best. "It's easy to *quit* smoking, I should know—I've done it dozens of times."

If you're ready to toss those cigarettes, *Clearing the Air: A Guide to Quitting Smoking,* available from the American Cancer Society, gives these recommendations:

- *Set a target date for quitting.* Then list all the reasons why you want to quit. Review these whenever you crave tobacco.

- *Before you quit,* change to a brand you find distasteful, then taper off a little more each day. Smoke only half of each cigarette. Smoke only during even hours of the day.

- *Involve friends and family.* Tell them when and why you are going to quit, and ask for their support.

- *On the day you quit,* toss out all cigarettes and matches. Go to the dentist to have your teeth cleaned. Keep very busy and concentrate on getting through that one day without tobacco.

- *After quitting,* change your normal routine. Spend as much time as possible away from places and situations which you associate with smoking. Go jogging, drink more fluids, get plenty of rest.

- *When you get the "crazies,"* chew on carrots, pickles, sunflower seeds, sugarless gum. Take a shower. Never allow yourself to think "One won't hurt." It will.

- *Mark progress.* Each month, celebrate the anniversary of your quit date. Put aside the money you've saved by not smoking and treat yourself to something special. You deserve it.

Marijuana

A drug that some people consider safe is marijuana. It is America's most widely used illegal drug and trails only alcohol and tobacco in popularity as a social or recreational drug.[33] Even though illegal, it has been used in medicine for over 2,000 years and has been proven somewhat effective in the treatment of glaucoma, epilepsy, multiple sclerosis, migraine headaches, and relief from side effects of chemotherapy.[34] **Marijuana** (sometimes called "pot" or "grass") is a psychoactive drug made from the leaves and flowers of the cannabis sativa plant. The leaves and flowers are dried and crushed, causing the marijuana to have a tobacco-like appearance. When marijuana is rolled in papers, the end product is a cigarette called a "joint." Although there are at least 421 ingredients in marijuana, **delta-9-tetrahydrocannabinol (THC)** is the psychoactive ingredient.

Marijuana is fat soluble and is stored in fatty tissues of the body, brain, and reproductive organs. Because the THC toxicity of marijuana has increased 300 percent since the 1960s, the effects of smoking a joint may last one to two hours, with the peak occurring 20 to 30 minutes after inhalation. Since THC is stored in the fatty tissues, it may stay in the body for 30 days. Also, THC has an accumulation effect. This means that if you smoke one joint a week, the body has not had enough time to rid itself of THC, which builds up. After a month of smoking marijuana every weekend, your body is saturated with THC.

Marijuana causes short-term memory loss, increased appetite, various respiratory conditions, increased heart rate, lowered sperm count, and abnormal menstruation. Because marijuana burns hotter than tobacco, it results in more lung and throat damage than cigarettes do. According to Robert Gilkeson, M.D., THC changes the cell membrane, causing it to be less efficient with less energy, particularly in the brain and testicles.[35] Amotivational syndrome is also linked to marijuana use. A person with **amotivational syndrome** experiences low energy, apathy, and little drive to do anything. Students exhibit this syndrome by not going to class, not completing assignments, "vegetating" on a chair, or appearing not to care about anything. Amotivational syndrome is thought to be linked to changes in the cell membranes.[36]

Drinking alcohol while smoking marijuana is dangerous. Marijuana inhibits vomiting, causing the alcohol to remain in your system. This increases the chance of alcohol poisoning.

Cocaine and Crack

Cocaine and **crack** (a cocaine derivative) are potent, rapid-acting drugs. Cocaine comes from the coca plant, which is mainly harvested in Central and South America. Cocaine is extracted from the coca leaf during a simple two-step chemical process involving sulfuric and hydrochloric acid. This process separates cocaine from the other chemicals in the coca leaf and results in cocaine hydrochloride (or "street cocaine"). Cocaine hydrochloride is the fine, opalescent, white, fluffy, odorless, and bitter-tasting drug that is sold for illegal, recreational use. It is the second most widely used illegal drug in the United States.[37] Until the early 1980s, cocaine was used mainly by the wealthy. Today it is truly an equal opportunity drug, used by members of all socio-economic groups.

Cocaine is a euphoriant and a central nervous system stimulant with its effects lasting from 20 minutes to several hours, depending on the drug's purity. There are several ways to take cocaine, and the speed with which the cocaine user achieves a "high" varies with each method. It may take 10–30 minutes to feel cocaine's effects when the drug is swallowed, three minutes when it is snorted, one-half minute when it is injected, and a few seconds when it is smoked. While it may be swallowed, this is not as effective as other methods because of poor absorption in the gastrointestinal tract. The most common method is to snort the drug (sniff it through the nose). The powder is first chopped fine with a razor blade and arranged into lines on a piece of glass. The user may then inhale the cocaine through a rolled-up dollar bill, straw, or "coke spoon." Injecting cocaine produces an intense and exhilarating rush, but one that is shortlived because of the drug's rapid metabolization by the liver. Cocaine may also be smoked in the form of either freebase cocaine or crack.

Freebase cocaine is separated from ordinary street cocaine (cocaine hydrochloride) in a process that results in a purer and more intense form that can be smoked. (Cocaine hydrochloride—the street, powder form—cannot be smoked.) In this process, the drug is freed from the parent compound by mixing it with water and ammonium hydroxide. The cocaine base is then separated from the water using a fast-drying solvent such as ether, leaving unadulterated cocaine freebase. Small amounts of the base are then placed in the neck of a specially designed water pipe and smoked at high temperature over a torch. The ether used in the process is extremely volatile and may explode. All of the freebase components are readily available in the retail marketplace. Smoking freebase cocaine creates a "rush" that is rapid, powerful, and shortlived, much like the high from injected cocaine. While the euphoria and feelings of energy last only a few minutes, the other effects (such as pupil dilation, increased blood pressure, and heart rate) are prolonged and can be dangerous.

Crack is crystallized freebase cocaine sold in the form of ready-to-smoke "rocks." The rocks of processed cocaine are smoked in a pipe, or placed in cigarettes or joints of marijuana. As a ready-to-smoke drug, crack spares the user the delay and bother of having to extract the potent freebase form of cocaine from cocaine hydrochloride. The rocks are nicknamed "crack" because of the crackling sound they make as they are smoked. Before crack came on the market, cocaine smokers had to make the freebase themselves, using dangerous, highly flammable chemicals such as ether. The extraction process was complicated and costly as well. Because crack is such a pure drug (about 90% pure cocaine), and approximately five times more potent than cocaine, smoking crack gives the user a far more intense and rapid euphoria than does snorting cocaine. One puff of a pebble-sized rock produces an intense high that lasts about 20 minutes. The user can generally get three or four "hits" off one rock. The high is always followed immediately by an equally unpleasant crash, characterized by irritability, agitation, and intense cravings for more of the drug.

Crack is usually purchased in small plastic vials containing two or three rocks. Crack, costing $5 to $20 per vial, is more affordable per dose than cocaine. However, most people cannot stop after one vial and may use five or more vials to keep the high. Even though crack is sold in inexpensive units, this has nothing to do with the actual price of the drug. Crack's price per gram is almost double that of cocaine powder. Crack only appears cheaper—much as buying a single cup of coffee for 50 cents seems cheaper, but is actually much more expensive, than buying a whole pound of coffee for $3.99. The deceptively low initial price of crack makes it possible for just about anyone to start using the drug. Some users go on a three-day crack binge, depleting their body and bankbooks. They quit only because they are out of money, out of crack, or because their bodies cannot take it anymore.

Addiction to crack takes less time to develop than addiction to snorting cocaine. Some users can become psychologically addicted after smoking it just a few times. Crack addiction is accelerated by the speed in which it is absorbed through the lungs (it hits the brain within 4–6 seconds) and by the intensity of the high.

Some people may start using cocaine to lose weight (it depresses the appetite) or to enhance alertness and relieve fatigue (it stimulates the central nervous system). As a stimulant, this drug also causes blood pressure, heart rate, and body temperature to rise. Because the heart and breathing are accelerated, and the fact that it acts as a vasoconstrictor (narrows blood vessels), cocaine can be dangerous to anyone with heart or respiratory problems. The increase in the number of strokes in the early 1990s has been linked to cocaine use.

Cocaine users develop tolerance and eventually need more and purer forms of the drug to get the same effect. If addiction occurs, withdrawal symptoms will develop. Eventually, the addict uses cocaine to avoid the unpleasant depression or crash that always follows the rush. How do you know if you are addicted to cocaine? Put simply, and as stated earlier in this chapter, continuing to use a drug (any drug) despite negative consequences constitutes addiction.

Consequences of using any form of cocaine may be severe. Since cocaine is an illegal drug, users risk arrests, fines, and jail terms. Some states are considering prosecuting women who take drugs during pregnancy and give birth to addicted babies.

Eventually, smoking crack and freebase cocaine may cause paranoia, other psychoses, lung and liver damage, depression, insomnia, impotence, nausea, vomiting, anxiety, and isolation. People who smoke crack (whether for the first or the fiftieth time) are risking their lives. The intense high can be too much for the body, causing respiratory arrest, heart attack, convulsions, and death. Snorting cocaine can lead to chronic rhinitis (runny nose), nasal congestion, perforation of the nasal septum, and greater vulnerability to upper respiratory infections. Injecting cocaine increases the risk of contracting AIDS, hepatitis, and other infectious diseases if needles are shared.

Crank and Ice

Crank, a term once used as a street name for cocaine, has emerged on the drug scene as an alias for methamphetamine (a synthetic form of amphetamine). Crank is a powerful stimulant, odorless, yellow or off-white in color, and sold in capsules, chunks, or crystals. "Eightballs," approximately one-eighth of an ounce, are considered to be a day's supply. Crank is often sniffed, inhaled, or injected to produce a greater "high." The "rush," an effect greatly desired by the abuser, is a highly pleasurable sensation experienced almost immediately after intravenous injection. It lasts from 2 to 4 hours. **Ice,** the street name for crystallized crank, sometimes called "crystal meth," is smoked, like crack cocaine. It is quickly overtaking crack cocaine as the drug of choice for many addicts. Experts claim that ice is more dangerous than crack cocaine because it is more addictive. The high caused by smoking crack lasts about 20 to 30 minutes, but ice users can feel a high lasting as long as 24 hours, followed by symptoms of depression and acute psychoses, including hallucinations. Ice costs about the same as crack, from $80 to $125 a gram, but is cheaper to use since each dose is smaller and the effects last much longer (between 8 to 24 hours).[38]

Ice, used in Asia for years, was imported to Hawaii in the early 1980s and has since spread to the West Coast. Both crank and ice are being manufactured and aggressively marketed by youth and motorcycle gangs and are quickly spreading eastward across the U.S. Crank can be easily manufactured in the home laboratory by a "cook" with a high-school education in chemistry and $500 worth of equipment by extracting pure methamphetamine from common industrial chemicals. Some law enforcement officials fear crank and its smokable form, ice, will be the basis for a national drug crisis during the 1990s. The aftereffects of crank and ice are similar to crack and cocaine—lethargy, severe depression, paranoia, and cardiopulmonary damage. Many users develop a tolerance for these drugs quickly and need larger and larger doses to gain the effect they seek.

Drugs Affecting Physical Performance

In the world of competitive athletics where the margin between winning and losing may be only a fraction of a second, athletes looking for an edge are tempted by illegal drugs. Anabolic steroids are taken to build muscle. Amphetamines may be taken to mask fatigue; caffeine to enhance performance. Diuretics may be used to cause rapid weight loss or to mask anabolic steroid use. All of these drugs can adversely affect your health.

Anabolic Steroids

Anabolic steroids are an artificial form of the male hormone **testosterone.** Testosterone is secreted by the testes of a mature male in quantities of 2.5 mg to 10 mg daily.[39] This hormone stimulates the bone, muscle, skin, and hair growth that are characteristically found in the adult male. Steroids were first developed in the 1930s to build body tissues and to prevent the breakdown of tissue that occurs in some diseases. In the 1950s, a few foreign countries experimented with giving testosterone to their male and female athletes. Because these athletes dominated many international competitions, an American doctor developed a form of

Overly aggressive behavior is a sympton of steroid use in males.

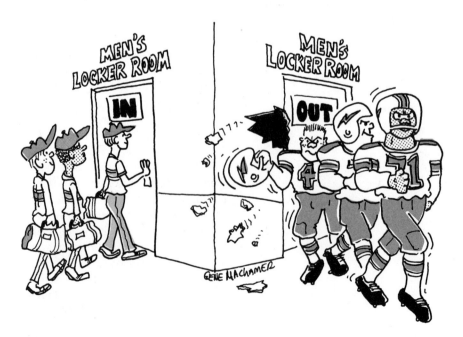

anabolic steroid that could help build muscle, yet minimize masculinizing size effects. Initially used only by weightlifters in small doses, athletes assumed that larger doses would build even more muscle. The race was on. Today, anabolic steroids are widely used and abused by both male and female athletes at all levels of competition, from young teens to professionals. Many "stack" them, that is, take a combination of brands in quantities of 100 mg or more daily.

While these drugs increase muscle mass and have some legitimate uses (i.e. treatment of anemia), they have numerous adverse side effects (table 12.11). When taken by men, steroids shut down the body's production of testosterone, causing breast growth, testicular atrophy, prostate enlargement, and premature cessation of bone growth. Large doses of anabolic steroids trigger masculine changes in women. Deepened voice, male pattern baldness, and increased facial and body hair are irreversible. Females experience loss of body fat, enlarged clitoris,

Table 12.11

The Bad News about Steroids

Sources: Physicians' Desk Reference, 1987; AMA Drug Evaluations, 1986; Death in the Locker Room by Bob Goldman, D.O. with Patricia Bush, PhD., and Ronald Klatz, D.O.; and U.S. Pharmacopeia Drug Index, Vol. 2, 1986. Used with permission. Department of Health and Human Services, HHS Publication No. (FDS) 88-3170/ "Athletes and Steroids: Playing A Deadly Game" by Roger W. Miller.

Established side effects and adverse reactions from anabolic steroids are:

- acne
- cancer
- cholesterol increase
- clitoris enlargement
- death
- edema (water retention in tissue)
- fetal damage
- frequent or continuing erections (mature males)
- HDL (which helps reduce cholesterol) decrease
- heart disease
- hirsutism (hairiness in women—irreversible)
- increased risk of coronary artery disease (heart attack, stroke)
- liver disease
- liver tumors
- male pattern baldness (in women—irreversible)
- priapism (painful, prolonged erections)
- prostate enlargement (which can result in blockage of the urinary tract)
- sterility (reversible)
- stunted growth
- testicular atrophy
- yellowing of the eyes or skin
- aggressive, combative behavior ("'roid rage")
- anaphylactic shock (from injections)
- breast development (sore or swelling—male)
- depression
- diarrhea
- fatigue
- feeling of abdominal or stomach fullness
- frequent urge to urinate (mature males)
- gallstones
- high blood pressure
- impotence
- increased chance of injury to muscles, tendons, and ligaments, plus longer recovery period from injuries
- insomnia
- kidney disease
- menstrual irregularities
- rash
- unnatural hair growth
- unpleasant breath odor
- unusual bleeding

decreased breast size, and changes in or absence of menstruation. The athlete who uses steroids faces a variety of other steroid side effects: acne, mood swings, changes in sex drive, and uncontrollable, aggressive behavior (**'roid rage**).

The popularity of anabolic steroids is attested to by the growth of a large black market and quack steroid products. Many of the black market brands come from underground labs and foreign countries and are of questionable quality and purity.

Steroids can be deadly dangerous. Unfortunately, to the high school junior trying to make first-string linebacker, the long-term effects of steroids may not seem important. However, steroid use can lead to sterility, kidney disease, liver tumors, bleeding ulcers, cancer, cardiovascular problems (high blood pressure, stroke, lowered number of high-density lipoprotein), and death. One surprising risk to the user who injects anabolic steroids is the exposure to acquired immune deficiency syndrome (AIDS).

Even though steroids may be easily accessible through health clubs and spas, they are illegal if purchased without a physician's prescription. Whereas some physicians have readily written prescriptions for athletes, this practice is decreasing as doctors become more aware of the drugs' dangerous side effects.

Amphetamines

Amphetamines ("speed," "uppers," "crank," "bennies," "meth," or "crystal") are powerful central nervous system stimulants. They are controlled drugs, meaning legislation has severely restricted even medical use. Currently amphetamines are legitimately used for short-term diet control in obesity and **narcolepsy** (uncontrollable attacks of deep sleep). They increase blood pressure, heart rate, respiratory rate, and metabolic rate, suppress the appetite, and place the body in a state of stress. The ability of amphetamines to relieve sleepiness and fatigue, to decrease appetite, and to increase alertness, confidence, and short-term performance has led to extensive nonmedical use, particularly by people involved in activities that demand stamina and long periods of wakefulness: long-distance truck drivers, pilots, flight attendants, and entertainers. They have also been used by students cramming for exams and by athletes to enhance their performance. These drugs do not increase maximal oxygen uptake. While they do enhance endurance by masking fatigue, their use without a prescription is illegal. Under the influence of amphetamines, an athlete may go out in a race too hard and burn out midway. Also, a person using amphetamines in competition may be seriously injured and not be aware of it.

Common side effects include headaches, mood swings, rapid heartbeat, restlessness, insomnia, and anxiety. Use of amphetamines over a prolonged time period increases tolerance of the drug and results in a need for larger doses. Large doses can lead to high blood pressure, anorexia, convulsions, and psychosis. Use of amphetamines during exercise in a hot environment may result in an elevated body temperature and death. Amphetamine injections, when needles are shared, may expose the user to needle diseases such as hepatitis and AIDS.

Diuretics

Diuretics cause the body to pass water by increasing urine output. They are useful in treating edema and mild hypertension. Diuretics are useless in producing true weight loss, since they result in loss of water, not fat. Any water lost is quickly regained over the next 24 hours. When used by wrestlers to temporarily decrease weight in order to compete, the resulting dehydration produces weakness and fatigue, along with increased susceptibility to heat illness. Diuretics have also been used, ineffectively, by some athletes attempting to mask anabolic steroid use. Urine tests for steroids are sufficiently sensitive to detect amounts as minute as a drop in a swimming pool of water.

Caffeine

Caffeine is probably the most common drug used by adults and children in our society. It occurs naturally in coffee, tea, colas, cocoa, and chocolate, and is added to some prescription and nonprescription drugs. Table 12.12 lists average amounts of caffeine found in commonly used drinks, food, and drugs. Caffeine is a powerful central nervous system stimulant. In healthy, rested people, a dose of 100 milligrams (about 1 cup of coffee) increases alertness, banishes drowsiness, quickens reaction time, enhances intellectual and muscular effort, increases heart and respiratory rates, and stimulates urinary output.

Table 12.12

Common Sources of Caffeine

	milligrams		milligrams
Coffee (5-oz. cup)		Vivarin	200
Brewed, drip method	115	NoDoz (1 Tablet)	100
Decaffeinated, brewed	3	Cold-allergy remedies	
Instant	65	Triaminicin	30
Decaffeinated, instant	2	Dristan A F	
Milk chocolate (1 oz.)	6	Decongestant	16
Chocolate-flavored		Pain Relievers	
syrup (1 oz.)	4	Excedrin	65
Soft drinks (12 oz.)		Anacin Maximum	
Mountain Dew	54	Strength	32
Mellow Yellow	52	Midol	32
Coca-Cola	45	Weight Control	
Diet Coke	45	Dexatrim Extra Strength	200
Mr. Pibb	40	Diuretics	
Dr. Pepper	39	Permathene H_2 Off	200
Pepsi-Cola	38	Aqua-Ban	100
Diet Pepsi	36		
Tea (5-oz. cup)			
Brewed	40		
Instant	30		

Ingestion of one to two cups of coffee an hour before prolonged exhaustive exercise produces a glycogen-sparing effect by promoting fat use, which may enhance performance in endurance activities.[40] It also tends to mask fatigue. This effect decreases as fitness increases, however, resulting in little or no benefit for highly trained athletes. If a competitive edge is desired, an athlete is wiser to drink plain water. Caffeine produces dehydration, and in some individuals, abnormalities in heart electrical function, both of which hinder performance.

While moderate use of caffeine is generally harmless, overconsumption can produce a toxic reaction known as caffeinism. A 300 mg dose for many people produces sleep disruption, nervousness, irritability, restlessness, muscle twitches, headaches, heart palpitations, and gastric disturbances. In addition, some women report increased incidence of premenstrual syndrome (PMS) or fibrocystic breast disease (noncancerous breast lumps) related to caffeine consumption. How much caffeine is too much? Although tolerance varies from one person to another, intake of less than 200 mg per day is a wise limit.

Caffeine use is habit forming, and those who try to abruptly stop a long-term pattern of heavy consumption often experience withdrawal symptoms. Headaches, lethargy, irritability, and difficulty concentrating are common symptoms that will gradually diminish over a few days to two weeks.

Over-the-Counter and Prescription Drugs

Legal drugs are often subdivided into over-the-counter drugs (OTCs) and prescription drugs. There are over 300,000 OTCs available in the United States. These are so named because they can be purchased without a prescription. Aspirin is the most common form, but most cold medicines, cough syrups, and laxatives also fall into this category. OTCs are not addictive if used correctly, and they must have clear warnings and instructions printed on labels for consumer use and protection. Still, there is a difference between safe and harmless. OTCs can do damage if used incorrectly, and some can lead to physical dependence if overused.

Four common kinds of nonprescription drugs are especially likely to produce adverse side effects or dependence.[41]

Nasal sprays. After several days' use, these can produce a "rebound" effect, making your nose more congested than ever. The "rebound" effect is the result of increased swelling of the nasal tissues. If you use one, limit it to one or two days.

Laxatives. The most habit-forming laxatives are the so-called "stimulants," which work by stimulating the walls of the intestines. A diet high in fruits, vegetables, and grains, plus two quarts of fluids a day will almost always eliminate constipation. Laxatives should not be used to induce weight loss.

Eyedrops. These blood vessel constrictors will whiten blood shot eyes, but like nasal sprays, they can produce a rebound effect.

Alcohol/Codeine Cough Syrups. Codeine, a narcotic, works directly on the part of the brain that controls coughing. In many drug stores, codeine-containing cough suppressants are available simply by signing at the cash register. Some of these medications contain substantial amounts of alcohol, which is dangerous for anyone with an alcohol problem.

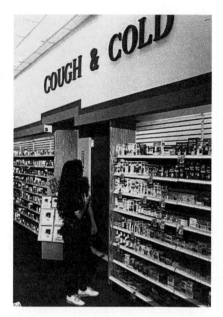

Over the counter drugs should be used with caution.

Most prescription drugs are put to good use (for example, antibiotics used for treating infection), but many are abused. Prescription drugs that are sometimes abused include amphetamines, barbiturates, narcotics, or tranquilizers. These drugs are used for a wide range of conditions such as to stimulate and/or depress the CNS, overcome fatigue, suppress hunger, induce sleep, deaden the senses, relieve pain, and control anxieties.

There seems to be a pill for every need. Unfortunately, once prescribed, drugs are often taken in amounts and combinations not anticipated by the prescribing physician. Some physicians prescribe drugs more readily than others, and some fail to stress the importance of reading labels carefully and taking drugs only as directed. Drugs prescribed to diminish physical or mental anguish are sometimes used for social purposes, leading to drug abuse.

Synergy, a major problem with drug use, is a phenomenon that occurs when various drugs are taken in combination, where the cumulative effect is greater than additive. Alcohol and tobacco act synergistically to increase the risk of oral cancer, and alcohol and oral contraceptives act synergistically to increase the risk of coronary heart disease. Two of the world's most widely prescribed drugs, Zantac and Tagamet (used by millions of people with persistent heart burn and ulcers) act synergistically with alcohol. One study reported[42] that in individuals who drank 1 1/2 glasses of wine with a meal and were taking Zantac, BAC increased 34 percent. For those taking Tagamet, BAC increased 92 percent. Especially hazardous is the combination of alcohol with barbiturates. This combination can kill a person or leave him or her in a persistent vegetative state.

Summary

The wellness journey does not include substance abuse. Before drinking alcohol, smoking, or using other drugs, consider what these substances do to you. Your mind and body are capable of handling stress, emotional and physical pain. You can feel happy, sexy, sad, angry, and joyous, and experience love without needing artificial chemicals to enhance feelings or cope with life's challenges. The fact is, these substances magnify your problems. The single biggest killer of young adults is not heart disease, stroke, or cancer. It is accidents. Over half of all fatal accidents are alcohol- or drug-related. Use of many substances leads to tolerance or addiction, as well as health problems. Drugs do not make you a better athlete, either. On the contrary, inappropriate substance use can ruin your health, relationships, and future.

Before using any substance, whether over-the-counter, illegal, or prescribed, remember that you have choices. What you do now will affect your future. Be responsible and choose wisely.

References

1. Nakken, Craig. *The Addictive Personality: Understanding Compulsion in Our Lives.* Hazelton Foundation, Center City, MN. New York: Harper and Row Publishers Inc., 1988.

2. Nakken Craig. *The Addictive Personality: Roots, Rituals, and Recovery.* Hazelton Foundation. Center City, MN 55012–0176, 1988.

3. *University of California, Berkeley, The Wellness Encyclopedia.* Boston: Houghton Mifflin Company, 1991.

4. Gibbons, Boyd. "Alcohol the Legal Drug." *National Geographic,* Vol. 181, No. 2, February, 1992.

5. Frezza, Mario, M.D., DiPadora, Carlo, M.D., Pozzato, Gabriele, M.D., Terpin, Madalesa, M.D., Barano, Enrique, M.D., and Lieher, Charles S., M.D. "High Blood Alcohol Levels in Women: The Role of Decreased Alcohol Dehydrogenase Activity and First-Pass Metabolism." *The New England Journal of Medicine* 322 (April 11, 1990): 95–99.

6. *PRIDE (Parents' Resource Institute For Drug Education)* Signal Press, 1730 Chicago Avenue, Evanston, IL 60201, 1990.

7. "Alcohol the Legal Drug"

8. "The Fact Is...." National Clearinghouse for Alcohol and Drug Information. Rockville, MD, 1990.

9. "The Fact Is...."

10. *PRIDE*

11. *The Wellness Encyclopedia*

12. *Healthy People 2000, National Health Promotion and Disease Prevention Objectives.* U.S. Department of Health and Human Services, Public Health Service, 1990.

13. Anna Lamb, Alcohol Education, Coordinator, Ball State Health Center, Ball State University, Muncie, IN

14. "Alcohol the Legal Drug"

15. "Alcohol the Legal Drug"

16. "The Effect of Ethanol on Fat Storage in Healthy Subjects." *The New England Journal of Medicine.* April 9, 1992, Vol. 326, No. 15.

17. *Healthy People 2000.*

18. Burgess, Donna. "Fetal Alcohol Syndrome and Fetal Alcohol Effect: Principles for Educators." *Phi Delta Kappan.* Vol. 74, No.1, September, 1993.

19. Gibbons, Boyd. "The Preventable Tragedy—Fetal Alcohol Syndrome." *National Geographic,* Vol. 181, No.2, February, 1992.

20. *Healthy People 2000*

21. U.S. Department of Health and Human Services. *The Health Consequences of Smoking: Cardiovascular Disease.* Washington, DC: U.S. Government Printing Office, 1983.

22. *1992 Heart Facts,* American Heart Association National Center, Dallas, Texas.

23. *1992 Heart Facts.*

24. *Healthy People 2000.*

25. U.S. Department of Health and Human Services. "If Your Kids Think Everybody Smokes, They Don't Know Everybody: A Parents Guide to Smoking and Teenagers." Washington, DC: U.S. Government Printing Office.

26. *1992 Heart Facts.*

27. New England Journal of Medicine. 1991. 324:739–745.

28. *Cancer Facts and Figures—1992,* American Cancer Society, New York, 1992.

29. *Cancer Facts and Figures—1992.*

30. *1992 Heart Facts.* American Heart Association National Center, Dallas, Texas.

31. *Healthy People 2000*

32. *Cancer Facts and Figures—1992.*

33. Sweeting, Roger. *A Values Approach to Health Behavior.* Champaign, IL: Human Kinetics Books, 1990.

34. *A Values Approach to Health Behavior.*

35. Gilkeson, Robert, M.D., "Effects of Drugs on Learning." Sixth Annual Conference of the Indiana Federation of Communities for Drug-Free Youth, Inc. Indianapolis, IN. October 30, 1987.

36. *A Values Approach to Health Behavior.*

37. Schlaat, Richard and Peter Shannon. *Drugs, 3rd. ed.* Englewood Cliffs, New Jersey: Prentice Hall, 1990.

38. Facts About Crank. Prevention Information Series. Indiana Prevention Resource Center for Substance Abuse, Indiana University, Bloomington, IN. 1990.

39. Miller, Roger W. "Athletes and Steroids: Playing A Deadly Game." FDA Consumer. Department of Health and Human Services, Washington, DC.

40. Costill, David L. *Inside Running: Basics of Sports Physiology.* Indianapolis: Benchmark Press, Inc. 1986.

41. *The Wellness Encyclopedia.*

42. *Journal of American Medical Association.* January, 1992.

Suggested Readings

"Alcohol Related Deaths of American Indians—Sterotypes and Strategies." March 11, 1992. *JAMA.* Vol. 267, No. 10.

Alcohol and Women. 1990. National Institute on Alcohol Abuse and Alcoholism. Rockville, Maryland.

Avis, Harry. 1990. *Drugs and Life,* Dubuque, IA: Brown & Benchmark Publishers.

Barnard, Charles. 1990. *Families With An Alcoholic Member.* New York: Human Sciences Press.

Blum, Kenneth. 1991. *Alcohol and the Addictive Brain: New Hope for Alcoholics from Biogenetic Research.* New York: Free Press.

Blumberg, Leonard. 1991. *Beware the First Drink.* Seattle, Washington: Glen Abbey Books.

Bruess, Clint and Glenn Richardson. 1992. *Decisions for Health.* Dubuque, IA: Brown & Benchmark Publishers.

Cahalan, Don. 1991. *An Ounce of Prevention; Strategies for Solving Tobacco, Alcohol and Drug Problems.* San Francisco: Jossey-Bass Publishers.

Cocores, James. 1990. *The 800-COCAINE Book of Drug and Alcohol Recovery.* New York: Villard Books.

Cox, Miles, editor. 1990. *Why People Drink: Parameters of Alcohol as a Reinforcer.* New York: Gardner Press.

Fields, Richard. 1992. *Drugs and Alcohol in Perspective.* Dubuque, IA: Brown & Benchmark.

Flynn, Laura. July/August 1992. "Beyond AA: Alternatives for Alcoholics Who Resist The Program's Religious Approach." *Health.* Vol. 23, No. 6.

Frances, Richard & Miller, Sheldon. 1991. *Clinical Textbook of Addicitve Disorders.* New York: Guilford Press.

Frankle, Mark and Leffers, David. June 1992. "Athletes on Anabolic-Androgenic Steroids, New Approach Diminishes Health Problems." *The Physician and Sportsmedicine.* Vol. 20, No. 6.

Giles, H.G. 1991. *Alcohol and the Identification of Alcoholics: A Handbook for Professionals.* Lexington, MA: Lexington Books.

Gold, Mark. M.D., 1990. *800-COCAINE.* Summit, NJ: The Pia Press, Bantam Books, Inc.

O'Brien, Robert and Chafetz, Morris. 1991. *The Encyclopedia of Alcoholism.* New York: Facts on File.

Rice, Dorothy. 1990. *The Economic Costs of Alcohol and Drug Abuse and Mental Illness:*

U.S. Department of Human Services, Public Health Service, Alcohol, Drug Abuse, and Mental Health Administration, Rockville, Maryland.

Scaffa, Marjorie, Crouse-Quinn, Sandra, Swift, Robert. 1992. *Making Choices: A Personal Look at Alcohol and Drug Use,* Dubuque, IA: Brown & Benchmark Publishers.

Schlaadt, Richard. 1992. *Alcohol Use & Abuse.* Guilford, CT: The Dushkin Publishing Group, Inc.

Schlaadt, Richard. 1992. *Drugs, Society, and Behavior.* Guilford, CT: The Dushkin Publishing Group, Inc.

St. Clair, Harvey. 1991. *Recognizing Alcoholism and Its Effects: A Mini Guide.* New York: Karger.

For Help or Information:

Al-Anon Family Group
Headquarters
P.O. Box 862
Midtown Station
New York, NY 10018
(212) 302–7240

Alcoholics Anonymous
175 Fifth Avenue
New York, NY 10010
(212) 473–6200

Alcoholics Anonymous World Services
P.O. Box 459
Grand Central Station
New York, NY 10163
(212) 686–1100

Boost Alcohol Consciousness Concerning the Health of University Students
(BACCHUS of the United States, Inc.)
c/o Campus Alcohol Information Center
University of Florida
Gainesville, FL 32611

1–800–COCAINE
The National Cocaine Hotline
Fair Oaks Hospital
Summit, NJ 07901

Gamblers Anonymous
National Service Office
P.O. Box 1713
Los Angeles, CA 90017
(213) 386–8789

Mothers Against Drunk Driving (MADD)
669 Airport Freeway
Suite 310
Hurst, TX 76053
(817) 268–6233

Narcotics Anonymous
P.O. Box 9999
Van Nuys, CA 91409
(818) 780–3951

National Association of Children of Alcoholics
P.O. Box 421691
San Francisco, CA 94142
(415) 431–1366

National Clearinghouse for Alcohol and Drug Information
P.O. Box 2345
Rockville, MD 20852
(301) 468–2600

National Council on Compulsive Gambling
444 West 56th Street, Room 3207S
New York, NY 10019
(212) 765–3833

National Council on Alcoholism, Inc.
12 West 21st Street
New York, NY 10010
(212) 986–4433

National Institute on Alcohol Abuse and Alcoholism
Parklawn Building
5600 Fishers Lane
Room 16–105
Rockville, MD 20857
(301) 443–3885

Remove Intoxicated Drivers (RID)
(518) 372–0034

Shoplifters Anonymous
P.O. Box 24515
Minneapolis, MN 55424

13
Preventing Sexually Transmitted Disease

Chapter Objectives

After reading this chapter, you will be able to:

1. Identify symptoms of AIDS and the five most common sexually transmitted diseases.
2. Differentiate between curable and incurable sexually transmitted diseases.
3. Identify four ways HIV is transmitted.
4. Recognize the latency period for AIDS.
5. List actions you can take to decrease risk of acquiring a sexually transmitted disease.
6. Identify four steps in correct condom use.
7. Give three out of seven ways to discourage unwanted sexual pressure.

Terms

- Acquired Immune Deficiency Syndrome (AIDS)
- Aids-Related Complex (ARC)
- Chancre
- Chlamydia
- Genital herpes

- Genital warts
- Gonorrhea
- Herpes simplex virus
- Human Immunodeficiency Virus (HIV)
- Human Papilloma Virus (HPV)
- Lymphocytes

- Opportunistic diseases
- Pelvic inflammatory disease (PID)
- Sexually transmitted disease (STD)
- Syphilis
- T-cells

Sexually Transmitted Diseases

Diseases that are spread through sexual contact were once called Venereal Diseases (VD), named for Venus, the Greek goddess of love, mother of Cupid. The terms VD and **Sexually Transmitted Disease (STD)** have often been used interchangeably. However, VD refers to diseases like gonorrhea, which are nearly always spread through sexual contact. The term STD refers to a broader category of diseases that are spread primarily through sexual intercourse but also through other intimate behavior, sex play, and occasionally, nonsexually.

Today, while **Acquired Immune Deficiency Syndrome (AIDS)** claims the spotlight as the most deadly and feared sexually transmitted disease (STD), we are experiencing a silent epidemic of STDs in the United States. As a group, STDs are the number one communicable disease problem, but many people are unaware of this because of our cultural reluctance to discuss STDs and fear of public embarrassment. Only colds and flu, which are not officially reported, occur more frequently. It is estimated that one in four Americans will acquire at least one STD in their lifetime.

Changing mores appear to be a major factor in the increasing rate of STDs. Increased rates of premarital sexual intercourse among young people offers more opportunity for the spread of disease.[1] Involvement with alcohol, a concern on many college campuses, is tied to increased sexual activity and lack of commitment to one's sex partner, which increase STD risk.[2] Another factor may be the development of the birth control pill, which has resulted in decreasing use of the

Condom machines are becoming more prevalent

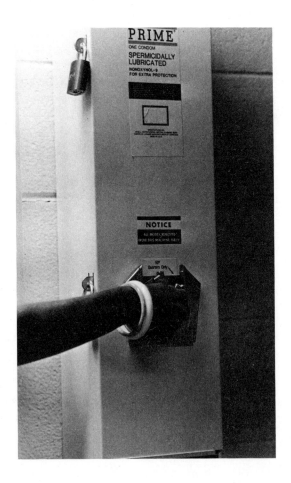

condom. With concern over AIDS, however, this is changing. Both male and female condoms not only prevent conception but serve as a barrier to transmission of STDs.

STDs are most common in people in their late teens to twenties: 86 percent of all STDs occur among persons ages 15–29.[3] Nevertheless, your risk of acquiring an STD is determined by your behavior, not by your age or sexual orientation. Risk can be reduced or increased by personal choices that you control. If you choose to be sexually active, you are at risk. Your chances of exposure to an STD increase with multiple sexual partners and with increased frequency of sexual activity. Risk of infection is low to zero in a mutually monogamous relationship or if you abstain from sex.

Unfortunately, many people, especially young people, feel that STDs aren't serious, or that "STDs only happen to others," and they fail to take precautions. A person may think, "If I get one, I'll just go get it taken care of." While some STDs are curable, some are not. Even some of the traditionally curable STDs are becoming antibiotic resistant, making treatment more difficult. STDs may not seem to be a serious problem because you can't tell by looking at your friends who is infected and who is not. Also, they're probably not going to discuss it with you like they would their last cold. Silence can be deadly. If you can't see it and don't hear about it, some think, the problem isn't real. They are wrong.

STDs are spread from an infected person to a partner during sexual intercourse, oral sex, or anal sex. Nonsexual infection is possible with some STDs, but uncommon. STDs are not spread on toilet seats, in hot tubs, or in swimming pools. The bacteria and viruses that cause STDs need the warmth and moisture of mucous membranes to live. That is why they infect the reproductive organs, rectum, and mouth. After transmission to a new host, the bacteria or virus quickly multiplies and may produce noticeable symptoms in two days to four weeks. Sometimes an infected person notices no symptoms, however.

Women are particularly vulnerable to STDs, including AIDS, because they have more mucous membranes in their genital tissue than men. Vaginal and cervical tissue can sustain microscopic tears through which viruses and bacteria, often transmitted by semen, can enter. In addition, women experience early warning signs of STDs much less frequently than men, resulting in more advanced disease before treatment is sought. STDs are serious and, if left untreated, can cause permanent damage. Early diagnosis and treatment is important both to prevent serious physical harm and to prevent spread of the disease to other sexual partners.

Symptoms of STDs vary with the type of infection, and may differ with males and females. Be aware of the warning signs that may indicate the presence of an STD (table 13.1).

Diagnosis and treatment of STDs is confidential. It is important to contact the STD clinic of your local county health department or see a doctor immediately if you suspect that you may have an STD. Your local family planning clinic can also give information on where to go for help, or you can call one of the hotlines at the end of this chapter. Wherever you are treated, your case will be kept private.

Table 13.1

Symptoms of Sexually
Transmitted Disease

Women

Pelvic pain
Bleeding from the vagina between periods
Burning or itching around the vagina
Pain deep inside the vagina during sexual intercourse

Women and Men

Abnormal discharge from the penis or vagina
A burning sensation during urination or bowel movements
Sores, bumps, or blisters near the mouth, rectum, or genitals
Flu-like feelings with fever, chills, or aches
Redness and swelling in the throat
Swelling in the groin

There are over 25 known STDs, some of which are incurable. Most STDs are either bacterial or viral. The most common bacterial STDs, which are treatable, are chlamydia, gonorrhea, and syphilis. Viral STDs, which are incurable, include genital herpes, genital warts, and AIDS (table 13.2). A person can have more than one STD at a time. Although less prevalent, AIDS is causing much concern because it is not only incurable, but fatal.

Table 13.2

Curable and Incurable STDs

Bacterial (Curable)	*Viral (Incurable)*
Chlamydia	Genital Warts
Gonorrhea	Genital Herpes
Syphilis	AIDS

Chlamydia

Chlamydia is one of the most widespread and damaging of all STDs. It is spread mainly through sexual intercourse but can be spread by the fingers from one body area to another such as from the genitals to the eyes. Chlamydia, the most common bacterial STD, is estimated to infect about 20 percent of college students.[4] It affects twice as many people as gonorrhea, although it mimics its symptoms, and both diseases often occur together. For this reason, physicians usually treat both infections if one is diagnosed. Early symptoms are usually mild, and if they occur, they appear within 1 to 3 weeks after exposure. Chlamydia causes an inflammation of the urethra, which produces a burning sensation during urination. In men, chlamydia can also infect the epididymis, causing painful scrotal swelling. About 80 percent of women and 10 percent of men have no noticeable symptoms and may not even know they are infected. This makes the disease even more difficult to diagnose and cure. As a result, the disease is often not diagnosed until it has done permanent damage.

Untreated chlamydia in women can produce a serious inflammation of the sexual organs called **pelvic inflammatory disease (PID).** PID is extremely damaging and can infect the lining of the uterus, fallopian tubes, and ovaries. This may cause fever and pain in the lower abdomen, scarring and blockage of the fallopian tubes, and sterility.

Chlamydial infections are most frequent among young people with multiple sexual partners. The preferred treatment for chlamydia is tetracycline.

Gonorrhea

Gonorrhea, the second most common bacterial STD, was named by Galen in 150 B.C. from the Greek meaning "flow of seed." At that time, the penile discharge was thought to be semen. Actually, the discharge was pus produced from inflammation of the urethra. The gonorrhea bacteria grows and multiplies quickly in mucous membranes such as in the cervix, mouth, rectum, or urinary tract. In women, the most common site of infection is the cervix, but it can spread to the ovaries and fallopian tubes, causing PID. It can be spread directly through sexual intercourse or from the genitals to the mouth with the fingers.

As with chlamydia, it often has no symptoms, or the symptoms go undetected as the infected individual continues to spread the disease. Men are much more likely to notice the symptoms than women. Up to 80 percent of women infected have no symptoms, compared to 20 percent of men. If they occur, symptoms usually appear within 2 to 14 days of infection. Gonorrhea often strikes the urethra, causing a burning sensation during urination. Males may notice an unusual penile discharge, as well as swollen lymph glands in the groin. Women may experience an abnormal vaginal discharge, abdominal pain, or vaginal bleeding. A rectal infection may produce anal itching or a discharge. Oral infections usually produce no symptoms, though a few may get a sore throat. Early symptoms may clear up on their own, but a person can still be infected and spread the disease to others.

If not treated, gonorrhea may cause permanent damage to the reproductive organs and sterility. In men, it may damage the penis, making urination difficult and erection impossible. It can also infect the epididymis, leaving scar tissue that can block the flow of semen from the infected testicle. In women, it can scar the fallopian tubes, making it impossible to bear children. In both sexes, the bacteria can spread to the bloodstream, producing a generalized bacterial infection. It can infect joints with gonococcal arthritis and irreversibly damage heart valves, spinal cord, or the brain. It can be spread from an infected mother via the birth canal to her baby, causing eye infection and blindness if not treated immediately.

Gonorrhea is usually treated with penicillin and antibiotics, although penicillin-resistant strains have developed. In fact, penicillin-resistant cases have doubled in each of the years since 1985, making treatment more difficult.[5] This increasing occurrence of penicillin-resistant gonorrhea underscores the need for taking protective measures during sexual activity and for being tested once or twice a year even if there are no symptoms.

Syphilis

> *"For when it has once been received into the body, it does not immediately declare itself; rather it lies dormant for a certain time and gradually gains strength as it feeds."*
>
> —Fracastoro (1483–1553): *Syphilis, the "French Disease"*

Syphilis was rampant in Europe in the late 1400s, spread during times of war by soldiers who frequented prostitutes, then returned home to their wives and mistresses. It was also reported spread by soldiers who sailed with Columbus to the New World and by many Renaissance explorers who took it beyond the boundaries of Europe. It was first known as the "great pox," in contrast to which "smallpox" was later named, and was at first thought to be a special divine punishment for sexual transgressions. In the eighteenth century, syphilitics wore wigs and high collars to hide hair loss and throat lesions. Many early treatments used mercury or arsenic but produced side effects that were as bad as the disease. Although syphilis has been a serious health problem during all major wars, it was not until after World War II began that the U.S. Public Health Service started using penicillin to combat it.

Syphilis cases in the United States have increased since 1985 to their highest rate in 40 years and occur mainly in the 20- to 24-year-old-age group.[6] Like other bacterial STDs, syphilis is easily spread because its symptoms are often unnoticed or confused with other diseases. In fact, syphilis is known as "the great imitator" because it mimics so many other diseases.

Syphilis occurs in four stages: primary, secondary, latent, and tertiary, depending on how long a person has had it and how far it has progressed. Each stage is described below.

Primary Syphilis

The first sign of syphilis is a **chancre,** or small painless sore, which appears within 1 to 12 weeks after sexual contact. It may appear on the penis, in the vagina, in the mouth, or any other area that contacted the bacteria, and lasts 1 to 5 weeks. It is often accompanied by painless swelling of the lymph nodes in the groin. The initial sore may go unnoticed and will disappear if left untreated. The disease then enters a secondary stage 2 weeks to 6 months later.

Secondary Syphilis

In the secondary stage, skin rash, fever, headache, sore throat, swollen lymph glands, flu-like symptoms, and patchy hair loss may occur. The symptoms are so general that the disease can be misdiagnosed even if medical help is sought. The rash may appear as pink spots or small raised bumps on the palms, soles of the feet, back, chest, arms, legs, face, or abdomen. Small, moist sores may appear in the mouth, and lesions may appear on the genital area. Secondary symptoms, if they occur, may clear up in 2 to 6 weeks without treatment but may recur for up to 2 years. During this time an infected individual can still spread the disease. If untreated, although the initial symptoms may subside and a person can feel perfectly normal, the disease progresses.

Latent Syphilis

In latent syphilis, the third stage, a person is generally no longer infectious to others unless there is a relapse of moist lesions or unless the disease is passed to a baby during pregnancy. This stage can last for several years with no symptoms, but the infecting bacteria can continue to multiply.

Tertiary Syphilis

While two-thirds of untreated people will have no more symptoms, the one-third who are affected may suffer permanent damage to the cardiovascular or nervous systems. Tertiary syphilis can occur anywhere from 3 to 40 years after initial infection. Complications include heart disease, blindness, brain damage, paralysis, insanity, and death.

Penicillin was discovered to be effective against syphilis in the 1940s. It is still considered the treatment of choice.

Genital Herpes

Genital herpes is another major contributor to human misery. It has no cure. Once you get it, you have it for life. Symptoms usually occur within 2 to 30 days after having sex. Early signs include itching, tingling, or burning on the genitals. This is followed by small painful genital sores or blisters that break open and crust over, causing intense itching and extreme pain. In addition, active herpes may be accompanied by fever, swollen glands, and general flu-like feelings. Herpes virus is shed from the sores, which are highly contagious. After the blisters appear, they last from 1 to 3 weeks, then heal and disappear. Once established, the herpes virus migrates into nerve cells, where it may lie dormant or reactivate to cause recurring outbreaks of sores from time to time. New attacks of the disease appear at intervals, triggered by lowered resistance, fever, sunburn, or even stress.

Genital herpes is caused by the **herpes simplex virus.** A virus invades body cells to live and reproduce. Nearly all herpes infections are caused by Herpes Simplex Type II, which is transmitted from one infected individual to another during intercourse. This is different from the common Herpes Simplex Type I, which causes cold sores to appear on or around the mouth. However, it is possible to spread Type I to the genitals or Type II to the mouth by touching the sores and scratching or rubbing somewhere else. You can also become infected by both types of herpes at the same time. It is important to avoid letting the lesions contact someone else's body through touching, kissing, or sexual contact. Touching an eye after touching a sore can cause a severe eye infection called ocular herpes. Simply washing the hands thoroughly after touching a sore can prevent transmission of the virus.

At least two-thirds of the infected individuals are not even aware that they have genital herpes—their symptoms are so mild that they go unnoticed. Because many unreported cases exist, experts estimate that the nationwide infection rate may be as high as 1 in 4 adult Americans.[7] In women, herpes sores can occur internally and cause no discomfort. However, these infected individuals can still spread the virus to others, and a mother with herpes can give it to her baby. Babies born to infected mothers can become infected with herpes at birth. In infants, the virus can cause blindness, brain damage, and death. For this reason, babies are usually delivered by caesarean section if the mother has genital herpes.

While a person was once thought to be contagious only during herpes outbreaks, current studies indicate that herpes can be spread, particularly from men to women, even if a person does not have symptoms. Women are four times as likely to get herpes from men as men are to get it from women, perhaps because of the greater exposure of vaginal and cervical mucous membranes to the virus during sexual contact.[8]

The severity and duration of symptoms can be decreased with Acyclovir, an antiviral drug. It can also be taken to prevent recurrence of symptoms, although it cannot cure the disease. Thus the joke: "What is the difference between love and herpes?" Answer: "Only herpes is forever."

Genital Warts and Other Human Papilloma Virus Infections

Human papilloma virus (HPV) infections are epidemic among young people of college age, and not all of them cause visible warts.[9] There are over 60 different types of HPV infections, and a person can have more than one type of HPV at a time.[10] Once HPV has invaded cells, depending on its type, it may produce genital warts, genital tract cancers, or there may be no symptoms at all. Both cervical cancer in women and penile cancer in men are associated with HPV, and these all too often occur in sexually active young adults.

HPV is passed through direct skin-to-skin contact through sexual activity. Nonsexual transmission is possible, though rare, since HPV can remain alive for several hours on wet towels or undergarments. HPV infections are more common in women than men, probably because the warmth and moisture of a woman's vagina provides an ideal place for viral growth.

Genital warts are caused by some types of HPV, are highly contagious, and take 1 to 8 months to appear after exposure. Until the warts appear, there are no symptoms that indicate presence of the HPV virus. Between the time of exposure and the appearance of warts, either partner can have the virus unknowingly and give it to the other. Genital warts may be flat or rounded bumps with a cauliflowerlike appearance. They are often painless but may itch or burn. On men, most genital warts occur on the outside of the penis. In women, they may appear around the vulva, inside the vagina and cervix. They may also appear in the mouth, throat, or around the anus, and they do not go away.

Warts can grow and spread, so they should be removed. Warts can be frozen with liquid nitrogen, burned off with an electric needle or laser, or removed surgically or chemically. While the external lesions can be eliminated, this does not eradicate the virus, which may become dormant and later reappear, or may be destroyed by the body's own immune system.

You can detect some genital warts by self-examination. Men should check the penis regularly. Women should use a mirror to examine the vulva and anus. Warts inside the vagina can be found by a doctor.

A genital wart infection is a major risk factor for cervical cancer, one of the leading cancer killers of women. In some cases, warts turn into precancerous growths called dysplasia and later become cancerous. Cervical cancer, thus, is considered a sexually transmitted disease.[11] This cancer infects far too many young women of child-bearing age and is not just a disease of the elderly. Other risk factors include initiating sexual activity at an early age and having unprotected sex with multiple sexual partners.

An abnormal Pap smear can detect an unseen HPV infection as well as precancerous cellular changes in cervical tissue. There is also a newly developed test that can both detect an HPV infection and indicate the strain of the virus. The Virapap test detects five strains of HPV linked to cancer. Since the Pap smear only detects abnormal changes in cells, it is a good idea to get a Virapap test along with the Pap test to detect latent HPV infections. Benign HPV infections that do not cause warts or cancer do not generally require treatment, but they do signal to the carrier the risk of both and the need for frequent checkups.

Having genital warts doesn't mean you will get cancer, but it does increase your risk. Not having warts doesn't mean you are safe. Since only about 10 percent of Human Papilloma virus cases have visible warts, it is possible to be infected and unaware of it.

Acquired Immune Deficiency Syndrome

AIDS is a threat to all men and women, heterosexual and homosexual alike. In the ten years since it first appeared, there were 206,000 cases of AIDS reported in the United States, and 133,000 of these people had died.[12] Most of these were infected before the virus was discovered in 1981. The toll continues to climb at an alarming rate. It took 6 years for the first 50,000 cases to be reported, 2 years for the next 50,000 cases, and 2 more years for the next 100,000 cases.[13] AIDS became the eleventh leading cause of death overall in the United States in 1992. It was projected to become the second leading cause of death in young men ages 25–44 by 1994.[14] Teens and young adults are particularly vulnerable to AIDS because they take risks when they may not appreciate the risks—of beginning sexuality or drug use, for example.

What Is AIDS? What Is HIV?

AIDS is a syndrome, or group of symptoms, caused by the **Human Immunodeficiency Virus (HIV).** The virus itself is not alive but is an infectious agent. It does not kill a person directly but attacks a particular type of **lymphocyte** (white blood cells) called **T-cells.** Lymphocytes control cell growth, transport nutrients to cells, and produce antibodies that protect the body against infection. They travel under their own power throughout the body and body fluids. When T-cells sense the presence of a disease, they send messages to other white cells to resist the infection. The virus penetrates T-cells and forces them to make copies of the virus. Then the cell dies. Gradually, over a period of years, when enough lymphocytes are destroyed, a person suffers from an impaired immune system, poor control of cell growth, and poor cell nutrition. A weakened immune system reduces the body's ability to defend itself against **opportunistic diseases** produced by common bacteria, viruses, parasites, and fungi that surround but do not usually have the opportunity to infect people with a healthy immune system. A person suffers infection after miserable infection, is susceptible to unusual cancers, and may become emaciated (Slim disease). Other STD infections, especially those that cause genital lesions, such as herpes and syphilis, may occur concurrently with AIDS and may speed the acquisition and transmission of the AIDS virus.

What Are Symptoms of an HIV Infection?

The disease appears to have three stages: incubation, AIDS-Related Complex, and AIDS. During the incubation period of the disease, many HIV carriers feel well and have no symptoms. As the disease progresses, victims may experience symptoms of **AIDS-Related Complex (ARC).** This is a pre-AIDS condition in which a person tests positive for the HIV virus and has symptoms somewhat less severe than classic AIDS. Symptoms include: chronic fatigue, swollen lymph glands, unexplained weight loss, fevers or night sweats. Poor appetite, diarrhea, and white spots in the mouth are also common. These symptoms are shared by many diseases and do not necessarily mean that you have AIDS.

For every person with AIDS, 20-30 are HIV infected

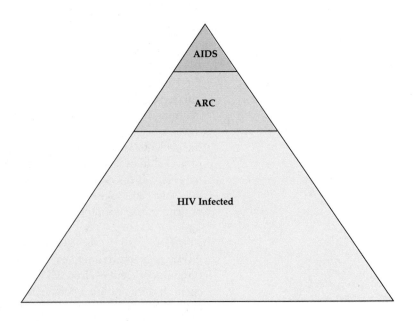

The third stage of an HIV infection is AIDS. The body's immune system is so weak that otherwise rare opportunistic infections may infect the AIDS victim causing life-threatening illness. A persistent cough and fever associated with shortness of breath may be related to pneumocystis carinii pneumonia, a parasitic lung infection, or tuberculosis. Kaposi's sarcoma, a cancer of the blood vessels, causes pink or purplish lesions on the skin and elsewhere. Women may suffer from persistent vaginal infections, severe pelvic inflammatory disease, and recurrent cervical cancers. In advanced stages of the disease, the virus may also damage the brain and spinal cord, causing memory loss, partial paralysis, or AIDS-related dementia.

Q. ***Can I tell if someone has HIV?***

A. You can't tell by looking. There are many HIV carriers who look and feel fine and don't even know they are infected. A blood test is necessary to detect presence of the HIV virus.

Q. ***If I get HIV, will I die?***

A. It is not known at this time whether 100 percent of HIV-infected individuals will develop AIDS. You can carry the HIV virus in your body for years and experience no symptoms as it gradually destroys your immune system. When enough of the immune system has been destroyed, a person may develop AIDS. Some people with AIDS alternate between periods of illness and periods of relatively good health. Generally, however, a person dies within 1 to 2 years after diagnosis of full-blown AIDS. It is felt that, given time, probably all HIV-infected individuals will develop AIDS.

How Does HIV Spread?

HIV is transmitted in body fluids such as blood and semen or vaginal fluid. It is most often spread in one of four ways (table 13.3):

Table 13.3
How HIV Is Transmitted

- Sexual intercourse with an AIDS carrier
- Sharing hypodermic needles
- By pregnant women to the fetuses they carry
- Rarely, a transfusion of infected blood

Some cases of AIDS from tainted blood and blood products occurred before 1985. Today, blood donors are screened, and blood is tested for HIV antibodies to ensure the safety of our blood supply.

HIV: What Is Safe?

AIDS is an infectious disease, but it is not spread through casual social contact with the general public or HIV carriers. You can share a classroom, dining area, or locker room with an HIV-infected individual without risk of transmission. It cannot be "caught" like a cold. It is not spread by insects. You cannot get HIV by shaking hands or by touching the clothes of a person infected with HIV. HIV is not spread through eating utensils, dishes, or food handled by a person with HIV. It is not spread through sweat or tears. It is impossible to get HIV by donating blood since clean needles are used for each donor. In studies of households where people with HIV were present, no case of HIV has been spread except through sexual contact or from infected mothers to their infants. You cannot get HIV from hugging, body massages, masturbation, nor other nonsexual contact. The AIDS virus is fragile. It cannot long survive outside the human body and is easily killed by common household bleach or disinfectant.

Q.   Can I get HIV from kissing?

A.   There is no risk in a kiss on the cheek, and no case of AIDS has been reported from kissing on the mouth. However, small amounts of the virus are present in saliva and could possibly be transferred to another person during deep kissing, especially if oral sores or cuts exist. To be safe, the Department of Health and Human Services recommends that you avoid deep or prolonged "French" kissing with someone who may be infected with HIV.

Q.   If mosquitoes can spread malaria, can they spread HIV?

A.   There has been no recorded case of transmission of HIV from mosquitoes. While a mosquito can pick up and carry HIV in its gut, the virus cannot reproduce there, nor travel to its saliva. Flies, lice, ticks, and other insects, likewise, cannot spread the virus.

Should I Be Tested for AIDS?

The Public Health Service recommends you be counseled and tested if you have had any STD, shared drug needles, had sex with a prostitute, or with a man who has sex with other men. Anyone who has had unprotected sex with 3 or more partners since 1981 is also at risk. People who have always practiced safe behavior do not need to be tested. For more information, call your local public health agency or the AIDS hotline at the end of this chapter.

Q.   Why doesn't a first test always detect AIDS?

A.   The test doesn't react to the HIV virus itself, but to antibodies the body produces to the virus. From the time a person is exposed to HIV to the time antibodies to the virus appear in the blood is 3 to 6 months. A person taking the test shortly after being infected may test negative, but the person can still spread HIV. Several months later, a test will show the infection.

What about an AIDS Vaccine?

There is no vaccine to prevent AIDS, and there is no cure. Drugs such as AZT are being tested to slow the progress of the disease, but results will not be available for many years, due to the long incubation period and slow progress of the disease. Another problem is that the virus rapidly mutates to produce new forms of the virus. A vaccine might be effective for only one viral strain. Scientists feel that an AIDS vaccine may be developed within 5–10 years, but it could take another 10–12 years to tell if it was effective in preventing AIDS. There is hope that treatments will be found, but the best way to prevent AIDS is to avoid exposure to the virus. We cannot depend on technology for a cure. Behavioral change to prevent infection is the only answer.

Why Should I Be Concerned about AIDS?

Too many young people feel that AIDS "can't happen to me." They think that it isn't in their peer group or neighborhood. But when you have sex with someone, you are, in a sense, having sex with all of that person's past partners. We have to face the fact that there are heterosexual students on campus who are HIV positive and are having sex. According to Dr. Richard P. Keeling of the American College Health Association Task Force on AIDS, blood samples tested from colleges across the USA revealed that 2 to 3 per 1,000 students tested HIV positive.[15] In a university of 20,000 this means 40 to 60 people may carry the virus. Keeling states "AIDS is a young person's disease. The average age of diagnosis is 32. The incubation period to diagnosis averages 10–12 years, so the highest risk time is ages 16–28. The problem doesn't seem real on most college campuses because people silently infected with HIV are not likely to appear ill." Many students who carry HIV look fine, and have no symptoms. They may not even know they are infected. However, during intercourse, they can spread the disease to others.

Among homosexuals, the group with the highest HIV infection rate, significant behavioral change is already dropping the rate of infection and diagnosis. There has been no behavioral change among the next two highest infected groups: IV drug users and their partners and young heterosexuals with multiple partners. Surveys of college students show that while most know how to prevent spread of HIV, over 60 percent report having sexual intercourse with more than one partner, and sporadic or no use of condoms.[16, 17] HIV infections among young heterosexuals has increased dramatically in the past 5 years.[18] Most students know the facts about AIDS, but many do not use condoms or know their sexual partners. Why? Keeling states that there are six reasons:

1. *They feel invincible.* They think, "Things like that don't happen to people like me."

2. *Lack of social skills and low self-esteem.* Many people don't feel comfortable with sexual feelings or behavior, don't feel

comfortable talking about these matters or negotiating with a sexual partner to take precautions.

3. *Unwanted sexual behavior.* They become involved in sex without really wanting to be—due to peer pressure, role expectations, or alcohol. Alcohol is involved in a tremendous amount of risky sexual behavior on campus. Alcohol increases risk taking, decreases ambivalence and judgment. It is impossible for sex under the influence of alcohol to be safe in terms of prevention of STDs.

4. *Sexual assault.* Date rape is a common unreported campus problem. If there is no consent; there are no precautions.

5. *Society sends mixed messages.* Our society may say, "Just say no," but in advertising and media, it screams "Just say yes. It will be O.K. Just try it."

6. *Sharing needles.* On campus, this is less a problem of recreational drugs than anabolic steroids. If needles are shared, it doesn't matter what's in them; they can still spread HIV.

Is sex under the influence worth it?

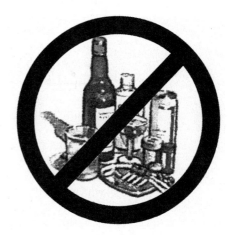

It doesn't matter who you are. It is not who you are that causes AIDS, but what you do. If you do things that can spread HIV, consider the risks. The problem with HIV is that if you make a mistake in judgment, it's irreversible. When you risk AIDS and lose, you lose it all.

How Can I Protect Myself from Sexually Transmitted Diseases?

While the facts about AIDS and other STDs are sobering, the good news is that you can reduce your risk of exposure to virtually zero by personal choices. The best prevention for any STD is sexual abstinence or a mutually monogamous sexual relationship with an uninfected partner. There is no "safe sex," only less risky sex. No orgasm is worth dying for. Unless you are willing to throw away your future, you must weigh the choices and consequences. If you are sexually active with more than one partner, there are steps that you can take to avoid becoming a victim of AIDS and other sexually transmitted diseases (table 13.4).

Table 13.4

How to Reduce Risk of STDs

1. Communicate assertively about sexual feelings, activities, partners, and STDs.
2. Choose lower-risk sexual activities that have less likelihood of transmitting STDs.
3. Separate alcohol and drugs from sexual activity. Drunk sex can't be safe sex.
4. Protect yourself. Use latex condoms and a spermicide containing nonoxynol-9.
5. Be selective. Limit the number of partners you have sex with. The fewer partners you have, the lower your risk. Do not have sex with someone who has several sex partners or with prostitutes. Prostitutes may also use IV drugs, increasing their chances of exposure to the AIDS virus.
6. Do not use intravenous drugs. If you do, do not share drug needles and syringes. Don't have sex with people who shoot drugs.
7. Observe a partner discreetly for discharge, sores, or rash. While it may not seem romantic, if you see anything that concerns you—**Don't have sex!**

In addition to these guidelines, you should also know the symptoms of STDs, and, if you notice a symptom that concerns you, see a physician. If you are sexually active, have an STD checkup every time you have a health exam. This is especially important for women who often have no signs of an STD. Have an STD checkup every 6 months if you have more than one partner. Abstain from sex if you think you have an infection, and see a doctor. If you do acquire an infection, make sure that all partners are notified and treated. To prevent infecting others, don't have sex until you have completed treatment and your doctor says you're cured.

How to Use Condoms

If abstinence or a mutually faithful, single-partner relationship is not your choice, the next best way to protect yourself from sexually transmitted diseases including AIDS is to use a condom during sex. While condoms are not 100 percent effective in preventing STDs or pregnancy, if used *correctly*, they can reduce risk by up to 99 percent. Unfortunately, few people know how to use them correctly, resulting in a failure rate of 15 percent to 20 percent.[19] If you are a woman, carry your own condoms, even if you don't plan to have sex (few young adults who have sex plan it). Do not store condoms in a hot place like a glove compartment nor carry them in a wallet for more than one week (they need to be fresh). Use a condom every time, including for oral or anal sex. Avoid skin condoms (i.e., lambskin)—they do not provide protection from all STDs, though they do prevent pregnancy.

To maximize condom effectiveness, follow these steps (figure 13.1):

1. Be careful when opening the package. Be especially careful not to tear the condom with a fingernail or teeth.

2. Put the condom on before penetration, even if ejaculation is not planned. Withdrawal is not effective in preventing STDs. Unroll the condom on the erect penis, leaving about 1/2-inch airspace at the tip. If there is no space at the tip, the force of semen coming out of the penis can break the condom.

3. Apply a water-based lubricant or spermicide with nonoxynol-9 onto the tip of the condom. Do not use an oil-based lubricant. Vaseline or baby oil quickly deteriorate latex.

4. Withdraw while the penis is still erect. Hold the rim of the condom to avoid spilling semen. Throw the used condom away. Do not reuse it.

Figure 13.1

How to use a condom

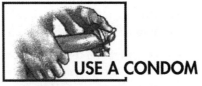
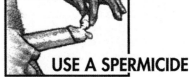
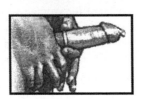
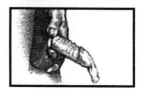

If you or your partner don't like male condoms, try a female condom, which works like an extra-large male condom inserted into a woman's vagina. It consists of a 6 1/2-inch long plastic tube with a large ring on each end. One ring holds it in the vagina, and the other ring fits outside the vaginal lips. It is as effective in preventing conception and STDs as the male condom.

Planning Ahead for Safer Sex

When you are in the midst of a passionate embrace, it may not seem convenient to discuss safe sex or learn how to use a condom. Before beginning a sexual relationship, plan ahead. Think about what you'll say to your partner about using condoms. It may help to use a news story about AIDS to bring up the subject of safe sex. Make your feelings about condom use clear. Tell your partner you want to take precautions because you care about both of you. If your partner won't agree to use condoms, don't have sex.

Choosing Lower-Risk Sexual Activities

There are a lot of ways to show someone you care besides having sex: respect, sharing, trust, commitment. Lasting relationships are built on alternative ways of expressing love and affection. Even if you have decided to have sex, there are lower-risk sex techniques you can use to protect yourself from STDs. Keep in mind that your skin is your largest sexual organ, and your imagination is your most important sexual asset.

No Risk
- Kissing with the mouth closed, hugging
- Touching, massage, masturbation
- Fantasy

Low Risk
- Vaginal or oral sex using a condom and spermicide
- Masturbating a partner using a latex barrier

Risky
- Wet kissing with your mouth open
- Anal sex with or without a condom
- Vaginal or oral sex without a condom

Coping with Unwanted Sexual Pressure

Dave and Sue were introduced by mutual friends and Dave has invited Sue to go out to a movie with him. They go to the movie, have a couple beers afterward, and Dave takes Sue home. It is very late. She wants to go to her apartment alone, but Dave has a long drive home and asks for a cup of coffee. This seems reasonable, so Sue invites Dave up. As soon as they are inside the door, he pins her to the wall with an aggressive kiss and starts taking off her blouse.

Joe is invited to a party at an off-campus apartment by Jill, whom he met at a football game. He doesn't know anyone there but doesn't want to miss the fun. The music is lively and the drinks are free so he has a few drinks and starts feeling relaxed. Jill shows up and invites him to go to her room so they can talk. He agrees. They take their drinks and head toward the bedroom.

Is a female "asking for it" if she has been drinking? Is consent implied if Sue invites Dave into her apartment? If Jill closes the bedroom door and sits on the bed? Unfortunately, the double standard is alive and well in the USA. Many people come to campus with little experience dealing with sexual matters. What can

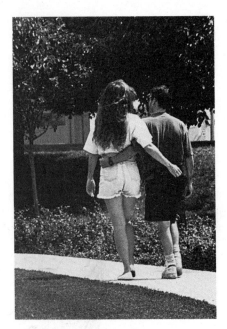

Serious relationships require serious decisions.

a person do to prevent unwanted sexual behavior? "We need to build skills in assertiveness, self-esteem, decision making, running a relationship, and dealing with intimacy. We need a personal commitment that says my life, my future, my potential are more valuable than what's going to happen in this relationship or on this date or in the next 10 minutes."[20] What do you do when he/she wants to have sex and you don't ? What do you do to avoid sexually pressured situations? Here are some tips from the Santa Monica Rape Treatment Center:[21]

- Attend parties with friends you can trust. Look out for each other. Leave together, rather than alone or with a new acquaintance. If you are attracted to someone you'd like to get to know better, agree to meet for lunch the next day.

- Communicate clearly. Don't lead someone on. Don't expect a person to know how you feel unless you speak up. Make your feelings and intentions clear. You have a right to say no to any unwanted sexual contact. If you are being pressured and feel uncertain, ask the person to respect your feelings.

- Listen closely to what a person is saying. If you think she/he is giving you a mixed message, ask for clarification. On a date when neither person stops to check out what the other person is feeling, the situation can get out of hand.

- Make sure *how* you say something agrees with *what* you say. Your body language, how

you say something, may come across louder than your words. If you say "No" with downcast eyes and a smile to soften the refusal, you may end up giving the other person a mixed message. You are more likely to get your message across if you look a person directly in the eyes and say "no" assertively.

- Rely on your gut instinct. If a situation doesn't feel right, exit as quickly as you can and go to a safe place.

- Speak up if you believe someone is at risk. If you see a woman in trouble at a party or if a friend is using force and pressuring a woman, don't be afraid to intervene. You may save the woman from the trauma of sexual assault and your friend from criminal prosecution.

- Be aware that having sex with someone who is intoxicated, passed out, drugged, or otherwise incapable of giving consent is rape.

Women:

- Realize that to some people, drinking heavily, dressing provocatively, or going to a private apartment or bedroom implies willingness to have sex. Be especially careful in these situations to make your feelings and intentions clear.

Men:

- Don't fall for the stereotype that when a woman says no she means yes. If she says no to sexual contact, believe her and stop.
- Don't make assumptions about a person's behavior. Just because a woman drinks heavily, dresses provocatively, or goes with you to your room, don't assume she wants sex. Just because she had sex with you once, don't assume she is willing now. Also, don't assume that because she willingly engages in kissing or other intimate behavior that she wants sexual intercourse.

Both men and women must be especially careful in situations involving drinking or drugs. These decrease reasoning ability, your ability to make a decision, and to communicate effectively. They increase willingness to take risks you wouldn't normally take. Alcohol, a social lubricant par excellence, sets you up for unwanted sexual behavior and STDs. It decreases ability to recognize an unsafe situation and to react appropriately. It also decreases likelihood that you will use a condom. Even if you have one, you may be too drunk to put it on.

Summary

Sexually transmitted diseases have reached epidemic levels in the nineties. Young adults are at greatest risk. Chlamydia, gonorrhea, syphilis, genital herpes, and human papilloma virus are the most common STDs. To reduce risk of STDs, people must take responsibility for their sexual behavior and take protective measures, for themselves and their partners. It is also important to learn skills in communication, assertiveness, negotiation, and relating to others. AIDS, a new and deadly STD, makes preventative measures more important than ever for those who are sexually active.

References

1. Abler, R. M. and Sedlacek, W. E. "Freshman Sexual Attitudes and Behaviors Over a 15-Year Period." *Journal of College Student Development,* 30 (May 1989): 201–209.

2. Murstein, B. I. et. al. "Sexual Behavior, Drugs, and Relationship Patterns on a College Campus over Thirteen Years" *Adolescence,* 24 (Spring 1989): 125–139.

3. Centers for Disease Control. "Sexual Behavior Among High School Students—United States, 1990." *Morbidity and Mortality Weekly Report,* 40 (51 & 52) (January 3, 1992): 885–887.

4. Centers for Disease Control. "1985 STD Treatment Guidelines." *MMWR Supplement,* (September, 1985).

5. Centers for Disease Control. "Summary of Notifiable Diseases, United States, 1990." *Morbidity and Mortality Weekly Report 1990,* 39 (53) (December, 1990): 24.

6. Centers for Disease Control. "Summary of Notifiable Diseases—United States, 1990." *Morbidity and Mortality Weekly Report,* 39 (53) (December 1990): 24.

7. Centers for Disease Control. "1985 STD Treatment Guidelines." *MMWR Supplement,* (September 1985).

8. Mertz, G. J. et. al., "Risk Factors for the Sexual Transmission of Genital Herpes" *Annals of Internal Medicine* 116 (Feb. 1992): 197–202.

9. Collison, Michele. "Dramatic Increase in Genital Warts Disease Among Students Worries College Health Officers." *Chronicle of Higher Education,* 35 (May 31, 1989): A23.

10. Ojanlatva, Ansa, "Human Papillomavirus Infections: The Next Epidemic?" *Health Education* 21 (5) (September/October 1990): 18–19.

11. Munoz, N. and Bosh, F. X. "Cervical Cancer—Second most Common Cause

of Cancer Death for Women." In Munoz, N.; Bosh, F. X.; and Jensen, O. M., Eds; *Human Papilloma Virus and Cervical Cancer*. (IARC Scientific Publication No. 94) Oxford, England: International Agency for Research on Cancer, 1989.

12. Centers for Disease Control. "The Second 100,000 Cases of Acquired Immunodeficiency Syndrome—United States, June 1981-December 1991." *Morbidity and Mortality Weekly Report 1992*, 41 (2) (Jan. 17, 1992): 28–29.

13. Centers for Disease Control, "The Second 100,000 Cases of Acquired Immunodeficiency Syndrome—United States, June 1981-December 1991.

Morbidity and Mortality Weekly Report 1992, 41 (2) Jan. 17, 1992; 28–29.

14. Curran, James, Centers for Disease Control, Atlanta, GA, Feb. 1992.

15. Keeling, Richard P., personal communication, September 15, 1992.

16. Ryan, Marilyn and Jones, Lorraine. "Survey of Sexual Attitudes and Practices on Campus." Ball State University, Muncie, IN, 1991.

17. Abler, R. M. and Sedlacek, W. E. "Freshman Sexual Attitudes and Behaviors Over a 15-Year Period." *Journal of College Student Development*, 30 (May 1989): 201–209.

18. Centers for Disease Control. "Summary of Notifiable Diseases—United States, 1990." *Morbidity and Mortality Weekly Report*, 39 (53) (December 1990).

19. Stone, K. M. "Avoiding STDs." *Obstetrics and Gynecology Clinics of North America*, 17 (4) (December, 1990): 789–799.

20. Keeling, Richard P., "Medical Issues." *AIDS In the College Community: From Crisis to Management*. Teleconference. Ohio State University. November 16, 1989.

21. Roden, M. and Abarbanel, G. *How It Happens*, Rape Treatment Center, Santa Monica Hospital Medical Center, Santa Monica, CA, 1987.

Suggested Readings

Baxter, Roger. "STDs—Sexually Transmitted Diseases." *Healthline* 8 (August 1989): 1–3.

Bogner, Jerry L. *Facts about AIDS & Other Sexually Transmitted Diseases: Sexual Decisions of Responsible Adults*. 1987. Goleta, CA: Bogners Limited.

Cox, Frank D. *The AIDS Booklet, 2nd ed.* 1992. Dubuque, IA: William C. Brown Publishers.

Holmes, King K. *Sexually Transmitted Diseases*. 1991. Winchester, MA: Faber & Faber.

Jackson, James K. *AIDS, STD, & Other Communicable Diseases*. 1992. Guilford, CT: Dushkin Publishing Group.

McIlhaney, Joe S., Jr. *Sexuality and Sexually Transmitted Diseases: A Doctor Confronts the Myth of "Safe" Sex*. 1990. Grand Rapids, MI: Baker Books.

Roden, M. and G. Abarbanel. *How It Happens*, 1987. Rape Treatment Center, Santa Monica Hospital Medical Center, Santa Monica, CA.

Resources

Nationally Sexually Transmitted Disease Hotline/American Social Health Association: 1–800–227–8922.

AIDS Hotline (U.S. Public Health Service): 1–800–342–AIDS.

National Gay Task Force—AIDS Crisis Line: 1–800–227–8922.

Teens Teaching AIDS Prevention: 1–800–234–TEEN.

National AIDS Information Clearinghouse: 1–800–458–5231.

AIDS Task Force for the American College Health Association, c/o Dr. Richard P. Keeling, Dept. of Student Health, Box 378, University of Virginia, Charlottesville, VA 22908, (804) 924–2670.

14
Planning Wellness for a Lifetime

Chapter Objectives

After reading this chapter, you will be able to:

1. Define quackery, and list five of the seven common characteristics of quackery.
2. Discriminate between a credible health product/discovery and a bogus or flimsy finding/promotion.
3. List the four premises on which corporate wellness programs are based.
4. Give ten examples of wellness programs that corporations might offer their employees.
5. List five of the seven key elements needed for a strong marriage.
6. Describe two ways parents can lessen the risk of their teen/preteen engaging in risky health behaviors.
7. Give two examples of behaviors within each dimension of wellness that parents can develop in a young child.
8. List six of the nine environmental concerns that may affect our wellness.
9. List three predictable trends, and describe how they will affect wellness in the future.
10. List and describe two future challenges we face in regard to wellness.

Terms

- Quackery

"May you live all the days of your life."

Jonathan Swift

The purpose of this book is to present wellness as a lifestyle where positive choices result in optimal functioning and enhanced living. You have gained knowledge that will help you to make informed decisions and have learned skills for making behavioral change. You are now "wellness educated." With knowledge comes responsibility, so you no longer have the luxury of saying, "I didn't know!" You know what choices contribute to wellness and those that do not. You can choose to eat right, exercise, and fasten your seat belt, or you can choose not to. And you know the possible consequences of such choices. The challenge for you is just beginning. Whereas wellness is ongoing, college days come to an end. A new career, a different living environment, marriage, and children will bring many changes to your life. During these changes, the wellness lifestyle can prevail. We hope it will grow. Wellness is a process, not a solution. It is a journey, not a destination. A major part of wellness is adapting to change and maximizing your potential amidst change.

Remember that wellness involves a balance and integration of all 6 dimensions of wellness. Too often physical fitness is used synonymously with wellness. Admittedly, being physically fit has a positive effect on the other dimensions. However, your job satisfaction, family relationships, social ties, emotional health, and spiritual health are equally linked to wellness. This final chapter focuses on a few important points for you to consider as you plan for the future.

Taking Charge

Following a performance of a great musician, an admirer said to him, "I'd give my life to play like that." The brilliant performer replied, "I did." We often view a performance of an athlete or artist with envy. Even seeing the volumes of handiwork and crafts at a festival brings thoughts of "How do they do it?" Accomplishment is often deceptive, because we don't see the perseverance that produces it. Pursuing wellness also involves a certain amount of perseverance and discipline. Many desire the benefits of wellness living but fail to make a commitment to its precepts. As you take charge of your lifestyle, focus on the positive outcomes of changing a health-robbing behavior, rather than the effort involved. Remember, you do not pay the price for having wellness; you pay the price for *not* having it.

Knowledge and good intentions are a good start. Then focus on self-management techniques and behavior-changing skills (chapter 1) that implement your knowledge into maintainable habits. Be aware of the power of cultural norms, the media, advertising, and sources of social support.

Partners in Prevention

The *Healthy People 2000* document sets high goals for the health and well-being of the American people. It emphasizes personal responsibility and self-empowerment as a means of increasing the quality and quantity of life. Some people need to know the facts in order to make informed decisions. Others need positive influences to motivate them toward appropriate choices. "Still others must have assistance in escaping the bonds of victimization and need support as they move toward self-empowerment . . . *Healthy People 2000* will become a reality by the year 2000 only through a change of culture in America."[1]

For the wellness lifestyle to permeate our culture, support systems within communities must be available. While emphasizing personal responsibility, we cannot overlook the importance of the collective burden of responsibility from governmental policies, wellness curriculum in the schools, corporate action, and the American family. Even though personal behaviors contribute to the leading causes of death, behaviors occur in and are influenced by the environment.[2] Advertisements, television programs, and popular songs that glamorize drinking, violence, sex, and immoral behavior undermine our nation's health and well-being. For example, cigarette ads show likable young people in upscale settings enjoying smoking. The subliminal message is that cigarettes must not be so bad if such bright, attractive people are not afraid to smoke. Of course, in these ads there is never a dirty ashtray, nicotine-stained teeth, or anyone coughing or getting chemotherapy. There is no dangerously underweight baby lying in intensive care. There is no one dying. An important part of wellness education is deciphering these messages and knowing what really does promote well-being.

Individuals, families, communities, corporations, and the government together share the task of enhancing the well-being of all Americans. Since you are "wellness educated," part of this challenge of culture change rests with you. Can you think of ways you can affect this change?

Understanding Quackery

The concept of wellness has widespread appeal. Most everyone is attracted to the thought of enhancing the quality of his or her life. The expanse of the wellness concept invites a considerable amount of quackery and short-cut schemes. **Quackery** is the promotion of a misleading and fraudulent health claim that is unproven. Most quackery products are foods, drugs, gadgets, or cosmetics that promote physical change—baldness cures, bust enhancers, wrinkle removers, cancer cures, eat-all-you-want weight-loss pills, instant strength devices, youth elixirs, arthritis cures. It is not uncommon to see other wellness-enhancing plans that also border on fraud—a two-hour course guaranteed to make you an all-A student, a videotape that shows you how to attract the perfect mate, an audiotape that promises to increase your yearly income, etc.

Many people erroneously believe that product advertisements are screened by government agencies and that claims on television or in print must be true. This is not so. It is hard to resist effortless, quick shortcuts to health and wellness. Many promoters are wealthy as a result of our willingness to spend money for miracle solutions. Unfortunately, the results are often shattered hopes, wasted money, and sometimes endangered health. Misconceptions and half-truths fuel these promotional fires. As an educated wellness consumer, you should be able to evaluate products and plans with intelligence and realism. See table 14.1 for common characteristics of quackery.

Table 14.1
How to Recognize Quackery

Some products use scientific jargon and carry professional logos and endorsements (many of which are bogus). Watch for the following characteristics common in quackery.
1. It sounds too good to be true.
2. It is quick and painless.
3. It has a "secret," "special," "foreign," "magical," "exclusive," or "ancient" formula.
4. It is available only through the mail (most often through a P.O. Box number) or telephone, and only from one supplier.
5. It is a scientific "breakthrough" or "miracle cure" that has been overlooked by the medical community.
6. It uses testimonials or case histories from "satisfied customers" as the only proof of its effectiveness.
7. It is a single product effective for a wide variety of ailments.

Remember, if it sounds too good to be true, it probably is! Sometimes television personalities or well-known celebrities write books, represent products in advertisements, or are portrayed as "experts" in the field of health and fitness. Be wary of the credibility of this type of product/information marketing.

Many hospitals, schools, corporations, community wellness centers, and health organizations offer legitimate programs that can assist you in pursuing a wellness lifestyle. Investigate references and sources before falling for any fly-by-night scheme. Your physician, the Better Business Bureau, local consumer office, or nearest office of the Food and Drug Administration (FDA) can offer professional advice if you suspect a product makes untrue claims.

Can you recognize quackery?

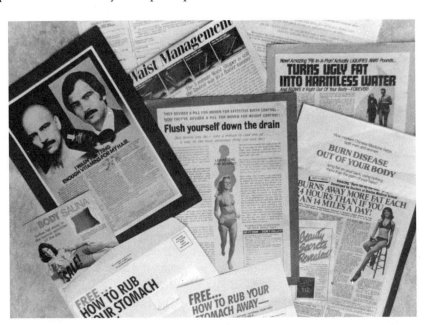

Also part of "well-informed wellness" is distinguishing good quality health research from flimsy or biased data. It seems like every day we hear contradictory information on health, fitness, or nutrition. Is coffee good or bad for you? Is the mega-trim diet safe or not safe? Will an aspirin a day prevent a heart attack? There is no easy answer to these and other questions. However, the more you know about the economics, politics, and methodology of research, the better able you are to form a sound opinion. Ask yourself the following questions as you weigh the evidence:

- Where is the work published? In a supermarket tabloid? In a homemaker's magazine? In a scientific journal that uses a board of experts to review the article?
- Who paid for the research? (Some companies and foundations might profit from certain outcomes.)
- Do my personal biases lead me to want to believe this information?
- Are advertisers using this information to sell a product?
- Is this only a preliminary finding that has not been fully tested?
- Are the researchers from respectable institutions?
- Was good scientific methodology used? Number in the study? Control group?

Remember, it takes more than headlines to draw a sound conclusion. Unfortunately, you cannot believe everything you read and hear!

Campus Wellness

Many colleges and universities have voiced a commitment to wellness and, as a result, offer a variety of wellness programs to students. Many programs are also available to faculty and staff. Realizing that the collegiate experience involves more than intellectual growth, universities are providing services and activities to promote self-discovery, psychological well-being, career planning, spiritual discovery, health risk assessment, and lifetime fitness. It is not uncommon to see programs for stress management, alcohol control, weight management, smoking cessation, eating disorders, and even investment counseling. Some universities have wellness residence halls, nutrition-controlled food services, academic wellness courses, and even fitness standards for all students. Investigate your campus for wellness resources. The variety of expertise and resources found at most universities not only prepares you for a lifetime career but can prepare you for lifetime wellness. Attending a wellness-oriented university is an example of how a supportive environment can enhance your quest for wellness.

Career Wellness

Your job will be a prominent facet of your adult life. You will spend approximately 50 percent of your waking hours at work, if you maintain a full-time job or career. This fact alone makes the workplace a likely place to receive information and support regarding personal health improvement. Leaders in business and industry are beginning to see employee wellness as an asset to be maintained and enhanced. When employees are happy and healthy, productivity increases. The promotion of wellness programs in business and industry is based on four related premises.

1. Prevention is preferable to curing.
2. Teaching people to stay healthy is generally less expensive than treating them when they are ill.
3. Healthful lifestyles offer a better quality of life, higher morale, increased productivity, and a possible increased longevity.
4. Health promotion programs promote a favorable corporate image and help attract prospective employees who see these programs as a valuable employee benefit.

Rising medical insurance costs, employee absenteeism, and sick leaves cut deeply into profits and lead to increases in the costs of doing business. As a result, corporate officials are experimenting with ways of incorporating wellness into the workplace. According to Michael O'Donnell, this exciting avenue for health promotion can bring about changes in behavior for an improved lifestyle, as well as enhance personal relationships.[3] Wellness in the workplace can be promoted in a variety of ways. Programs can involve diagnosis (assess current health and habits), education (give information about health enhancement), and/or behavior modification (give help and support in making a specific behavior change). According to a national survey conducted by the Public Health Service, nearly two-thirds of the nation's private worksites with 50 or more workers have at least one wellness promotion activity.[4] These programs include, among others, smoking cessation, health risk appraisals, back care, stress management, fitness classes, nutrition education, weight management, and cholesterol screening.

Employers realize that the work and nonwork parts of our lives are interactive. That is, job satisfaction is also dependent on family happiness, leisure pursuits, and feelings of worth. Knowing this, employers are actively pursuing a multidimensional approach to supporting employee wellness. Examples are flexible work hours, child care, on-the-job retraining, sports team participation, job sharing, smoke-free work sites, parental leaves, family hikes and picnics, and even children's fitness classes. Several forward-thinking companies are even responding to the needs of employees with elderly parents (by providing elder care), as well as providing substance abuse and marital counseling. Since spouses and children of employees account for 40 percent to 60 percent of company's health-care expenditures, such multidimensional programs can be cost-effective.[5]

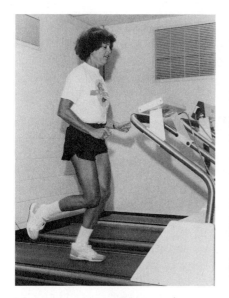

Many companies support employee wellness.

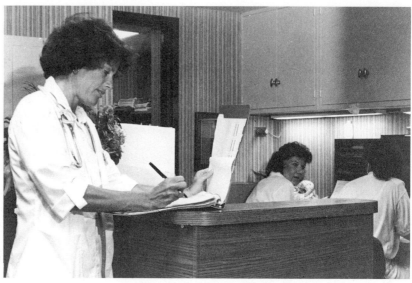

Due to the growing interest and emphasis on wellness in business and industry, many employers prefer hiring personnel who have already adopted a wellness lifestyle—nonsmoking, physically fit, reasonable weight, etc. This knowledge is added incentive for you to continue a wellness lifestyle. As a potential employee, your confirmed dedication to wellness may also influence your final selection of a job. You may favor a company that is highly supportive of wellness and provides wellness programs for employees. Remember how important a supportive environment is in the maintenance of positive lifestyle choices.

Many college students, pressured by school demands, feel they will have more time to exercise and eat right once they graduate. Your life will most likely be just as busy, if not more so once you begin your career. Time restraints and demands will always be with you. Making wellness living an important part of your current lifestyle will help you to maintain it after graduation, as a habit.

Wellness in the Family

It is likely that you will marry and have children someday. Perhaps you are already a spouse and/or parent. In all cultures, the family unit is the primary transmitter of values and attitudes in the society. You and your spouse come together with values, norms, and expectations derived from your own families. As partners you continue to grow, interact, and develop a value framework. When children come along, the parental role of maintaining the culture from generation to generation is created. The interacting dynamics of your family unit promote physical, psychological, and social growth of each member. Just as wellness is a dynamic state, the family unit is also everchanging. Throughout all ages and stages of development, family nurturance is essential for all members to strive toward full potential.

It is important to find time to play together as a family

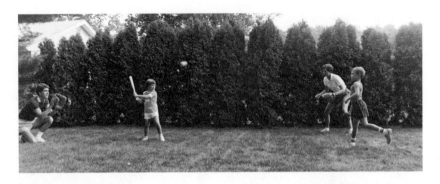

The Well Marriage

Many romantic fairy tales conclude with . . . "and they lived happily ever after." Whereas these words end these fantasies, marriage is the beginning of the story in real life. Who you marry is one of your most important life decisions. Much of your happiness and life satisfaction will be based on the success of this marriage. Like the wellness lifestyle, a marriage demands conscious effort, commitment, and even personal sacrifice. It is a partnership that involves change and growth. Many factors influence the success of a marriage relationship. Consider the following key elements that help build a strong and lasting marriage relationship:

1. Communication—be able to share your true feelings with your partner.

2. Compromise—each partner must be willing to give a little. Sometimes it's 50–50, sometimes 100–0!

3. Values—common values and shared goals help maintain a focus during tension-filled times.

4. Likability and respect—enjoying each other's company and respecting each other's needs is essential.

5. Shared responsibilities—in a world where the two-parent career is the norm, each partner must be willing to share in the responsibilities of home and child care.

6. Space—each partner needs to have his or her own identity and be allowed to grow individually.

7. Sense of humor—laughing and having fun are ways to keep daily problems in proper perspective.

You probably wonder why "sex" is not on the list. If you have the other seven keys, a great sex life will most likely occur!

Just as in wellness growth, marriage growth is a process. It doesn't happen all at once. Enjoy each step along the path!

The Well Child

It will be your challenge as a parent to initiate wellness living within your growing family. All dimensions (emotional, social, physical, intellectual, spiritual, and occupational) demand your attention. If you as a parent favor behaviors that promote wellness, your children will follow your example. Family wellness patterns can set

Exercise habits start young

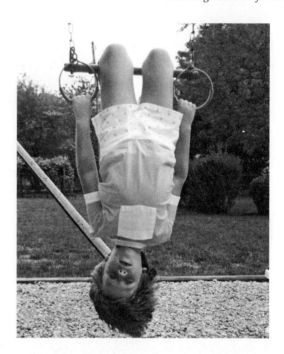

the stage for a lifelong pattern of self-responsibility. Since self-responsibility relies on learning and practicing skills, you can be the master teacher of wellness and help your child grow as a decision maker. Children do not learn just in school. They learn by watching you, too. If you exercise, eat nutritiously, read instead of watch television, handle stress, communicate your feelings, and display attitudes of cooperation and respect, your child will, too. Since the personality and self-concept of most children is formed by the time they start kindergarten, you as parents will be prime molders of this self-concept. A positive self-esteem is an important foundation as the child moves into larger social spheres beyond the family. The child with a high degree of self-worth is able to confront life's situations with confidence. "A most fundamental ingredient of enduring happiness is confidence in our own ability . . . Self-confidence gives rise to optimism and hope."[6] Optimism and self-confidence are the building blocks for wellness living.

Although it is popularly believed that risk-taking behavior among teenagers and preteens is most strongly influenced by peer pressure, new research by adolescent medicine specialists concludes that family closeness plays a key role. Young people who have a balance of strong attachment to family and parental encouragement to be independent are least likely to take part in high-risk activities (alcohol and drug use, sexual activities, cigarette experimentation) that could seriously affect their well-being.[7]

Even though the broad concept of wellness is difficult for young children to understand, they can become aware and learn the value of specific wellness choices. Their capacity to understand the cause and effect of certain choices depends on their age and maturity level. Can children learn to habitually fasten their seat belts?

Table 14.2

Wellness Behaviors That Can Be
Developed by the Young Child

Physical Dimension

Forms habits of regular, vigorous exercise
Establishes healthy eating habits and preferences
Forms self-care habits (personal hygiene, dental care, etc.)
Forms safety habits (seat belts, fire, bike riding, etc.)
Establishes attitude about smoking, drug use, alcohol

Social Dimension

Seeks companionship with others
Senses responsibility for behavior
Shows concern and respect for others
Displays willingness to share work responsibilities with others

Emotional Dimension

Forms feelings of self-worth and self-confidence
Talks freely about feelings
Develops appropriate coping behaviors for a variety of situations
Displays capacity to give and receive love

Spiritual Dimension

Develops an awareness of life versus death
Develops a sense of the importance and expanse of life
Begins establishing a value system—right versus wrong
Begins showing compassion and forgiveness

Intellectual Dimension

Develops creativity and curiosity
Establishes listening skills
Learns "cause-and-effect" concepts
Recognizes the expanse of the world by a variety of experiences

Occupational Dimension

Identifies a variety of jobs/careers
Understands the importance of work and effort
Begins developing work habits
Begins understanding the importance of money

Select fruits for snacks? Show respect for others? Appreciate nature? Enjoy vigorous exercise? Of course, they can! Look at table 14.2 for examples of wellness behaviors that parents are instrumental in developing in their children.

You face the challenge of pursuing wellness both as an adult (striving for full potential), and also as a parent (fostering optimal child development). The American family is changing. We face a growing trend toward single-parent households and increasing numbers of working mothers. Such changes affect the balance between work life and family life, often creating role conflicts, stress, and changing values.[8] Regardless of the makeup of the family unit, everyone, young and old, can achieve high-level wellness. Hopefully, the "Memo" in table 14.3 will stimulate your thoughts concerning the awesome responsibility of parenting.

Table 14.3

Memo

Source: Unknown

To: *Parents*
From: *A Child*

1. Don't spoil me, I know quite well that I ought not to have all I ask for—I'm only testing you.
2. Don't be afraid to be firm with me. I prefer it. It makes me feel secure.
3. Don't let me form bad habits. I have to rely on you to detect them in the early stages.
4. Don't make me feel smaller than I am. It only makes me behave stupidly "big."
5. Don't correct me in front of people if you can help it. I'll take much more notice if you talk quietly with me in private.
6. Don't make me feel that my mistakes are sins. It upsets my sense of values.
7. Don't protect me from consequences. I need to learn the painful way sometime.
8. Don't be too upset when I say, "I hate you." Sometimes it isn't you I hate, but your power to thwart me.
9. Don't take too much notice of my small ailments. Sometimes they get me the attention I need.
10. Don't nag. If you do, I shall have to protect myself by appearing deaf.
11. Don't forget that I cannot explain myself as well as I should like. That is why I am not always accurate.
12. Don't put me off when I ask questions. If you do, you will find that I stop asking and seek my information elsewhere.
13. Don't be inconsistent. That completely confuses me and makes me lose faith in you.
14. Don't tell me my fears are silly. They are terribly real, and you can do much to reassure me if you try to understand.
15. Don't ever suggest that you are perfect or infallible. It gives me too great a shock when I discover that you are neither.
16. Don't ever think that it is beneath your dignity to apologize to me. An honest apology makes me feel surprisingly warm toward you.
17. Don't forget I love experimenting. I couldn't get along without it, so please put up with it.
18. Don't forget how quickly I am growing up. It must be very difficult for you to keep pace with me, but please do try.
19. Don't forget that I don't thrive without lots of love and understanding, but I don't need to tell you, do I?
20. Please keep yourself fit and healthy. I need you.

Environmental Wellness

Environmental policy has long been a mainstay of public health. Regulations regarding safe food, water, and sewage management have substantially improved our well-being.[9] However, rapid technological changes have resulted in new environmental hazards, many whose effects on the body may be unrecognized for years.[10] This opens new opportunities for you to make an impact on your wellness—and that of others. "For the first time in history, human beings are in the position of creating the world in which they live (including pollution of the environment)."[11]

Being apathetic or becoming accustomed to environmental pollution is a very serious matter. There is a lot you can do to limit, or at least minimize, the pollution in your "own little world." Recall the "tools" necessary for growth in wellness (chapter 1)—*awareness* and *knowledge* are paramount in forming a plan to combat environmental hazards. Look at the following list of environmental concerns, and consider ways you could make changes in your daily living in order to make the world a better place in which to live.

1. The earth's protective ozone layer—our shield against the sun's hazardous ultraviolet rays—is being eaten away by man-made chemicals. The result is damaged food crops and ocean plants, increased skin cancer and cataracts, and decreases in human immunities. Aerosol sprays, refrigerants, plastic foam, and cleaning fluids contain chlorofluorocarbons (CFCs)—the chief agents of ozone destruction.

2. Our excesses of paper, plastic, glass, and aluminum continue to pile up in our landfills. Recycling can decrease the need for more landfills and cut down on the pollution from the manufacture of new products.

3. Residues of harmful pesticides can be found in the air, on crops, in the ground, and in water supplies. Lawn and garden chemicals are significant contributors to this.

4. Water and air, essentials for life, face increasing contamination. Fish caught in polluted waters may be contaminated.

5. Loud rock music is associated with hearing loss.

6. Traffic sounds, aircraft noise, and noisy industrial areas are associated with stress and stress-related physical symptoms.

7. Radon gas and asbestos have been linked to cancer. Radon is a naturally occurring radioactive gas emitted by soil and rocks. Radon is diluted to safe levels outdoors but can be dangerously concentrated if trapped in poorly ventilated basements, houses, and buildings. Asbestos, a commonly-used insulating material, has been linked to a variety of lung diseases. The U. S. government has ordered an end to the production of nearly all asbestos in the country by 1997.

8. Exposure to high levels of lead is toxic to the central nervous system and can be fatal. In our country, nearly 3 million children are at some risk from elevated lead levels.[12] House paints used before 1980 often contained lead. Also, those that live near airports, battery factories, and landfills are at risk.

We often take too many things for granted. Part of your challenge in wellness living will be to assume some responsibility for preserving the environment.

Wellness Trends and Challenges for the Future

Whereas some regard wellness as a passing fad, we disagree. In his highly acclaimed book, *Megatrends*, John Naisbitt predicted: "The focus of health care is shifting from the short-term treatment of illness to the long-term attainment of wellness. Regarded by some as fad, wellness is a trend that is here to stay."[13] We have already seen the wellness trend give impetus to societal changes. Designated smoking areas, seat belt laws, shopping mall wellness screenings, and the emergence of alcohol treatment centers are all examples of positive wellness changes. What else is down the road for wellness? What other changes and trends will you see in your lifetime? What are the challenges that will continue to demand attention? The remainder of this chapter addresses these questions.

Predictable Trends

One of the biggest trends is the changing focus in hospitals and the health-care profession. Medical care is shifting from the sickness business to the wellness business. Many community hospitals now offer a variety of wellness programs with the intention of preventing individuals from becoming ill and needing hospitalization. Cholesterol testing, nutrition workshops, family counseling, drug rehabilitation, weight management classes, and exercise prescription are examples of such programs. Some health facility administrators have found that a simple name change attracts clients to some of their programs. For example, a "mental health" center renamed to be a "stress" center has an easier time drawing individuals searching for help in dealing with personal problems. The counseling services of such a center may not be altered at all. But the connotation of learning ways to handle personal stress, rather than dealing with mental health (often erroneously linked to mental illness), better attracts individuals needing such services.

Another change in medical care deals with the medical education of physicians. Medical schools are expanding their physician training to include studying lifestyle and preventive influences on health and disease, rather than solely learning to identify and cure illness. There is compelling evidence showing that physicians exert a strong influence on their patients' behavior patterns. By incorporating preventive services and counseling into their patient encounters, physicians can dramatically affect the well-being of the nation.[14] In this way, the physician can become a prime force in advocating a wellness lifestyle.

The high cost of medical care and the rising cost of health insurance have initiated another trend. Insurance companies are beginning to provide incentives for staying well. Insurance benefits are being expanded and costs lowered to those who actively strive for optimal well-being by refraining from smoking, participating in periodic health screenings, fastening seat belts, exercising regularly, etc. Group health benefits at reduced rate will be sought by companies that promote wellness in their workplaces and have predominantly healthy employees.

Americans are living longer

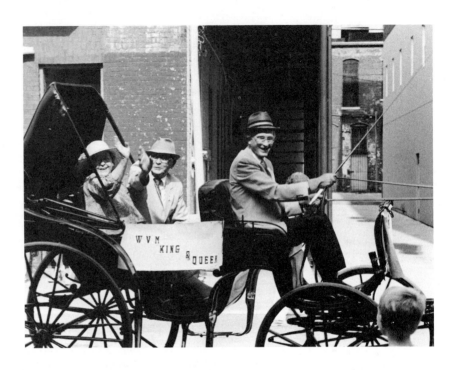

Another trend affects all of us. More Americans are living longer, and, as a result, we have an expanding population of elderly. By the year 2000, people over the age of 65 will represent about 13 percent of the American population. And, the "oldest old"—those over age 85—will have increased by about 30 percent to a total of 4.6 million.[15] The majority of this population is not, as many would think, senile or confined to nursing homes. Many older Americans are healthy, self-sufficient, and physically capable. They have money to spend and desire to continue as active contributors to society. They want and need programs for nutrition education, exercise, personal enrichment, and financial management. The elderly group is one of the top markets perceived by health promotion analysts to be important during the next 10 years.[16] As wellness becomes a way of life, you, too, will want programs as you reach older adulthood, whether they be special exercise classes, social activities, or living environments.

Research has already begun and will continue in an exciting new area—the link between mind and body. The field of mind/body research explores the unconscious interactions between our bodies and our minds, moods, and spirit. Consider the following:

- You have to get up extraordinarily early tomorrow morning to catch a flight. You set your alarm for 5:15 a.m. The next morning you wake up with a jolt at 5:12, before the alarm has sounded!

- You have not spoken with your distant brother for several months. Just as you are thinking about him, the phone rings. It is your brother calling.

- A mother feels a sharp pain in her right leg. At that same moment, hundreds of miles away, her daughter breaks her right leg while skiing.

These phenomena accentuate the power and complexity of the human brain.

Studies suggest there is a direct link between states of mind and the immune system.[17] That is, emotional states affect us right down to our cells. Mental states, such as loneliness, depression, and pessimism, alter the responses in the immune system. Having close relationships, hope, and social support enhance the body's ability to fight diseases. Owning a pet has even been found to have a positive effect on health. This confirms the power of positive thinking! The explosion of research in this area may soon confirm that the mind-body connection is a major key to high-level wellness.

Challenges We Face

The biggest challenge we face is spreading the word, making wellness information available to everyone. Research shows that blue collar workers, low socio-economic and low education groups, and persons with the most risk for coronary heart disease (particularly smokers) are the individuals most resistive to public health promotion.[18] This group cannot afford health club memberships and specialized medical screenings. Many of these people are more concerned about maintaining decent housing and feeding their families than about their cholesterol levels. However, they, too, deserve a higher level of functioning and well-being. Showing how small lifestyle changes can enhance well-being, providing wellness information, and changing attitudes toward self-responsibility in this particular population is difficult. Nevertheless, making wellness available to all Americans is in itself a wellness issue. In today's world, television is a common learning environment, especially for the uneducated. While there is considerable amount of health-related information in television programming and commercials, many of these images are in serious conflict with realistic guidelines for wellness (nutrition, sexual activity, alcohol use, violence, body image, etc.).[19] This presents a considerable challenge to those in health promotion. Perhaps the biggest payoff would be to integrate wellness information, behaviors, and attitudes into all segments of primary and secondary school curricula, reaching all youth before unhealthy life habits develop.

The notion of teaching wellness in the schools leads to another enormous challenge. Our children are fatter and less fit than ever before. Computer games, television, and home videos have made this generation quite sedentary. The health profile of the American child is frightening: 50 percent do not get enough exercise to develop healthy cardiorespiratory systems; 98 percent have at least one heart disease risk factor; 13 percent have 5 or more risk factors; 20 percent to 30 percent are obese; and 75 percent consume diets with excess fat.[20] Combine this with the fact that only about 36 percent of American school children have daily physical education (but only 1 state requires daily physical education from kindergarten through grade 12).[21] The average American child spends as much time watching television each year as she or he does attending school.[22] "Childhood and adolescent obesity now represent the most prevalent nutritional problem in children and adolescents in the United States."[23] This picture does not speak well for building a fit and healthy adult population. It is obvious that a comprehensive wellness package must be delivered to school-age children. This package should include information and skills for growth in all dimensions of wellness, including self-management and self-regulation skills for carryover to adulthood. It is unfortunate that many people wait until middle age to lose weight, change their diets, or begin exercising (often only after a heart attack or experiencing a life-threatening health problem). Wellness in an adult begins with wellness in a child.

A Parting Thought

Suppose you are the owner of a very fine show dog. To make this dog a champion, you handle it in very special ways: you make sure it gets proper exercise everyday, its coat is brushed and groomed, and its diet is carefully monitored (at the grocery store you walk past the doggie treats and junk food to "Lean and Win Dog Food"). Its living environment is regulated to make it the best show dog possible. Do you treat yourself as you would a champion show dog? Do you walk past the treats and junk food to the "lean and win" food? Are you managing your environment in such a way that it makes you the best you can be? You have 24 hours a day, 365 days a year to make choices. Our society provides you the opportunity to make many positive choices. Our society also allows for choices that are not in your best interest. You now have the knowledge and skills to make choices that enhance your well-being.

Remember, wellness is a journey in which the benefits are gained along the trip. It is not a life of self-sacrifice and delayed gratification. It is being the most you can be every day of your life. It is reveling in the fact that you have considerable control over your own well-being and happiness. Go to it! We wish you well.

Summary

Everyone is born with a genetic blueprint. However, personal lifestyle choices have a great impact on whether you maximize your potential. You, as an educated citizen, know the choices that enhance wellness. You, as an informed consumer, must be able to evaluate wellness products and programs. No doubt your campus offers activities and facilities that can support your quest for wellness. The business world has also discovered the value of wellness in the workplace, in terms of increased productivity, lessened health insurance costs, and enhanced employee morale. Knowing how important a supportive environment is in pursuing wellness, you may want to consider working for a company that supports and values employee wellness. After all, you will spend approximately one-third of your life at work.

Wellness is an integral part of a productive family life. Family wellness involves meeting the various physical, psychological, and social needs of all family members, regardless of ages, as they strive toward full potential. You, as a parent, will be the master teacher of lifestyle habits to your children. Your example will have a strong influence on your children's ability to make responsible wellness choices.

Wellness is not a passing craze. The wellness trend is revolutionizing medical care and the health insurance system. The broad scope of wellness creates opportunities for life enhancement for everyone—young, old, poor, rich, black, and white. Wellness becomes a global issue as we work together to protect the environment. The ultimate challenge is to get the word to everyone (especially to those who need wellness the most), and get it to them while they are young. "Wellness is, as much as anything else, an opportunity, perhaps the best opportunity we have had, both as a society and as individuals. Let us not miss it."[24]

References

1. Sullivan, Louis W., M. D. "Partners in Prevention: A Mobilization Plan for Implementing *Healthy People 2000.*" *American Journal of Health Promotion* 5 (March/April 1991): 291–97.

2. Eddy, James M., Daniel L. Bibeau, Elbert D. Glover, Barry P. Hunt, and R. Carl Westerfield. "Wellness Perspectives Part I: History, Philosophy and Emerging Trends." *Wellness Perspectives* 6 (Winter 1989): 3–19.

3. O'Donnell, Michael P. "Definition of Health Promotion." *American Journal of Health Promotion.* 1 (Summer 1986): 1–4.

4. "Employees See Worksite Benefits in Health Promotion and Disease Prevention." *Public Health Reports* 102 (July/August 1987): 457–58.

5. "Businesses Promote Family Health." *The Futurist.* 24 (November/December 1990): 48.

6. Friedman, Myles I., and George H. Lackey, Jr. *The Psychology of Human Control: A General Theory of Purposeful Behavior.* New York, NY: Praeger Publishers, 1991.

7. "Teen Risk-Taking Behavior." *Healthline* 9 (August 1990): 9.

8. Zedeck, Sheldon, and Kathleen L. Mosier. "Workplace Wellness: Work in the Family and Employing Organization." *American Psychologist.* 45 (February 1990): 240–51.

9. Department of Health and Human Services, Public Health Service. *Healthy People 2000: National Health Promotion and Disease Prevention Objectives.* Washington, DC: Department of Health and Human Services, 1990.

10. Johnson, Jerry A. *New Dimensions in Wellness: A Context for Living.* Thorofare, NJ: SLACK Incorporated, 1986.

11. *New Dimensions in Wellness.*

12. Agency for Toxic Substances and Disease Registry. *The Nature and Extent of Lead Poisoning in Children in the United States: A Report to Congress.* Washington, DC: U.S. Department of Health and Human Services, July 1988.

13. Naisbitt, John. *Megatrends.* New York: Warner Books, 1982.

14. "Education for Health: A Role for Physicians and the Efficacy of Health Education Efforts." *The Journal of the American Medical Association.* 263 (April 4, 1990): 1816–19.

15. Spencer, G. "Projections of the Population of the United States, by Age, Sex, and Race: 1988 to 2080." *Current Population Reports, Population Estimates and Projections.* Series p-25, No. 1018. Washington, DC: U.S. Department of Commerce, Bureau of the Census, 1989.

16. Miller, Cheryl, and Ray Tricker. "Past and Future Priorities in Health Promotion in the United States: A Survey of Experts." *American Journal of Health Promotion.* 5 (May/June 1991): 360–67.

17. Ornstein, Robert, and Charles Swencionis. *The Healing Brain: A Scientific Reader.* New York: The Guilford Press, 1990.

18. Dishman, Rod K. *Exercise Adherence: Its Impact on Public Health.* Champaign, IL: Human Kinetics Publishers, 1988.

19. Signorielli, Nancy. "Television and Health: Images and Impact," *Mass Communication and Public Health.* Edited by Charles Atkin and Lawrence Wallack, 96-113. Newbury Park, CA: Sage Publications, 1990.

20. Haydon, Donald F. "The Family and Health/Fitness." *Health Values* 11 (March/April 1987): 36–39.

21. U. S. Department of Health and Human Services. "National Children and Youth Fitness Study II." *Journal of Physical Education, Recreation and Dance* 58 (November/December 1987): 50–96.

22. Haydon. "The Family and Health/Fitness."

23. Dietz, William, M. D. "Increasing Child Obesity Raises Concerns Over Available Treatments." *Obesity and Health.* 5 (May/June 1991): 41.

24. Ardell, Donald B. *The History and Future of Wellness.* Dubuque, IA: Kendall/Hunt Publishing Co., 1985.

Suggested Readings

Atkin, Charles, and Lawrence Wallack (eds.) 1990. *Mass Communication and Public Health.* Newbury Park, CA: Sage Publications.

Barrett, Stephen, M. D. 1990. *Health Schemes, Scams, and Frauds.* Mount Vernon, NY: Consumer Reports Books.

Boss, Pauline. 1988. *Family Stress Management.* Newbury Park, CA: Sage Publications.

Brammer, Lawrence M. 1991. *How To Cope With Life Transitions: The Challenge of Personal Change.* New York: Hemisphere Publishing Corporation.

Bricklin, Mark, Mark Golin, Deborah Grandinetti, and Alexis Lieberman. 1990. *Positive Living and Health.* Emmaus, PA: Rodale Press.

Brown, H. Jackson, Jr. 1991. *Life's Little Instruction Book.* Nashville, TN: Rutledge Hill Press, Inc.

Chen, Moon S. "Wellness in the Workplace: Beyond the Point of No Return." *Health Values* 12 (January/February 1988): 16–22.

Cowan, Philip A., and Mavis Hetherington (eds.) 1991. *Family Transitions.* Hillsdale, NJ: Lawrence Erlbaum Associates, Publishers.

Crooks, Catherine E., Nicholas K. Iammarino, and Armin D. Weinberg. "The Family's Role in Health Promotion." *Health Values* 11 (March/April 1987): 7-12.

Dishman, Rod K., ed. 1988. *Exercise Adherence: Its Impact on Public Health.* Champaign, IL: Human Kinetics Publishers.

Dychtwald, Ken and Joe Flower. 1989. *Age Wave.* Los Angeles: Jeremey P. Tarcher, Inc.

Eddy, James M., Daniel L. Bibeau, Elbert D. Glover, Barry P. Hunt, and R. Carl Westerfield. "Wellness Perspectives Part I: History, Philosophy and Emerging Trends." *Wellness Perspectives* 6 (Winter 1989): 3–19.

Elias, Maurice. "The Role of Affect and Social Relationships in Health Behavior and School Health Curriculum and Instruction." *Journal of School Health* 60 (April 1990): 157–63.

Fish, Helen T., Ronald B. Fish, Lawrence A. Golding. 1989. *Starting Out Well: A Parent's Approach to Physical Activity and Nutrition.* Champaign, IL: Human Kinetics Publishers, Inc.

Foege, William H. "Closing the Gaps: Ensuring the Application of Available Knowledge in the Promotion of Health and the Prevention of Disease." *Journal of School Health* 60 (April 1990): 130–32.

Gebhardt, Deborah L., and Carolyn E. Crump. "Employee Fitness and Wellness Programs in the Workplace." *American Psychologist* 45 (February 1990): 262–72.

Gelman, David. "Body and Soul." *Newsweek* (November 7, 1988): 88–97.

Gurin, Joel and Daniel Goleman. 1993. *Mind/Body Medicine: How to Use Your Mind for Better Health.* New York: Consumer Reports Books.

Halpern, Charles R. "The Political Economy of Mind-Body Health." *American Journal of Health Promotion* 6 (March/April 1992): 288–91, 279.

Heath, Douglas H. and Harriet E. Heath. 1991. *Fulfilling Lives: Paths to Maturity and Success.* San Francisco: Jossey-Bass Publishers.

Jaffe, Michael. 1991. *Understanding Parenting.* Dubuque, IA: Wm. C. Brown Publishers.

Kain, Edward L. 1990. *The Myth of Family Decline: Understanding Families in a World of Rapid Social Change.* Lexington, MA: Lexington Books.

Kuntzleman, Charles T. 1988. *Healthy Kids for Life.* New York: Simon and Schuster, Inc.

Lau, Richard R., Marilyn Jacobs Quadrel, and Karen A. Hartman. "Development and Change of Young Adults' Preventive Health Beliefs and Behavior: Influence from Parents and Peers." *Journal of Health and Social Behavior* 31 (September 1990): 240–259.

Marrone, Robert. 1990. *Body of Knowledge: An Introduction to Body/Mind Psychology.* Albany, NY: State University of New York Press.

Miller, Cheryl, and Ray Tricker. "Past and Future Priorities in Health Promotion in the United States: A Survey of Experts." *American Journal of Health Promotion.* 5 (May/June 1991): 360–67.

Neilson, Elizabeth. "Health Values: Achieving High-Level Wellness—Origin, Philosophy, Purpose." *Health Values.* 12 (May/June 1988): 3–5.

O'Donnell, Michael P. "Definition of Health Promotion: Part II: Levels of Programs." *American Journal of Health Promotion.* 1 (Fall 1986): 6–9.

Opatz, Joseph P. 1985. *A Primer of Health Promotion: Creating Healthy Organizational Cultures.* Washington, DC: Oryn Publishers.

Ornstein, Robert, and David Sobel. 1987. *The Healing Brain.* New York: Simon and Schuster, Inc.

Ornstein, Robert, and David Sobel. 1989. *Healthy Pleasures.* New York: Addison-Wesley Publishing Co., Inc.

Ornstein, Robert, and Charles Swencionis. 1990. *The Healing Brain: A Scientific Reader.* New York: The Guilford Press.

Peck, M. Scott. 1978. *The Road Less Traveled.* New York: Simon and Schuster, Inc.

Pelletier, Kenneth R. "Mind-Body Health: Research, Clinical, and Policy Applications." *American Journal of Health Promotion.* 6 (May/June 1992): 345–58.

Rothman, Howard. 1991. *The Employee Handbook for Building a Healthier Lifestyle.* Brookfield, WI: International Foundation of Employee Benefit Plans.

Taylor, Robert L. 1990. *Health Fact, Health Fiction.* Dallas, TX: Taylor Publishing Co.

Zedeck, Sheldon, and Kathleen L. Mosier. "Workplace Wellness: Work in the Family and Employing Organization." *American Psychologist.* 45 (February 1990): 240–51.

Appendix

1

Aerobic Dance

Advantages/Disadvantages

Aerobic dancing is a popular fitness activity. Usually performed under the leadership of an instructor, it combines the cardiovascular benefits of jogging with the joy of dancing. The variety of movements not only strengthens the cardiorespiratory system but also increases flexibility, tones muscles, and enhances body composition. It is a total body workout. The upbeat music tempo creates an atmosphere of excitement; exercising in a group is fun and emotionally stimulating. The popular music and group comraderie help prevent boredom and can keep you motivated. Aerobic dancing can be so much fun, you often forget you are exercising. Because the participants focus on the instructor, aerobic dance classes are good for the beginning or self-conscious exerciser. Aerobic dance allows for individualization of a workout. The same movement sequence or exercise can be done by both a well-conditioned participant and a beginning exerciser by varying the intensity or number of repetitions. Because aerobic dance is done indoors, the environment provides security and comfort.

Aerobic dance has excellent potential for developing all components of physical fitness, but it can have some drawbacks. Even though participants are urged by instructors to work at their own pace, some exercisers overdo it. These exercisers try to keep up with the group or work as hard as the instructor, even though they may not be ready for this intensity. Many times the result is excessive soreness or fatigue. Performing aerobic dance on a hard, unyielding surface (like cement) or while wearing poor shoes also increases the risk of injury. Some overzealous aerobics participants attend classes one or more times a day,

leading to overuse. Excessive impact may cause leg and foot problems. Also, not all aerobic dance instructors have had training in exercise instruction and safety, and may teach improper technique. Unless good body mechanics and reasonable progressions are emphasized in a class, the result can be discomfort rather than exhilaration and a desire to continue exercising. Having to join or travel to a fitness facility to take an aerobics class may be viewed as a disadvantage to some exercisers. Others find it motivating to have a set time, financial investment, and a group of friends to exercise with. Aerobic dance videotapes are available for the home exerciser. They allow exercising in private but lack the spontaneity, instruction, and enthusiasm available in a live class.

What to Wear

Even though some aerobic dancers have color-coordinated leotards and fancy exercise apparel, any loose-fitting and comfortable clothing will do. A t-shirt and shorts are fine. More important than the clothing are supportive shoes. Shoes specially designed for the impact and movement of aerobic dance are recommended. A good aerobic shoe has a well-cushioned, resilient midsole to aid in shock dispersion, and a sturdy heel counter to hold the foot in place. The shoe should allow for lateral movement and, as a result, not have a wide heel flair that is often seen in a jogging shoe. Like the jogger, the aerobic participant should replace old shoes when their cushioning ability has decreased.

Techniques and Safety Tips

Many injuries and discomforts can be avoided in aerobic dance with proper shoes, gradual progression, and exercising on a resilient surface. Chapter 5 gives several general suggestions for preventing injury in fitness activities. In aerobic dance, careful attention to technique and body mechanics further eliminates chance for injury and heightens the enjoyment of the activity.

1. *Always warm up with low-intensity, whole body movements. Your warm-up should include slow, full range-of-motion joint movements. Static stretching should also be included in the warm-up.*

2. *Keep abdominals pulled in and buttocks tucked under.*

3. *Avoid twisting the spinal column excessively (windmill toe touches, elbow-to-knee lunges, etc.).*

4. *Limit the hopping on one foot to a maximum of 4 consecutive times.*

5. *Soften your jumps and bounces by maintaining a slightly bent-knee landing position.*

6. *Try to make your heels go all the way to the floor when landing from jumps.*

7. *Never fling or throw arms or legs. Maintain control of limbs throughout movements.*

8. *Avoid hyperextending elbows, knees, or lower back.*

9. *Listen to your body. If a stretch, exercise, or position causes pain or a burning sensation, do not do it.*

The amount of concern for technique and safety depends on your instructor. A wise wellness consumer chooses a knowledgeable, trained instructor. The popularity of aerobic dance has skyrocketed very quickly, and the number of qualified instructors has not kept pace. While standards and certification programs have now been established, it is still up to you to select a class. Do not be shy. Check the instructor's qualifications. Is she certified by a national fitness organization? Does the instructor have knowledge in anatomy, exercise physiology, kinesiology, and first aid? Is she currently certified in CPR (cardiopulmonary resuscitation)? Does the instructor do some health screening or fitness assessment of students? Is the class supervised effectively? Does the instructor monitor the intensity of the workout with periodic heart rate checks? Does the class begin with a good warm-up and end with a cool-down period? Does the instructor give corrective cues and technique suggestions throughout the workout? Does she consider the variances in fitness levels in the class by showing how to modify the intensity of the workout? Is she

easy to follow? Looking good in a leotard and being a fluid dancer are not requirements for being a quality aerobic dance instructor. Most important is the ability to conduct a safe, yet invigorating, workout from which all participants can benefit.

How to Begin and Progress

Like any other fitness activity, begin slowly. Attend no more than 3 classes per week for several weeks. Start with 5 to 10 minutes of the aerobic phase, and progress gradually. If the aerobic portion of the class is 30 minutes, do low-impact moves or walk in place while the experienced exercisers continue. Monitor your pulse and stay within your target heart rate range. You should be able to talk or sing with the music throughout the entire workout. Gradually add a few minutes weekly to the aerobic phase until you can exercise aerobically for 20 to 30 minutes.

Some exercisers prefer the low-impact style of aerobics instead of high-impact. Low-impact aerobics reduces the strain on knees and ankles by minimizing jumping and bouncing movements. In low-impact aerobics, one foot contacts the ground at all times. Low-impact does not necessarily mean low-intensity. To maintain a training heart rate, move your arms vigorously and travel along the floor by wide-stride walking, sliding, and side-stepping. Beginners and even well-trained exercisers with joint problems can benefit from low-impact aerobics. Or you may want to combine low-impact and high-impact moves. Most jumps and steps can be modified to become low-impact steps.

Most aerobic dance classes incorporate a body toning segment to the workout. Once again, use common sense. Do not try to do as many repetitions as the teacher, unless you are equally fit. Stop and stretch if you feel pain or a burning sensation in the muscle. Aerobic dance participants often tend to compare themselves or compete with others in the class. Avoid falling into this trap. Work to be the best you can be without shame or guilt.

Variety

It is easy to add variety to aerobic dance. Vary the music. Use pop, jazz, country, or classical music. Try some holiday or theme music when appropriate. Vary the routines or steps. Aerobics can be taught by using set routines (repetitive movements in a programmed format) or in a freestyle format (participants mimic the instructor and change accordingly). Varying between learned routines and a freestyle approach helps keep interest high. Try circuit aerobic dance. Set up exercise stations around the room. Do different aerobic movements 1 to 2 minutes per station, then jog to the next station to sustain your training heart rate. There are many other ways to add variety to aerobic dance. One- to two-pound hand weights can be used during aerobic routines to increase upper body endurance and to maintain a training heart rate. Heavier hand weights are often used during stationary power moves to tone arms and legs. To prevent knee injuries, do not wear ankle weights while doing aerobic dance steps. Weights are, however, an effective way to add resistance while doing floor toning. Thick rubber bands and elastic tubing can also be used to increase the efficiency of body toning exercises.

Step Aerobics

Also known as bench/step training, step aerobics is an innovative activity that involves stepping up and down on a 4- to 12-inch platform. Combining a variety of stepping patterns with kicks, turns, and upper body movements results in a brisk workout. Step aerobics appeals to a wide range of exercisers for several reasons: it can be a high-intensity workout with low-impact force; it is adaptable to different fitness levels by adjusting the bench height, adding jumps, varying arm gestures, and adding light hand weights; and it is easy to do! Step aerobics has become especially popular with men, who may be put off by "dance-like" aerobics classes. As with all aerobic exercise activities, proper form and technique are necessary to prevent injury.

To prevent injury while stepping:

1. *As much as possible, keep your shoulders aligned over your hips.*

2. *Step up lightly, making sure the whole foot lands on the platform.*

3. *Keep your knees aligned over your feet when they're pulling your body weight onto the platform.*

4. *At the top, straighten your legs, but don't lock your knees.*

5. *Do not pivot a bent, supporting knee.*

6. *As you step down, stay close to the platform.*

If you are a beginner to step aerobics, start with the lowest bench, and keep your eyes on the bench until you adjust to the activity. Once you learn the stepping patterns, you can add arm movements and light hand weights, or challenge yourself by raising the height of the bench. (However, never use a height that flexes your knees to an angle less than 90 degrees.)

Step aerobics is a great workout for the lower body and, when combined with a variety of arm movements, is an exciting new variation in aerobic exercise.

Common Discomforts

As in most fitness activities, mild soreness can be anticipated by the beginning exerciser. Some discomforts may be avoided by emphasizing stretching and toning the first 3 to 4 weeks to condition muscles and connective tissue for the stress of impact and the new movements. Veteran exercisers can suffer pain or injury by increasing frequency, time, or intensity too rapidly. Since most aerobic dance discomfort is found in the legs, be sure to warm up and stretch this area. Refer to chapter 5 for further information about prevention and treatment of injuries. If you use hand weights, elbow and shoulder strain can be avoided by not flinging the weights. Always move them with control. Having a towel or exercise mat with you provides additional comfort and padding while doing floor exercises.

Resources

International Dance-Exercise Association (IDEA)
6190 Cornerstone Court East, Suite 204
San Diego, CA 92121–3773
(619) 535–8978 or 1–800–999–IDEA

National Dance-Exercise Instructor's Training Association
  (NDEITA)
1503 S. Washington Ave., Suite 208
Minneapolis, MN 55454
1–800–237–6242

Aerobics and Fitness Association of America
15250 Ventura Blvd., Suite 310
Sherman Oaks, CA 91403
(818) 905–0040

The Aerobic Center
12200 Preston Road
Dallas, TX 75230

Casten, Carole, and Peg Jordan. 1990. Aerobics Today. *St. Paul, MN: West Publishing Co.*

Francis, Lorna, Peter Francis, and Gin Miller. 1990. Step-Reebok: The First Aerobic Training Workout with Muscle. Instructor Training Manual. *Stoughton, MA: Reebok International Ltd.*

Kan, Esther, and Minda Goodman Kraines. 1992. Keep Moving! It's Aerobic Dance, 2nd ed. *Palo Alto, CA: Mayfield Publishing Co.*

Kennedy, M. S., Carol Legel, and Deb Legel. 1992. Anatomy of an Exercise Class: An Exercise Educator's Handbook. *Champaign, IL: Sagamore Publishing Inc.*

Mazzeo, Karen. 1992. Aerobics: The Way to Fitness. *Englewood, CO: Morton Publishing Co.*

McIntosh, Matthew. 1990. Lifetime Aerobics. *Dubuque, IA: Wm. C. Brown Publishers.*

Van Gelder, Naneene, (ed.). 1987. Aerobic Dance-Exercise Instructor Manual. *San Diego, CA: IDEA Foundation.*

Wilmoth, Susan K. 1986. Leading Aerobic Dance-Exercise. *Champaign, IL: Human Kinetics Publishers.*

Music

Aerobics Power Mix
Power Productions, Inc.
P.O. Box 3812
Gaithersburg, MD 20878
1–800–777–BEAT

Ken Alan Associates
7985 Santa Monica Blvd. #109
Los Angeles, CA 90046
(213) 659–2503

Mix Music International, Inc.
P.O. Box 2452
Kankakee, IL 60901
1–800–733–3049

Muscle Mixes Aerobic Music Service
2934 Northwood Blvd.
Orlando, FL 32803
1–800–52–MIXES

Resource for evaluating aerobic videotapes:

Complete Guide to Exercise Videos
available from Collage Video Specialists
5390 Main St., N.E.
Dept. 6
Minneapolis, MN 55421
1–800–433–6769

Appendix

2
Bicycling

Advantages/Disadvantages

Cycling is a popular choice for people of all ages. You can fit in a cycling workout while running errands, going to work, or at home in front of the TV (on rollers or a stationary bike). You can cycle alone, with family, or with friends. If you have a small child, you can take him along in a bike seat instead of having to hire a sitter while you get a workout. It is nonimpact, minimizing stress to the back, shins, and ankles.

Of course there are a few drawbacks. You must have a bicycle, keep it in good working condition, and store it securely to prevent theft. Cycling in traffic requires alertness and use of defensive driving skills to prevent accidents. Cycling in rain, snow, or icy conditions is uncomfortable and hazardous. Also, bicycles are so efficient that they can do most of the work for you. Most people don't work hard enough to do themselves much good. Cycling to class or short distances is fine for transportation, but if you want to get in shape, you will need to put in more effort. Nevertheless, cycling produces cardiorespiratory benefits without impact, making it the third most popular activity in the United States. It can be enjoyed throughout a lifetime.

What to Wear

In order to be clearly visible to vehicles, wear bright-colored clothing during the day and light-colored clothing at night. Fancy bicycling gear is not necessary, although if you really get into cycling, you might find that a pair of bicycling shorts makes long rides more comfortable. Hard-soled, athletic, or bicycling shoes are fine.

Equipment

Always wear a helmet, one approved by the American National Standards Institute, even if you're just going across campus. The sidewalk is just as hard there as anywhere else. There are plenty of bike-pedestrian as well as bike-car accidents on campus, and usually it is the bicyclist who is at fault. You may lose some skin in a slide or break some bones, but they will heal. Brains don't. Head injuries account for over 75 percent of deaths and permanent disabilities in cycling crashes. If you hit something and go flying head first, wearing a good helmet is the best way to prevent serious injury.

A water bottle is essential for workouts, particularly in the heat. Because sweat evaporates so quickly while you are riding, you may not realize how quickly water is lost. Dehydration, leading to heat illness, can easily occur. Drinking regularly from a water bottle to maintain an adequate level of hydration during a workout is a necessity, not a luxury.

It doesn't matter what type of bike you ride—one-speed, ten-speed, mountain—the important thing is that it be kept in good working order. If you are not mechanically inclined, your local bicycle shop can help. Most people ride with the bike seat too low, which is inefficient and can make the knees hurt. The bike seat should be high enough that when you sit centered on the seat with your heel on the pedal at its lowest point, your knee is straight. That way, when you move the ball of your foot to its proper position on the pedal, your knee will be almost fully extended at the bottom of the stroke. If the seat is too high, on the other hand, the rider tends to rock side to side with each footstroke and may develop a sore crotch. A sore crotch can also be caused by improper seat tilt. Start with the nose of the seat level. If it bothers you, tilt it down slightly. Pedals, wheels, and steering should turn or spin freely with no binding, catch, or click. The derailleur should shift smoothly. Brakes should close and release easily. Brake shoes should be one-eighth inch or less from and level with the rim of the bike. If they are badly worn, replace them. The air in the tires usually needs to be topped off weekly to keep them hard and rolling smoothly, but use caution when filling them. The air pumps at service stations are designed for cars, and it's easy to explode a bicycle tire by overfilling it. If a bike wheel is badly out of true and wobbles, it may hit your brake shoe with each revolution. A bike shop can true a wheel, lubricate sticky brake cables, adjust the derailleur, and show you how to keep your machine running smoothly, which makes riding safe and enjoyable.

Technique and Safety Tips

Shifting

On ten-speeds, the gears overlap slightly and you have to shift by feel. To shift, continue pedalling, but ease up on the pedal pressure. Shifting without pedalling can cause a bent or broken chain or gear teeth. You should not hear a loud "clunk" as you shift, nor a constant rubbing sound, if you are shifting smoothly and getting it into gear correctly.

Most beginners gear too high and pedal too slowly. They feel like they're not getting any exercise unless they're pushing against resistance. This is inefficient and can increase fatigue and cause knees to ache. It is better to pedal quickly against light resistance.

If your bike has several gears, practice using them. Gearing is a matter of maintaining an even cadence regardless of terrain, weather, or wind conditions. If you're going uphill, shift before you have to slow your cadence so that you can go up smoothly. Also practice downshifting before stop signs so that you don't have to stand on the pedals to get going again.

Pedalling

Ride with the ball of your foot on the pedal. If you have toe clips, you can try ankling–pulling up as well as pushing down on the pedal each stroke–which doubles your efficiency.

Braking

Use your brakes as little as possible. Look ahead, signal, slow down, and learn to anticipate problems instead of simply reacting to them. Be careful not to jam on your brakes too suddenly or you can pitch head first over the handlebars. The front brake is the most powerful because as you decelerate,

your weight shifts forward, lessening the weight over the back tire. For a most efficient stop, keep the body weight back, gradually increase pressure on the front brake, and hold pressure on the back brake just below the point where the wheel will skid. In wet conditions, brakes lose up to 90 percent of their braking ability. It is good to frequently apply the brakes lightly to wipe water off the rims and to allow extra stopping distance. When going downhill, pump on-off-on-off to avoid overheating the wheel rims or brake shoes. When in doubt, favor the rear brake. It may skid the bike, but at least you won't land on your face.

Bumps

When you come up to bumps, holes, and railroad tracks, don't sit on the seat like a sack of potatoes. Shift your weight to pedals and handlebars to absorb the shock. It's better for you and for your bike.

Safety Tips

1. *Wear brightly colored clothing, wear a helmet, and carry water.*
2. *Keep to the right side of the road, and ride in a straight line. Always ride in single file with traffic.*
3. *Do not make sudden turns or swerves. Signal all turns and stops.*
4. *Keep alert. Look out for cars pulling out into traffic or turning. Listen constantly for traffic approaching out of your line of vision.*
5. *Observe all traffic regulations—red and green lights, one-way streets, stop signs. Slow down at all street intersections and look right and left before crossing.*
6. *Be sure your brakes are operating efficiently, and keep your bicycle in perfect running condition. Keep hands on or near the brakes at all times.*
7. *Keep speed under control, especially on long downhill runs. Speed should be low enough that you can stop quickly.*
8. *In rainy weather, allow much more distance for stopping, and don't take corners too fast.*
9. *Watch for sudden door openings from parked cars. Ride at least 3 feet away from them.*
10. *Avoid sewer grates that parallel your direction.*
11. *Railroad tracks—If rough, walk your bike (to prevent blowout or other damage to the bicycle). If you choose to ride over the tracks, cross them at a 90 degree angle.*
12. *Make sure you are at least 3 feet off the traveled portion of the road when you stop or park.*
13. *Hug the right-hand shoulder of the road on all curves.*
14. *Give pedestrians the right-of-way. Avoid sidewalks.*

15. *Watch out for child cyclists. Children on bicycles usually weave from side to side, turn unpredictably without signaling, and can run into you even when you are passing them.*

16. *All dogs are potential adversaries. If he is far enough away, you probably outrun him. Water from your bottle or a bike pump may scare him off. If you stop, keep the bike between you and the dog. Walk slowly away. Generally, he will leave you alone, but watch him carefully before you get under way again. You can also buy a small can of "dog repellent," which will shoot a thin stream of chemical about 10 feet. Although the effects are potent, there is no permanent damage done to the animal.*

17. *Don't wear headphones—they block out street sounds that enable you to anticipate traffic.*

18. *Don't wear a heavy backpack. It can throw off your balance. Carry packages in baskets or bags attached to the cycle.*

19. *Learn to shift gears while keeping your eyes on the road.*

How to Begin and Progress

First, measure your fitness level using the 5-mile timed ride test in chapter 4. Begin at the step indicated by your current fitness level. If you cannot complete the test, begin at level 1. Exercise 3 to 5 days a week at your training pulse. (An appropriate pulse for bicycling appears to be about 5 percent lower than other exercise, so subtract 5 percent to adjust for this difference.) You may work at one level until you can comfortably handle the recommended distance and intensity, then move to the next step. To develop balanced fitness, add 25–30 pushups, a minute of abdominal curls, and 5–15 minutes of stretching to each workout.

Bicycling Program

Fitness Category	Starting Level
Very poor	1 or 2
Poor	3
Average	4
Good	5
Excellent	6

Level	Cycling	Total Distance
1	20–30 min. (8–10 mph)	3–5 miles
2	20–30 min. (10–12 mph)	4–6 miles
3	30–45 min. (12 mph)	4–8 miles
4	30–60 min. (15 mph)	7–15 miles
5	40–75 min. (15 mph)	10–18 miles
6	40–90 min. (15 mph)	10–22 miles

Variety

Part of the appeal of bicycling is exploring an area and seeing things you wouldn't normally notice as you whiz past enclosed in a car. Try cycling to a park, a lake, a scenic spot, or merely exploring. Plan an outing with a picnic or refreshment break halfway. Ride to a nearby small town and back. Plan a bike rally, similar to a car rally with checkpoints, or a bike scavenger hunt in which you gather bits of information from certain locations (i.e., what is the name of the store at 21 Oak Street?). If you are interested in more, consult your local bicycle shop for bicycling organizations in your area and find out what rides and tours are planned.

Common Discomforts

Bicyclists beginning a conditioning program often experience a sore crotch the first week or two. As you and your saddle adjust to each other, the syndrome should disappear. It may help to tilt the nose of the saddle down a bit (not so much you slide off!) or to try a different saddle, one with padding under the "sit bones."

If your fingers feel numb after cycling, you need to change hand position more frequently. The ulnar nerve runs across the palm, and constant pressure on the hands can temporarily cut off sensation to the area. Wearing padded cycling gloves or cushioning your handlebars with foam grips may also help.

Do your toes tend to go numb on long rides? It may be because pedalling tends to push the foot forward into the shoes until the toes touch the end, reducing blood flow to the area. Try lacing your shoes snugly enough so that they hold your foot back in the heel of the shoe, but not so tightly that circulation is hindered.

Resources

Bicycle Federation of America
1506 21st St., NW
Washington, DC 20036
(202) 332-6986
promotes bicycle transportation, recreation, and programs.

League of American Wheelmen
19 South Bothwell
Palatine, IL 60067
(708) 991–1200
bicyclists and clubs

The Bicycle Institute of America
1506 21st St., NW
Washington, DC 20036
1-(800) 251-2453

Bicycling Magazine
33 E. Minor Street
Emmaus, PA 18049

Ballantine, Richard. 1987. Richard's New Bicycle Book. *New York, NY: Ballantine Books.*

Bicycling Magazine Editors. 1990. Bicycling Magazine's New Bike Owners Guide. *Emmaus, PA: Rodale Press, Inc.*

Bicycling Magazine Editors. 1992. Bicycling Magazine's Training for Fitness & Endurance. *Emmaus, PA: Rodale Press, Inc.*

Cuthbertson, Tom. 1988. Anybody's Bike Book. *Berkeley, CA: Peter Smith.*

Sloan, Eugene. 1988. The Complete Book of Bicycling. *St. Louis, MO: Fireside Books.*

Van der Plas, Rob. 1989. Bicycle Fitness Book: Riding Your Bike for Health and Fitness. *Mill Valley, CA: Bicycle Books, Inc.*

Van der Plas, Rob. 1991. Mountain Bike Magic. *Mill Valley, CA: Bicycle Books.*

Basic Bicycle Tool Kit:

If you wish to save money and time by doing much of your own maintenance, the following tools are recommended: Tire patch kit, tire irons, adjustable wrench or set of crescent wrenches (best), third hand (for brakes), screwdriver, tire gauge, silicone lubricant, tire pump.

How to Fix a Flat Tire

1. *Remove wheel. Caliper brakes may need to be loosened to permit wheel removal. Loosen axle nuts and remove wheel from forks. In rear, you must also press tension roller forward to wiggle wheel out.*

2. *To remove tire, push tire irons between rim and bead. Pry up tire carefully so as not to pinch and further damage tube. Work around tire.*

3. *Push valve stem into rim and pull tube out of tire. Locate source of puncture and remove from tire. Feel inside tire to check for foreign objects. Also check rim to make sure a spoke is not protruding. Mark puncture on tube. If source of leak is not readily apparent, slightly inflate tire and listen for hiss or put tube in water and look for bubbles. Dry tube and mark hole with chalk. Deflate.*

4. *Read and follow patch kit directions. Rough around puncture with roughing tool. Apply thin layer of cement and let dry thoroughly. Apply patch, pressing out air bubbles.*

5. *Replace tube in tire, valve first.*

6. *Replace bead of tire in rim, being careful to avoid pinching tube between bead and tire. Use tire irons to replace last few inches of tire bead.*

7. *Inflate tire. Replace, center between forks, tighten axle nuts and, if necessary, brakes.*

Bicycle Inspection Checklist

Name _____

Bicycle make & model _____ Serial No. _____

Note: Proper bicycle fit and maintenance is essential for comfort, safety, and riding efficiency. Any problems must be identified and corrected before the first ride.

	OK	FIX
Frame Size		
Can you straddle frame with both feet flat on the ground? (Need 1"–2" space between crotch and top bar.)	____	____
Horizontal Adjustment—nose of the saddle should be 1" to 3" behind a vertical line drawn through the crank hanger. A cyclist 5'6" tall would position saddle 1" back, 5'10", 2" back, and 6'3", 3" back.	____	____
Vertical adjustment—Sit on bike with heel on pedal at lowest position. Knee should be straight.	____	____
Tilt—horizontal or slightly downtilted	____	____
Is saddle tight and in good condition?	____	____
Handlebars		
Vertical adjustment—Top bar level with nose of saddle.	____	____
Horizontal adjustment—Place elbow on nose of saddle. Outstretched fingertips should just touch center of handlebars. (Length of stem may need to be changed.)	____	____
In line with wheel and symmetrical	____	____
Tight, no horizontal or vertical movement	____	____
Tubing ends plugged, grips tight	____	____
Tire Pressure		
Check. Correct pressure for this bike is _____ .	____	____
(Correct tire pressure is embossed on side of tire.)		
Check once a week.		
Bolts		
Check bolts for looseness. Re-check monthly.	____	____

	OK	FIX
Hand Brakes		
Adequate space between lever and handlebar when engaged?	____	____
(If not, tighten cable.)		
Cable: Should be taut, with no kinks, rust, or frayed ends.	____	____
Brake shoes: Tight? Openings face rear?	____	____
Level with and no more than 1/8" from rim?	____	____
At least 3/16" rubber remaining? (Replace if needed.)	____	____
Test operation of each brake separately. Must hold without catching: Front	____	____
Rear	____	____
Wheels		
Spin each wheel. It should run true (no wobbles).	____	____
Should have no binding or looseness (bearings).	____	____
Centered between forks (and chain stays in rear).	____	____
Rim: Not dented or kinked?	____	____
Spokes: All intact and tight	____	____
Tire: Properly seated? At least 1/8" of tread remaining?	____	____
Derailleurs		
Turn bike upside down or have partner lift rear wheel while you crank pedal and shift through first the front then rear gears. (Shift only while pedal is turning!) Derailleur should shift chain smoothly from one sprocket to the next without skipping a gear, catching, or throwing chain off.	____	____
Chain condition (Clean with silicone spray if dirty.)	____	____
Sprocket teeth intact, not bent or broken	____	____
Pedals intact and tight	____	____
Tread intact and tight	____	____
Press down on both pedals at once. Tight?	____	____
Remarks:		

Appendix

3
Fitness Swimming

Advantages/Disadvantages

Swimming is a superb form of exercise. It is a total body workout using major muscle groups of both the upper and lower body. Other forms of aerobic exercise, jogging for example, use mainly large muscles of the lower body. In addition, water exercise is a natural form of strength training. Resistance of the water against the body's movements enhances muscle strength. Swimmers are also subject to fewer injuries than participants in many other activities. Joint and muscle injuries are not common among swimmers because of water buoyancy. Water supports the body, alleviating the jarring effects of weight-bearing exercise such as aerobics or jogging. Swimming is ideal for the overweight, arthritic, injured, older student, or the individual prone to joint problems.

Another advantage of swimming is the rare occurrence of heat exhaustion and heat stroke. This can be a concern when exercising in hot, humid weather. If you don't like to sweat, you will probably prefer to exercise in water.

Swimming does have its drawbacks. You must have some swimming ability and have access to a pool at a time convenient for you. That first plunge into the water may be difficult for some, but after a brief warm-up period, the cool water temperature will be invigorating. Warm water quickly becomes uncomfortable during a vigorous workout.

Although the injury rate is very low, you may experience some minor annoyances as you train in water. Eye irritations and "swimmers ear" are the most common.

A few women complain about having to redo makeup and hair. This inconvenience is minor when you measure the positive outcomes of aquatic exercise. After the workout, an efficient hair and makeup routine develops quickly.

What to Wear

Swimming is an inexpensive sport since the only equipment needed is a comfortable swimming suit. Many swimmers wear goggles to protect their eyes and, for added comfort, you may wish to use ear plugs and a swim cap. Swimmers can exercise indoors or outside, making it a year-round sport.

Technique and Safety Tips

Learn to swim the following 5 basic strokes efficiently: sidestroke, elementary backstroke, breast stroke, back crawl, and front crawl. Incorporate stroke mechanics sessions on these strokes into each workout. The butterfly stroke is too strenuous for most fitness swimmers.

Learn and practice the front crawl flip turn and the back crawl spin turn. These will make lap swimming more enjoyable. Construct your daily training program to include water warmup, conditioning bout, and water cooldown. Monitor your heart rate, and do not allow it to exceed your swimming target zone. Use hand paddles, kick boards, pull-buoys, and swim fins to increase muscular strength and stroke efficiency. Hyperextension of the lower back (arching) is natural in water exercise. It is important to strengthen the abdominal muscles and always stretch the lower back area to counteract this tendency.

Other safety tips:

1. *Never swim alone. A lifeguard should be present. Safety equipment, such as a ring buoy and reaching pole, should also be available.*

2. *Do not dive into the pool at the shallow end. The risk is too great. Even experienced swimmers have misjudged the depth of the water and hit the bottom, resulting in serious injuries.*

3. Stay to the right of the lane, and make your turns counterclockwise.

4. If resting at the pool edge, keep to one side of the lane to allow other swimmers to turn easily.

5. Be careful with electrical equipment around the pool (radios, pace clocks, etc.). Make sure electrical outlets are grounded.

6. Telephone and emergency rescue numbers should be in the pool area.

7. All doors going into the pool area should be locked unless there is a lifeguard on duty.

Heart Rate During Swimming

Do not use the same target heart rate range when you swim as when you perform land sports. Weight-bearing activities such as running, aerobic dance and fitness walking cause the heart to beat faster. Thus, to avoid risk of overtraining and for more comfortable workouts, reduce your swimming THR by approximately *10 percent* (see chapter 2).

For example, if your THR for land activities is 150–170 bpm your swimming THR would be 135–153.

Example:

1. $150 \times .10 = 15$ $170 \times .10 = 17$

2. $150 - 15 = 135$ $170 - 17 = 153$

3.   Swimming THR = 135–153 bpm

How to Begin and Progress

Assess your aerobic swimming fitness on the 500-yard swim as described in chapter 4. Based on your fitness category, begin on the appropriate Starting Level. Progress through each level, one step at a time. Do not skip steps, and stay on each as long as necessary to adapt to that workload. Remember to monitor your pulse, and do not exceed your swimming target heart rate range. When you have completed level four, you may want to swim continuously for distance or time, or continue with the routine of four lengths and a brief rest for the measured distance or time. Keep in mind the FITT prescription factors covered in chapter 2.

Note: In this program, swim the number of lengths suggested, but if the workout feels too hard, rest a few seconds by climbing out of the pool and walking back to the starting point, or rest at the end of the pool for a few seconds before continuing the workout. Swim the front crawl, if possible, or any stroke that allows you to reach the prescribed swimming target heart rate. For your information see the pool distance table.

Pool Distance

Most standard pools are 25 yards in length

One length = 25 yards
One lap = two lengths

18 lengths = 1/4 mile	(approx. 450 yds.)
35 lengths = 1/2 mile	(approx. 875 yds.)
53 lengths = 3/4 mile	(approx. 1325 yds.)
70 lengths = 1 mile	(approx. 1750 yds.)

Fitness Swim Program

Fitness Category	Starting Level
Very poor	I
Poor	I
Average	II
Good	III
Excellent	IV

Level I

Lengths		Repeats		Distance
1	×	4	=	100 yds.
1	×	6	=	150 yds.
1	×	8	=	200 yds.
1	×	10	=	250 yds.

Level II

Lengths		Repeats		Distance
2	×	4	=	200 yds.
2	×	5	=	250 yds.
2	×	6	=	300 yds.
2	×	7	=	350 yds.
2	×	8	=	400 yds.
2	×	9	=	450 yds.
2	×	10	=	500 yds.
2	×	11	=	550 yds.

Level III

Lengths		Repeats		Distance
3	×	7	=	525 yds.
3	×	8	=	600 yds.
3	×	9	=	675 yds.
3	×	10	=	750 yds.
3	×	11	=	825 yds.
3	×	12	=	900 yds.
3	×	13	=	975 yds.
3	×	14	=	1050 yds.

Level IV

Lengths		Repeats		Distance
4	×	7	=	700 yds.
4	×	8	=	800 yds.
4	×	9	=	900 yds.
4	×	10	=	1000 yds.
4	×	11	=	1100 yds.
4	×	12	=	1200 yds.

Variety

To add variety to your swimming workouts, practice stroke mechanics on the 5 basic strokes. This will allow you to use a variety of strokes in your workouts instead of being limited to one or two. Swim for time instead of distance for a change, or vice versa. Use swim fins, pull-buoys, swim trainers, hand paddles, kick boards, webbed gloves, or a tethering system to add interest to your workouts. These devices also improve strength and stroke efficiency. For a complete change of pace, try a swimnastics or water running session in shallow water or a deep water jogging workout using some type of flotation device. See appendix 6.

Discomforts

While swimmers are less susceptible to injuries, they may experience a few minor discomforts. Eye irritations are caused by an imbalance in the pH of the water (balance of acidity and alkalinity) or excessive amounts of chlorine. Wear goggles and you will have no problem. "Swimmers ear" refers to a rashlike inflammation of the ear canal that is caused by frequent exposure to moisture. Dry your ears thoroughly with a towel to prevent this nuisance. If you have frequent ear infections, it would be wise to purchase a pair of ear plugs. See a specialist to get a good fit; those purchased over the counter do not fit well enough to keep water out of the ear canal. A few swimmers complain of sore shoulders. A certain amount of soreness is normal during the first weeks of training. But if pain persists, you may be developing tendinitis. Shoulder tendinitis may be caused by an inherent structural shoulder problem, use of hand paddles, or improper stroke mechanics. See an orthopedic specialist if shoulder pain persists, and use strokes with an underwater recovery (i.e., breaststroke, sidestroke, and elementary backstroke). Some swimmers experience knee pain, especially along the inner borders of the knees when swimming the breaststroke and elementary backstroke. This is caused by the kick used in these strokes. Do not swim the breaststroke or elementary backstroke until the pain subsides, or avoid them altogether. It is a common myth that you are more susceptible to colds if you participate in aquatic activities, especially during the winter. Colds and respiratory infections are caused by viruses and are spread by contact with infected individuals. You are more likely to catch a cold in a warm, dry, crowded room than in a swimming pool. Another myth is that swimming during menstruation is prohibited. Minor discomfort during this period may be alleviated by exercise. If cramps are severe, use your judgment.

Resources

Aquatic Exercise Association (AEA)
Ruth Sova, President
Box 497
Port Washington, WI 53074
(414) 284–3416

Council for National Cooperation in Aquatics (CNCA)
901 W. New York Street
Indianapolis, IN 46223
(317) 638–4238

International Swimming Hall of Fame
1 Hall of Fame Drive
Ft. Lauderdale, FL 33316
(305) 462–6536

United States Water Fitness Association (USWFA)
John Spannuth, Executive Director
P.O. Box 3279
Boynton Beach, FL 33424

Colwin, Cecil. 1992. Swimming Into the 21st Century. *Human Kinetics Publishers, Inc. Box 5076, Champaign, IL 61825–5076.*

Costill, David, Ernest Maglischo, and Allen Richardson. 1992. Swimming. *Human Kinetics Publishers, Inc. Box 5076, Champaign, IL 61825–5076.*

Thomas, David. 1990. Advanced Swimming. *Human Kinetics Publishers, Inc. Box 5076, Champaign, IL 61825–5076.*

Appendix

4
Jogging

Advantages/Disadvantages

Running is a simple way to develop cardiorespiratory endurance. You can do it alone, with a partner, or with a group. A good pair of running shoes is the only equipment you need. Finding a place to run is as simple as walking out your front door. It takes less time than many other aerobic activities to get a full workout. It can be done in most types of weather, on vacation, or squeezed into a lunch break. Drawbacks to running include traffic, uneven pavement, and an occasional aggressive dog. Trying to progress too quickly may cause impact problems such as shin splints, sore knees, or other discomforts. For individuals who are overweight or very out of shape, it may be best to start with a less intense activity, such as walking. With a carefully planned program of progressive activity, running can be enjoyed by almost everyone.

What to Wear

You can run in almost any kind of weather if you dress appropriately. On hot days, wear as little as decently possible—shoes, socks, shirt, and shorts. For cooler weather, add layers—a long-sleeved t-shirt and tights or long pants. In cold weather, add a jacket or a turtleneck sweater, and to protect ears and hands, a stocking cap and mittens. In wet weather, wear a cap with a brim to keep rain out of your eyes, and rain-repellent clothing, if desired. Keep in mind that when you are running, you generate a great deal of body heat. When you are warmed up, it will feel about 20 degrees warmer than the actual temperature. A hot day would be 70 degrees or higher, a warm day 50 to 60 degrees, a cool day 30 to 40 degrees, and a cold day is below freezing. High humidity on hot days and the wind chill factor on cold days also should be considered (see chapter 8).

A good pair of properly fitted running shoes is important in preventing injuries. When running, your foot strikes the ground with an impact approximately three times your body weight. A well made running shoe fitted by a trained salesperson can absorb shock and support the foot. A cheap pair of poor quality shoes is no bargain if it leaves you with blisters or shin splints.

Technique and Safety Tips

Good running form is relaxed and mechanically efficient. Your energy goes into moving you forward and is not dissipated in extraneous movements. Maintain a relaxed, erect posture, head up, eyes looking ahead. Keep your shoulders relaxed and level, arms swinging freely from the shoulder, hands unclenched, traveling between the hips and lower chest. Avoid hunching forward, eyes watching feet, arms held stiffly or swinging across the midline of the body. Knees and feet should aim ahead, not to the center or side. Foot contact should be heel to ball or midfoot, not on the toes like a sprinter. Keep your stride length comfortable and effortless, with the foot landing under the center of gravity. Be careful not to overstride or bounce when you run. Stride length is a product of speed and leg strength. Unless you increase one of these elements, attempts to increase your stride length will waste energy. Breathe through mouth and nose. It is hard to get enough air breathing through the nose alone.

While you are working on your running form, there are some safety guidelines you need to keep in mind.

1. *Before leaving home, let someone know your route and when you expect to return. Carry identification.*

2. *If you wear a headset, keep the volume low enough so you can hear approaching traffic.*

3. *Keep alert.*

4. *If there is a sidewalk, jog on it.*

5. *If there is no sidewalk, run facing traffic on the extreme left edge or shoulder of the road.*

6. *Respect private property. Do not run across lawns.*

7. *Obey traffic signs and signals. When crossing a street at the light, cross with the green light only.*

8. *Maintain eye contact with motorists whenever you cross in front of them.*

9. *Give the right of way to cars. Don't antagonize drivers, even if they try your patience.*

10. *If you run at night, wear light-colored clothing with reflective strips.*

11. *At night, do not run in unfamiliar areas.*

12. *Do not wear a rubber sweat suit while exercising, ever!*

How to Begin and Progress

Begin at the level indicated by your cardiorespiratory fitness assessment (chapter 4), and progress slowly. If you cannot complete a mile in 15 minutes, then begin with walking briskly 15 to 30 minutes until your heart rate stays within the target range. When you can comfortably handle two miles in 30 minutes, you may begin the jog/walk program. As in all activities, follow the FITT guidelines.

Run/Walk Program

Fitness Category	Starting Level
Very poor	1, 2, or 3
Poor	4
Average	5 or 6
Good	7 or 8
Excellent	9 or 10

Level	Run	Walk	Repeats
1		15–20 min.	1
2		20–30 min.	1
3	30 sec.	30 sec.	8–12 plus 10- to 15-min. walk
4	1 min.	30 sec.	6–10 plus 10-min. walk
5	2 min.	30 sec.	4–10 plus 5- to 10-min. walk
6	4 min.	1 min.	4–6
7	6 min.	1 min.	4–5
8	8 min.	1–2 min.	3–4
9	12 min.	2 min.	2
10	20–30 min.	5 min.	1

Directions: Start at the level appropriate for your fitness category. For each run-walk interval, begin with the lowest number of repeats indicated, and each successive workout, add one repeat. When you can do the maximum number of intervals at one level, move to the next level. A 5-minute warm-up and 5-minute cool-down should accompany each workout. You may stay at one level as long as you need to, or even move back a step if the beginning level is too difficult. If the workout has been appropriate, you should feel refreshed and relaxed, not exhausted, after exercise.

Variety

Much of the variety in running comes from running different routes and from observing the changing scenery and seasons. If you run alone, you may wish to occasionally run with a partner, or vice versa. Instead of a long run at a continuous pace, you might try fartlek, a Swedish term for speed-play. Fartlek mixes fast-paced runs, brief all-out sprints, and slow-paced recovery intervals. It is best done on uneven or hilly terrain such as a park or golf course. Interval training done once or no more than twice a week can add a change of pace. This alternates a fast-paced run over a predetermined distance with walking or a slow recovery jog. An example might be running 220 yards, four to six times in 40 to 50 seconds with a 220-yard walk between each. With interval training, you may vary the distance run, recovery interval, number of repetitions, and time or pace of the run. These workouts are usually done on the track but can be done on the road by running, then walking, a set amount of time, by running a certain number of telephone pole intervals, or by selecting a long hill on your route and running up it several times. A fitness trail, or parcour, with exercise stations linked by a running trail, may be available at a local park or university, or you can make your own. To simulate a parcour, on a regular running route, stop every two to four minutes to do a stretching or toning exercise (i.e., hamstring stretch, run two minutes, calf stretch, run three minutes, push-ups, run three minutes, abdominal curls ...).

Some activities are suitable for a small group. You can take a tennis or foam ball along to toss among some friends. You'll get quite a workout, because it mixes sprinting and upper body exercise into the run. This is safer if your route has little traffic. Hashing is a popular club sport in the southern United States, Europe, and Russia. The idea is for a group to follow a marked course through an unfamiliar area. Elected group members meet at an earlier time to mark the route, usually with flour. Local fun-runs give you a chance to run and meet other runners in a noncompetitive atmosphere. If you like competition, you can get information on road races from your local running club or athletic shoe store.

Common Discomforts

Most aches and pains in running do not occur suddenly. They are often from overuse—a long steady erosion that wears down the body. Many general complaints are addressed in chapter 5. Specific to running, two additional discomforts, easily avoided, occasionally occur. If you run with shoes that are too short or that don't fit well, in addition to developing blisters, you could injure a toe. The toenail may turn black and possibly even fall off. While painful, the condition is not permanent. The nail will grow back. If your thighs rub together when you run, you may suffer an abrasion. The solution is to apply vaseline to the area and to wear tights or shorts that cover your thighs.

Resources

American Running and Fitness Association
9310 Old Georgetown Road
Bethesda, MD 20814–1111
Phone (301) 897–0197

Runner's World Magazine
Box 366
Mountain View, CA 94042

The Runner
Ziff-Davis Publishing Co.
P.O. Box 2702
Boulder, CO 80321

Campbell, Dale. 1990. Jogging: A Successful Guide to Aerobics. American Press.

Corbin, David. 1988. Jogging. Glenview, IL: Scott, Foresman and Company.

Cooper, Kenneth. 1986. Running Without Fear. New York: Bantam Books.

Costill, David. 1986. Inside Running: Basics of Sports Physiology. Indianapolis: Benchmark Press, Inc.

Heinonen, Janet. 1989. Sports Illustrated Running for Women: A Complete Guide. New York: NAL-Dutton.

Henderson, Joe. 1991. Think Fast: Mental Toughness Training for Runners. New York: NAL-Dutton.

Higdon, Hal. 1990. The Masters Running Guide. Van Nuys, CA: Gain Publications.

Johnson, Alice. 1989. Half a Mind: Hashing: The Outrageous New Running Sport. Camden, ME: Yankee Books.

Murphy, Ray. 1990. If You Felt Like I Did ... You'd Start Running. Boston: Stethophonics

Rosato, Frank. 1988. Jogging for Health and Fitness. Englewood, CO: Morton Publishing.

5

Fitness Walking

Advantages/Disadvantages

Walking is simple, enjoyable, and probably the safest form of aerobic exercise known. It is inexpensive and can be done by almost anyone, any place, any time. There is no need to join a club or to find partners or opponents. It is a wise exercise choice for the overweight, older adult, the very out-of-shape, postsurgical patient, or the individual in a cardiac rehabilitation program. Appropriate shoes and comfortable clothes are the only equipment you need. Walking is excellent for weight control. In fact, you use as many calories walking a mile as you would jogging the same distance. The difference is that walking takes longer. Even though the injury rate is very low, some walkers who try to increase distance and pace too quickly may experience sore muscles and knees or other discomforts. Another disadvantage to walking is that the already physically fit may not be able to elevate the heart rate into the target zone. In this case, one of the advanced forms of fitness walking can be tried, such as power walking (with hand weights) or race walking. Dogs and inclement weather present other problems to the walker. Many shopping malls have opened their doors for early morning walking and also to provide a safe, weather-controlled environment year round.

What to Wear

You don't have to buy special clothes; anything loose and comfortable will do. It is a good idea for your exercise clothes to have a pocket, for carrying identification, keys, and a handkerchief. For suggestions on dealing with weather, read the tips for hot and cold weather dressing provided in the jogging appendix.

Studies show that walking generates a downward force of about 1.5 times your body weight, so wearing appropriate shoes is important in helping you progress smoothly and injury free. You may save a few dollars on inexpensive shoes, but a good pair of shoes will help protect your feet, legs, and back. When purchasing new shoes, go to a reputable store and ask for a trained salesperson. Look for shoes with a cushioned heel, flexible sole, firm heel support, and arch supports that fit your feet. The toe box must provide room for the toes to work to prevent blisters. Several companies manufacture shoes designed for the sport of walking. Try one of these or one made for jogging, but be sure it fits your foot. The shoe should never feel like it needs to be "broken in." It should feel comfortable from day one.

Do you replace your worn-out shoes soon enough? A study at Tulane University found that all shoes, regardless of brand, price, or type of construction, lose about 30 percent of their shock absorbency after 500 miles of use. This is a good reason for keeping records of your mileage. Take your old shoes with you when shopping for a new pair so that a knowledgeable salesperson can evaluate the wear pattern to help you choose a suitable shoe.

Technique and Safety Tips

Walking posture is erect, but relaxed. To alleviate tension, the abdomen should be pulled in, the rib cage lifted, and the shoulders pulled down. This will help you keep relaxed and increase your endurance. Your arms should be bent at about a 90-degree angle, and the hands (loose fist) should swing slightly above the waist. Your arms counterbalance your leg motion. You may discover during your walk that the arms have dropped, resulting in a slower pace. Visualize that you are walking in a straight line. Hold your head up with eyes focused ahead, watching the ground but not the feet. Your foot contact should be a heel roll to the ball of the foot and toes for push off. Resist the tendency to lean forward at the waist.

While you are walking, keep in mind these simple tips for a safe workout.

1. *Always carry some form of identification (include pertinent medical information).*

2. *Choose a safe time and place to exercise. Take keys with you, and lock the car and/or house.*

3. *Plan your route carefully. Use well-populated, well-lighted areas. Avoid areas that are dark and have dense shrubs and alleys.*

4. *Know where you can get help along your route.*

5. *Use sidewalks or walk facing oncoming traffic and in single file.*

6. *Obey traffic signals and signs. Do not jaywalk.*

7. *Keep alert at all times. Give the right-of-way to cars. Don't assume the driver sees you.*

8. *Wear bright, reflective clothing at dusk or night.*

9. *Tell someone where you are going and when you think you will return. Better yet, use the "buddy" system. It's more fun to walk with someone.*

10. *Avoid dogs by selecting routes that are free of them. The best advice is to ignore a barking dog, and never walk between a barking dog and its owner, especially if the owner is a child.*

11. *For the cleanest air, walk in the morning. The air is more polluted at midday, and pollution drops after rush hour in the evening.*

12. *Don't wear a headset; you are losing one of your most valuable sensory aids. If you wear a headset, keep volume low so you can hear traffic or approaching strangers.*

13. *Avoid walking on snow/ice-covered roads and walks.*

14. *Avoid peak traffic hours unless you can use a jogging path or a sidewalk.*

How to Begin and Progress

Test your fitness using the 1-mile Walk Test described in chapter 4 (Fitness Assessment). Then follow the appropriate level on the W.A.L.K.S. Program. After completing the "S" level continue on the W.A.L.K.S. Maintenance Program for a lifetime of fitness.

Always check your heart rate to be sure it stays within the target zone. Listen to your body, and progress slowly for optimal results. Take each step on the chart, and don't skip ahead. If the increase is too difficult, go back to the preceding level for awhile. You should feel energized after your workout, not exhausted.

Fitness Category	Starting Program
Very Poor	"W" Level
Poor	"A" Level
Average	"L" Level
Good	"K" Level
Excellent	"S" Level

The W.A.L.K.S. Program

"W" Level

Week	1–2	3–4	5–6	7–8	9–10	11–12	13–14
Warm-up (min)	5–10	5–10	5–10	5–10	5–10	5–10	5–10
Conditioning Bout (mileage)	1.0	1.25	1.5	1.75	2.0	2.25	2.5
Intensity (target heart rate)	60–75	60–75	60–75	60–75	60–75	60–75	60–75
Cool-down (min)	5–10	5–10	5–10	5–10	5–10	5–10	5–10
Frequency	3	3	3	3	4	4	4

"A" Level

Week	1–2	3–4	5–6	7–8	9–10	11–12	13–14
Warm-up (min)	5–10	5–10	5–10	5–10	5–10	5–10	5–10
Conditioning Bout (mileage)	2.0	2.25	2.5	2.75	3.0	3.25	3.50
Intensity (target heart rate)	60–75	60–75	60–75	60–75	60–75	60–75	60–75
Cool-down (min)	5–10	5–10	5–10	5–10	5–10	5–10	5–10
Frequency	3	3	3	4	4	4	4

"L" Level

Week	1–2	3–4	5–6	7–8	9–10	11–12	13–14
Warm-up (min)	5–10	5–10	5–10	5–10	5–10	5–10	5–10
Conditioning Bout (mileage)	3.0	3.25	3.25	3.5	3.75	3.75	4.0

Intensity (target heart rate)

60–75	60–75	60–75	60–75	60–75	60–75	60–75

Cool-down (min)

5–10	5–10	5–10	5–10	5–10	5–10	5–10

Frequency

3	3	4	4	4	4	4

"K" Level

Week	1–2	3–4	5–6	7–8	9–10	11–12	13–14

Warm-up (min)

5–10	5–10	5–10	5–10	5–10	5–10	5–10

Conditioning Bout (mileage)

3.5	3.75	3.75	4.0	4.0	4.0	4.0

Intensity (target heart rate)

60–75	60–75	60–75	60–75	60–75	60–75	60–75

Cool-down (min)

5–10	5–10	5–10	5–10	5–10	5–10	5–10

Frequency

4	4	4	4	5	5	5

"S" Level

Week	1–2	3–4	5–6	7–8	9–10	11–12	13–14

Warm-up (min)

5–10	5–10	5–10	5–10	5–10	5–10	5–10

Conditioning Bout (mileage)

4.0	4.0	4.0	4.25	4.25	4.5	4.5

Intensity (target heart rate)

60–75	60–75	60–75	60–75	60–75	60–75	60–75

Cool-down (min)

5–10	5–10	5–10	5–10	5–10	5–10	5–10

Frequency

5	5	5	5	5	5	5

W.A.L.K.S. Maintenance Program
(For a lifetime of fitness)

Warm-up:	5–10 minutes
Conditioning Bout:	3–5 miles per workout
Intensity:	At Target Heart Rate Range
Cool-down:	5–10 minutes
Frequency:	3–5 times per week
Weekly Mileage:	9–25 miles

Variety

Adding variety to your walking workouts can keep you enthused about the sport for many years. Varying your walking routes gives you a change of scenery. Drive the car to a new area, park, and explore the surroundings during your workout. Mailing a letter, walking an errand, window shopping walks, and shopping mall workouts can be fun.

Walk with a friend, in a group, or by yourself for a change. Get a dog; they make excellent walking companions. For a challenge, try an advanced exercise walking technique such as race walking, power walking, hill walking, or walking a fitness trail. Participate in a volksmarch, a competitive walking event, or join a Hashing Club (described in the jogging appendix). Water walking (walking in waist-deep water) is popular in many areas; give it a try. Some people enjoy listening to music while exercising in a traffic-free area. You won't become stale or bored with exercise if you vary your workouts.

Common Discomforts

As in running, most aches, pains, and injuries occur from overuse. Listen to your body. Don't attempt to work through an injury. It will only aggravate the condition. The two most common walking complaints are shin splints and back-of-the-knee soreness. Refer to chapter 5 for information about shin splints. Cut back on pace and distance until all soreness subsides. Comfortable well-fitting shoes will help prevent blisters. Consult a sports podiatrist if you suffer from foot problems such as calluses, bunions, heel spurs, ingrown toenails, high arches, flat feet, or an overly pronated foot. These conditions can be remedied and, if not corrected, may prevent you from fully enjoying your walking program.

Resources

The Rockport Walking Institute
P.O. Box 480
Marlboro, MA 01752

Walkers Club of America
445 E. 86th
New York, NY 10028

North American Race-Walking Foundation (NARF)
Box 50312
Pasadena, CA 91105–0312
(818) 577–2264

The Walking Magazine
11 Harcourt St.
Boston, MA 02116
(617) 266–3322

Reebok Walking Program
Reebok International Ltd.
100 Technology Center Dr.
P.O. Box 9116
Stoughton, MA 02072–9801

American Heart Association Walking Program
American Heart Association
National Center
7320 Greenville Ave.
Dallas, TX 75231

Heart and Sole Newsletter
National Organization of Mall Walkers
P.O. Box 191
Hermann, MO 65041

Walk Ways
Walk Ways Center
733 15th St., NW
Washington, DC 20005

Balboa, Dean. 1990. Walk for Life, The Lifetime Walking Program for a Healthy Body and Mind. *New York: Perigee Books.*

Decker, June. 1989. Y's Way to Fitness Walking. *Champaign, IL: Human Kinetics Publishers, Inc.*

Ford, Normal. 1992. Walk to Your Hearts Content: The Way to Fitness, Health and Adventure. *Woodstock, VT: The Countryman Press, Inc.*

Hawkins, Jerald and Sandra Weigle. 1992. Walking for Fun and Fitness. *Englewood, CO: Morton Publishing Co.*

Least Heat-Moon, William. 1991. Prairyerth. *Boston: Houghton Mifflin.*

Seiger, Lon and James Hesson. 1991. Walking for Health *and* Walking for Fitness. *Dubuque, IA: Wm. C. Brown Publishers.*

Sweetgall, Robert, James Rippe and Frank Katch. 1990. Fitness Walking. *New York: The Putnam Publishing.*

Thoreau, Henry David. 1991. Nature Walking. *Beacon Press.*

Yanker, Gary. 1990. Walking Medicine. *New York: McGraw Hill.*

Appendix

6

Water Exercise/Aqua Aerobics

Advantages/Disadvantages

You don't have to know how to swim to get a vigorous workout in the water. You don't even have to get your head wet! As more and more people are discovering, exercising against water resistance in shallow water is a fine workout and great fun, especially with a group. Water exercise can be a social activity because you can carry on a conversation while working out. It is low impact, so joint problems are rare. The supportive effect of water buoyancy makes water exercise enjoyable and relaxing for individuals who have concerns about other forms of exercise. In chest-deep water, a person weighs only about one-tenth what he does on land. People who have arthritis or joint problems find that this buoyancy decreases stress to the joints, allowing a fuller range of motion than on land. It is easy to individualize intensity levels so that you get a good workout, whatever your level of fitness. Inclement weather is not a problem. Water exercise is cool, even on the hottest summer days, so heat stress is eliminated. It is also a comfortable indoor workout for rainy or cold winter days. If you are overweight and sensitive about exercising in public, the water covers you up so that you don't feel so obvious. Water exercise is also beneficial during pregnancy because of both decreased joint stress and decreased heat stress as compared to other forms of exercise.

The drawbacks are few. You need access to a pool at a time when you can have a lane separate from lap swimmers. It is probably best to first join a class to learn the exercises and activities. Then you can work out on your own.

What to Wear

A comfortable swimsuit is all that is required. Some people also like to wear pool shoes to protect their feet when doing water running and walking workouts.

Technique and Safety Tips

Workouts may have a muscle toning emphasis, an aerobic emphasis, or a combination of the two. In constructing workouts, maintain muscle balance by exercising all major muscle groups. Particularly emphasize stretching tight muscle groups (i.e., lower back, hamstrings, calves) and toning weak areas (i.e., abdominals, upper body). To overload, keep in mind that as in weight training, water adds resistance. The harder you push and pull, the more resistance you create, and the more benefit you receive. In any activity, it is important to limit back hyperextension by keeping abdominals firm while exercises are being performed. In the water, like on land, workouts must maintain a training heart rate for 20–30 minutes to produce aerobic benefit. Training heart rates for swimmers appear to be about 10 percent lower than for land exercisers. This may also be true for other cardiorespiratory water exercise. In order to calculate an appropriate exercise intensity for water exercise, subtract 10 percent from your training pulse on land. Jogging in the water, aqua aerobics, or other vigorous activities can all provide aerobic benefit if an adequate overload occurs. Several books that give examples of water exercises are available.

Whenever you exercise in the water, a few safety guidelines must be followed.

1. *Never work out in the water alone. A lifeguard or workout partner, preferably one who can swim, should be present. Safety equipment, such as a life ring or reaching pole, should also be available.*

2. *Shower before entering the pool.*

3. *Do not go into the deep water unless you can swim.*

4. *Water and electricity don't mix. If you like to exercise to music, keep electrical equipment away from the water, and make sure that all electric outlets have ground-fault circuit interruptors that shut off the electricity if it contacts water. Better yet, use battery-powered equipment.*

5. *Do not enter the pool if you have an open sore, infection, or rash.*

6. *Do all exercises through a full range of motion with slow, controlled movements. Swinging or flinging movements can injure joints.*

7. *Maintain good body alignment in walking and jogging. Keep abdominals tight, hips tucked under, and avoid excessive forward lean.*

How to Begin and Progress

Water exercise may involve many different activities—aerobic, muscle toning, and stretching. Recommendations on how to progress are given for the aerobic portion of the workout, in terms of length of time at a training heart rate.

Water Exercise Program

Fitness Category	Starting Level
Very poor	1
Poor	2
Average	3
Good	4
Excellent	5 or 6

Level	Vigorous	Easy	Sets	Total Time
1	1 min.	30 secs.	8–12	10–18 mins.
2	2 mins.	30 secs.	6–8	15–20 mins.
3	4 mins.	30 secs.	4–6	18–27 mins.
4	6 mins.	30 secs.	3–4	19–26 mins.
5	8–10 mins.	1 min.	3	26–32 mins.
6	continuous		1	30 min.

Variety

Exercise with friends or with music (see appendix 1 for music resources). After mastering the exercises with only water resistance, use kickboards, pull-buoys, or empty plastic milk jugs to increase resistance. Vary the exercises and activities so that you don't do the same workout two days in a row. For example, an aerobic workout may involve, on different days, running widths, aqua-aerobics, water games, treading and kicking drills, or circuit training. There are so many different things to do in the water, it is easy to add variety. Some examples of different types of workouts follow.

Muscular strength and endurance is built by performing repeats of exercises against resistance: side leg swings to tone inner thigh and outer hip, straight arm raises to tone deltoids, back leg kicks to strengthen hamstrings and gluteus. A series of 8–12 exercises covering all major muscle groups can be performed one minute each and repeated 2–3 times for a thorough muscular workout.

Water walking involves walking in waist- to chest-deep water fast enough to produce a target heart rate. Variations include walking forward, backward, or sideways, and adding different arm variations such as forward pulls, breaststroke, or backstroke.

Shallow water jogging is similar to water walking but is more intense, using a faster, bounding stride.

Deep-water jogging is a nonimpact workout. Exercisers wear a flotation vest or belt and run, varying directions and arm movements.

Interval training alternates high- and low-intensity workout segments. For example, alternating 4 laps of shallow-water running with 2 laps of water walking.

Water aerobics, like land aerobics, puts exercise to music. Workouts may be either choreographed or freestyle. Bench step workouts have also made the transition into the aquatic environment, with similar benefits as in land workouts.

Plyometrics are vigorous jumping and bounding exercises that increase muscle strength and power. They are also very aerobic! Examples include high jumps in place, bounding across the pool, and a series of high two-foot hops. Because these are impact exercises, they should be avoided if you have ankle, knee, or back problems.

Flexibility exercises are often used as a part of a water exercise program. A static stretch is held 20 to 30 seconds or more for each major muscle group in order to increase range of motion.

In circuit training, a series of exercises are performed for a certain number of repetitions or a given amount of time (i.e., 1 minute each of side leg circles, jumping jacks, pushups, forward kicks, etc.). Exercises may be written on numbered cards placed around the pool edge, and as each exercise is completed, participants move quickly to the next exercise station. Exercises may stress one fitness component or several. A set of exercises can be repeated, or time at each station can be increased to produce overload.

Occasionally, it is fun to try a water game for variety. Examples include shallow-water polo, inner-tube water polo, water baseball, freeze tag, sharks and minnows, water basketball, or volleyball.

Common Discomforts

The most common discomforts water exercisers encounter are tight calves and blisters from running barefoot on the pool bottom. Blisters can be avoided by starting with only a few minutes of running in the pool and giving the feet time to toughen as you gradually progress in workouts. You could also wear pool shoes or clean sneakers during workouts. Calves tend to get tight because, due to buoyancy, most running and walking in the pool is done on the ball of the foot. Simply take care to stretch calves before and after the workout to maintain flexibility.

Resources

The Aquatic Exercise Association
Ruth Sova, President
Box 497
Port Washington, WI 53074
(414) 375–2503

US Water Fitness Association
John Spannuth, Executive Director
P.O. Box 3219
Boynton Beach, FL 33424

IDEA Resource Library: Aqua Exercise
IDEA: The Association for Fitness Professionals
6190 Cornerstone Court E., Suite 204
San Diego, CA 92121-3773

Huey, Linda, and R. R. Knudson. 1986. The Waterpower Workout. *New York: New American Library.*

Katz, Jane. 1985. The W.E.T. Workout. *New York: Facts on File Publications.*

Krasevec, Joseph, A., and Diane C. Grimes. 1985. HydroRobics. *Champaign, IL: Leisure Press.*

Spitzer, Terry-Ann and Hoeger, Werner. 1990. Physical Fitness the Water Aerobics Way. *Englewood, CO: Morton Publishing Company.*

Sova, Ruth. 1992. Aquatics: The Complete Reference Guide for Aquatic Fitness Professionals.

Sova, Ruth. 1993. Aquatics Activities Handbook. *Boston: Jones and Bartlett.*

Chapter

1

Activities

Name _____   Class/Activity Section _____

Assessing Your Wellness

Read each statement carefully and respond honestly by using the following scoring:

Almost always	= 2 points
Sometimes/Occasionally	= 1 point
Very Seldom	= 0 points

Physical Dimension

_2_ **1.** I exercise aerobically (vigorous, continuous) for 20–30 minutes at least 3 times per week.

_2_ **2.** I eat fruits, vegetables, and whole grains everyday.

_2_ **3.** I avoid tobacco products.

_1_ **4.** I wear a seat belt while riding in and driving a car.

_0_ **5.** I deliberately minimize my intake of cholesterol, dietary fats, and oils.

_2_ **6.** I avoid drinking alcoholic beverages, *or* I consume no more than 1 drink per day.

_0_ **7.** I get an adequate amount of sleep.

_2_ **8.** I have adequate coping mechanisms for dealing with stress.

_1_ **9.** I maintain a regular schedule of immunizations, physical and dental checkups (including pap smears, blood pressure and cholesterol checks), and monthly self-exams of breasts or testicles.

_2_ **10.** I maintain a reasonable weight—avoiding extremes of overweight and underweight.

_14_ *Physical Total*

Social Dimension

_0_ **1.** I contribute time and/or money to community projects.

_1_ **2.** I conserve energy in my place of residence *and* practice recycling.

_2_ **3.** I exhibit fairness, justice, and concern in dealing with people.

_2_ **4.** I have a network of close friends and/or family.

_2_ **5.** I am interested in others, including those from different backgrounds than my own.

_1_ **6.** I am able to balance my own needs with the needs of others.

_2_ **7.** I am able to communicate with and get along with a wide variety of people.

_2_ **8.** I obey the laws and rules of our society.

_2_ **9.** I try to help others when I can.

_1_ **10.** I am committed to cleaning up the environment (air, water, noise, soil, etc.).

_15_ *Social Total*

Spiritual Dimension

_1_ **1.** I feel comfortable and at ease with my spiritual life.

_2_ **2.** There is a direct relationship between by personal values and daily actions.

_1_ **3.** When I get depressed or frustrated by problems, my spiritual beliefs and values give me direction.

_2_ **4.** Prayer, meditation, and/or quiet personal reflection is/are important in my life.

_1_ **5.** Life is meaningful for me, and I feel a purpose in life.

_2_ **6.** I am able to speak comfortably about my personal values and beliefs.

_2_ **7.** I am consistently striving to grow spiritually and see it as a lifelong process.

_2_ **8.** I am tolerant of and try to learn about others' beliefs and values.

_2_ **9.** I believe that it will be easy to maintain my values within my selected career field.

_2_ **10.** I appreciate the natural forces that exist in the universe.

_17_ *Spiritual Total*

Emotional Dimension

__2__ 1. I am able to develop and maintain close relationships.

__2__ 2. I accept the responsibility for my actions.

__1__ 3. I see challenges and change as opportunities for growth.

__1__ 4. I feel I have considerable control over my life.

__2__ 5. I am able to laugh at life and myself.

__1__ 6. I feel good about myself.

__2__ 7. I am able to appropriately cope with stress and tension and make time for leisure pursuits.

__1__ 8. I am able to recognize my personal shortcomings and learn from my mistakes.

__2__ 9. I am able to recognize my feelings and express them.

__1__ 10. I enjoy life.

__15__ *Emotional Total*

Intellectual Dimension

__2__ 1. I am interested in learning new things.

__1__ 2. I try to keep abreast of current affairs—locally, nationally, and internationally.

__0__ 3. I enjoy attending special lectures, play, musical performances, museums, galleries, and/or libraries.

__1__ 4. I carefully select movies and television programs.

__2__ 5. I enjoy creative and stimulating mental activities/games.

__0__ 6. I am happy with the amount and variety that I read.

__1__ 7. I make an effort to improve my verbal, writing, and expression skills.

__1__ 8. A continuing education program is/will be important to me in my career.

__2__ 9. I am able to analyze, synthesize, and see more than one side of an issue.

__0__ 10. I enjoy engaging in intellectual discussions.

__10__ *Intellectual Total*

Occupational Dimensions

__1__ 1. I am happy with my career choice.

__1__ 2. I look forward to work.

__2__ 3. My job responsibilities/duties are consistent with my values.

__2__ 4. The payoffs/advantages in my career field choice are consistent with my values.

__0__ 5. I am happy with the balance between my work time and leisure time.

__1__ 6. I am happy with the amount of control I have in my work.

__1__ 7. My work gives me personal satisfaction and stimulation.

__1__ 8. I am happy with the professional/personal growth provided by my job.

__2__ 9. I feel my job allows me to "make a difference" in the world.

__1__ 10. My job contributes positively to my overall well-being.

__12__ *Occupational Total*

Scoring

Add your total score for each dimension of wellness.

15–20 points: Excellent strength in this dimension.

9–14 points: There is room for improvement. Look again at the items in which you scored 1 or 0. What changes can you make to improve your score?

0–8 points: This dimension needs a lot of work. Look again at this dimension and challenge yourself to begin making small steps toward growth here. Remember . . . the goal is balanced wellness.

Take your score in each dimension of wellness and shade it in on this wheel. How smoothly will your "wellness wheel" roll? A smooth ride indicates *balanced* wellness, and the LARGER the wheel, the better!

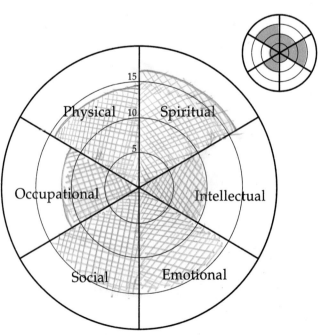

	Chapter **1** *Activities*	
Name _____		*Class/Activity Section* _____

How Are You Doing? (on your wellness contract)

Briefly discuss and evaluate your use of the wellness contract.

What was your goal?

1. General reactions to the contract:

2. Obstacles and setbacks encountered:

3. Support sought, gained, needed:

4. Methods of maintaining commitment:

5. Discuss outcomes in terms of personal growth:

6. Where will you go from here? What is your next step?

	Chapter
Name _____	**2**
	Activities
	Class/Activity Section _____

Exercise/Activity Log Sheet

	S	M	T	W	Th	F	Sa
Week 1							
Week 2							
Week 3							
Week 4							

Goals: _____

_____

Comments: _____

Name _____

Chapter
3
Activities

Class/Activity Section _____

Strength Training Log

Exercise											

┌─────────────────────┐
│   Chapter   │
│   4   │
│   *Activities*   │
└─────────────────────┘

Name _____   *Class/Activity Section* _____

Exercise Clearance Form

This form must be ___ to the Health Center or to your personal physician for a signature. It must be returned to your instructor b_ _____.

_____ _____ is presently enrolled in _____ .

He/she has identified th_ _llowing health problems that may affect participation in the activities of the course:

_____

_____

_____

_____

The class will include the follow_ _ctivities: _____

_____

_____

After examining _____ , I recommend the following level of participation in the course described above.

_____ Full participation

_____ May not participate in this class**

_____ Modified participation as indicated _ _w.

The student may participate in the classes wi_ _e following modifications to activity: _____

_____

** If the student may not participate in this class, _ activities in which the student may participate.

_____   _____   _____   _____
Signature of physician   *Phone*   *Date*

Name _____

Chapter

6

Activities

Class/Activity Section _____

How to Mend a Broken Heart

Directions: Read the opening scenario concerning "Rob" on page 2 in your text. You were the physician on call when he was brought in. Please complete a medical history on this patient, and answer his wife's questions (Use back if needed).

1. List Rob's 3 primary risk factors for heart disease given in the scenario.

2. List Rob's 5 secondary risk factors for heart disease.

3. What 3 lifestyle changes will you tell Rob to make to reduce his heart disease risk?

Rob's wife has read the chart. She is distraught and has several questions for you. Please respond (You may use back of sheet).

4. "Doctor, I really don't understand some of the words used on the chart." What is angina? Myocardial infarction? What is atherosclerosis, and will it ever go away?

5. "I saw that his cholesterol was 280, and his HDL level was 28. What does that mean? What is normal?"

6. "Rob doesn't want to quit smoking—since he's smoked for 20 years. Why is smoking bad for his heart?

7. "A nurse said Rob needs a special exercise program to aid in recovery. Won't exercise strain the heart? What good will it do?" (Give three benefits.)

8. "Rob enjoys having an occasional beer. Will he have to give this up?"

```
                    Chapter
                       7
                   Activities
```

Name _____   *Class/Activity Section* _____

Becoming Stress Resistant and Hardy

List two ways your "hardiness" can be strengthened in each of the following traits:

A. **Commitment (Task Involvement):** How can you build commitment in your life (i.e., family, friends, studies, work, community)?

List two ways to improve commitment.

Example: I will complete my nursing degree by 19___.

Control: Do you feel you are in control of your life? List two ways you gain more control.

Example: Today, I am plotting out all the courses I need to complete my degree, semester by semester. It is apparent that I will need to go one summer session. I am now aware of the courses that I must take in sequential order.

C. **Challenge:** Do you see change and/or setbacks as challenges instead of stumbling blocks? Give two examples that have occurred recently, list two strategies you can use in the future.

Example: So I didn't do very well on this anatomy pop quiz . . . now I know how much work I need to do in this course.

D. **Choices in Lifestyle (Personal Health Practices):** How healthy is your current lifestyle? List two improvements you can make in your lifestyle.

Example: I will get at least eight hours of sleep every night for two weeks.

E. **Connectedness:** Do you feel "connected" with at least one other person or group? Do you have "close" friends and family? List two ways to improve connectedness.

Example: Twice a week I will either telephone or write a note to a friend to keep in touch with friends I rarely get to see.

Chapter
7
Activities

Name _____

Class/Activity Section _____

Relaxation

There are many ways to relax—meditation, progressive relaxation, autogenic training and imagery, hatha yoga, massage, abdominal breathing and flotation tanks—all are excellent tension relievers. You cannot simply "wish" to become a more relaxed person. It is a **skill** that takes *commitment* and *practice!* Make a commitment:

Choose any relaxation technique in the chapter, and practice it for **twenty minutes** every day for **one week.** Then respond to the questions below. Before you begin, rate your current ability to relax. How good are you at relaxing? Put an "X" on the line where you would rate your current skill.

Very Poor	Poor	Average	Good	Excellent

1. How often do you practice relaxation now? Circle one: never . . . once in a while . . . everyday
   Explain: (i.e., why don't you practice relaxation? What method do you use? How often? etc.)

2. Do you believe you could benefit by improving your ability to relax? Explain your response.

3. Which relaxation technique did you choose to practice?

Why did you select this technique? Describe your experience with this technique (i.e., how you felt before and after, etc.).

4. Did this technique help you feel relaxed? Why or why not?

5. Is this a skill you feel you can use to manage the stress in your everyday life? Explain:

6. Would you like to try any of the other techniques? If so, which and why?

7. Do you think relaxation is important in the management of your stress? Why or why not?

8. Take the Holmes and Rahe Life Event Scale or the Life Event Scale for the College Student. What was your score?_____ What was your implication for illness?_____

9. What role does diet play in the total stress picture of your life? List three ways you can improve the diet-stress connection in your everyday life.

10. List the top three daily hassles and top three daily uplifts in your life.

	Chapter **7** *Activities*	
Name _____		*Class/Activity Section* _____

Measuring Your Stress and Coping Skills

This is a four-part test. The first three parts are designed to give you an indication of how vulnerable you might be to certain types of stress and to make you aware of how they might affect you. The last part of the test will provide you with information on how to cope with stressful situations.

Test One

Choose the most appropriate answer for each of the 10 questions as it actually pertains to you.

	a. Almost always true	b. Usually true	c. Usually false	d. Almost always false
1. When I can't do something "my way," I simply adjust and do it the easiest way.	_____	_____	_____	_____
2. I get upset when someone in front of me drives slowly.	_____	_____	_____	_____
3. It bothers me when my plans are dependent upon others.	_____	_____	_____	_____
4. Whenever possible, I tend to avoid large crowds.	_____	_____	_____	_____
5. I am uncomfortable when I have to stand in long lines.	_____	_____	_____	_____
6. Arguments upset me.	_____	_____	_____	_____
7. When my plans don't flow smoothly, I become anxious.	_____	_____	_____	_____
8. I require a lot of space in which to live and work.	_____	_____	_____	_____
9. When I am busy at some task, I hate to be disturbed.	_____	_____	_____	_____
10. I believe that it is worth waiting for all good things.	_____	_____	_____	_____

To score: 1 and 10, a = 1 pt., b = 2 pts., c = 3 pts., d = 4 pts. 2 through 9, a = 4 pts., b = 3 pts., c = 2 pts., d = 2 pts.

This test measures your vulnerability to stress from being frustrated or inhibited. Scores in excess of 25 seem to suggest some vulnerability to this source of stress.

Total Scores _____

Test Two

Check or mark the letter of the response that best answers the following 10 questions. How often do you . . .

	a. Almost always	b. Very often	c. Seldom	d. Never
1. Find yourself with insufficient time to complete your work?	_____	_____	_____	_____
2. Find yourself becoming confused and unable to think clearly because too many things are happening at once?	_____	_____	_____	_____
3. Wish you had help to get everything done?	_____	_____	_____	_____
4. Feel your boss/professor expects too much from you?	_____	_____	_____	_____
5. Feel your family and friends expect too much from you?	_____	_____	_____	_____
6. Find your work infringing on your leisure hours?	_____	_____	_____	_____
7. Find yourself doing extra work to set an example to those around you?	_____	_____	_____	_____
8. Find yourself doing extra work to impress your superiors?	_____	_____	_____	_____
9. Have to skip a meal so that you can get work completed?	_____	_____	_____	_____
10. Feel that you have too much responsibility?	_____	_____	_____	_____

To score: a = 4 pts., b = 3 pts., c = 2 pts., d = 1 pt.

Total your score for this exercise.

This test measures your vulnerability to "overload," that is, having too much to do. Scores in excess of 25 seem to indicate vulnerability to this source of stress.

Total Score _____

Test Three

Answer each question as it is generally true for you.

	a. Almost always true	b. Usually true	c. Usually false	d. Almost always false
1. I hate to wait in lines.	____	____	____	____
2. I often find myself racing against the clock to save time.	____	____	____	____
3. I become upset if I think something is taking too long.	____	____	____	____
4. When under pressure I tend to lose my temper.	____	____	____	____
5. My friends tell me that I tend to get irritated easily.	____	____	____	____
6. I seldom like to do anything unless I can make it competitive.	____	____	____	____
7. When something must be done, I'm the first to begin even though the details may still need to be worked out.	____	____	____	____
8. When I make a mistake it is usually because I've rushed into something without giving it enough thought and planning.	____	____	____	____
9. Whenever possible, I try to do two things at once, such as eating while working, or planning while driving or bathing.	____	____	____	____
10. When I go on a vacation, I usually take along some work to do just in case I get a chance.	____	____	____	____

To score: a = 4 pts., b = 3 pts., c = 2 pts., d = 1 pt.

This test measures the presence of compulsive, time-urgent, and excessively aggressive behavioral traits. Scores in excess of 25 suggest the presence of one or more of these traits.

Total Score _____

Test Four

This scale was created largely on the basis of results compiled by clinicians and researchers who sought to identify how individuals effectively cope with stress. This scale is an educational tool, not a clinical instrument. Its purpose, therefore, is to inform you of ways in which you can effectively and healthfully cope with the stress in your life. At the same time, through a point system, it will give you some indication of the relative desirability of the coping strategies you are currently using. Simply follow the instructions given for each of the 14 items listed. Total your points when you have completed all of the items.

Points

1. Give yourself 10 points if you feel that you have a supportive family.   _____

2. Give yourself 10 points if you actively pursue a hobby.   _____

3. Give yourself 10 points if you belong to some social or activity group that meets at least once a month (other than your family).   _____

4. Give yourself 15 points if you are within five pounds of your ideal body weight, considering your height and bone structure.   _____

5. Give yourself 15 points if you practice some form of deep relaxation at least three times a week. Deep relaxation exercises include meditation, imagery, yoga, and so on.   _____

6. Give yourself 5 points for each time you exercise thirty minutes or longer during one average week.   _____

7. Give yourself 5 points for each nutritionally balanced and wholesome meal you consume during one average day.   _____

8. Give yourself 5 points if you do something just for yourself that you really enjoy during an average week.   _____

9. Give yourself 10 points if you have some place in your home that you can go in order to relax and/or be alone.   _____

10. Give yourself 10 points if you practice time management techniques in your daily life.   _____

11. Subtract 10 points for each pack of cigarettes you smoke during one average day.   _____

12. Subtract 5 points for each evening during an average week that you take any form of medication or chemical (including alcohol) to help you sleep.   _____

13. Subtract 10 points for each day during an average week that you consume any form of medication or chemical substance (including alcohol) to reduce your anxiety or just to calm you down.   _____

14. Subtract 5 points for each evening during an average week that you bring work home—work that was meant to be done at your place of employment.   _____

Now calculate your total score. A "perfect" score would be 115 points or more. If you scored in the 50–60 range you probably have an adequate collection of coping strategies for most common sources of stress. You should keep in mind, however, that the higher your score, the greater your ability to cope with stress in an effective and healthful manner.

Total Score _____

Chapter

8

Activities

1. Your sister's gynecologist just told her she is pregnant. Knowing you were taking a college fitness/wellness course, she asks you for advice concerning the fitness walking program she began 2 months ago to help her get back into shape and lose a few pounds. Give her 3 or 4 tips.

2. At dinner 2 of your friends were debating whether to use a popular sports drink to replace all the sweat they expected to lose in the July 4th six-mile run. The July 4th festivities are tomorrow with the race beginning at noon in Old Town and ending at the top of Heartbreak Hill. What advice will you give them?

3. Your grandparents (age 65) were advised by their next-door neighbor to stop all that "foolish" exercising, to slow down, and to start acting their age. They ask you your opinion of this advice. What can you tell them about the benefits of staying physically active?

4. In Speech 101, your topic for the final exam speech is "The Difference between Men's and Women's Exercise Performance Levels. Are They More Alike Than Different?" List 3 similarities and differences you want to highlight in your speech.

5. Your friend signed up for a fitness class, and, while he was demonstrating one of the workouts, you noticed he was doing standing toe-touch with legs crossed and double leg-lifts. Explain to your friend why those 2 exercises are contraindicated (how they can hurt him) and give him safe alternatives for them.

Chapter

9

Activities

Name _____   Class/Activity Section _____

Analyze your Diet

Using the food log on the following page, write down everything you eat and drink for 3 to 5 full days. Make copies of the food log as needed. Be sure to note the approximate quantity of food, and assess combination foods (e.g., pizza, casseroles, tacos, salads, etc.) to be able to list the foods in them. Keep track of the number of servings in each food group. (Use the blank columns at the right to record calories, sodium milligrams, fat grams, iron milligrams, etc., as desired.)

1. Looking at the 7 "Dietary Guidelines for Americans," how does your diet measure up within *each* guideline?

2. Look at the "Food Guide Pyramid". Do you meet the daily criteria for recommended servings in each food group? Explain.

3. Identify 2 positive dietary changes that you could implement that would enhance your nutritional wellness. Include *what* you will do and a *specific strategy* of how you will do it.

	Chapter
	9
	Activities

Name _____   Class/Activity Section _____

Food Log

Date _____
(12:01 A.M. to 12:00 midnight)

Major Food Groups—Servings

Time	Food	Amount	Bread Cereal Rice Pasta	Vegetable	Fruit	Meat Poultry Fish Beans Eggs&Nuts	Milk Yogurt Cheese	Fats Oils Sweets				
Totals =												

Vitamin Supplements:

Name _____   *Class/Activity Section* _____

82%
FAT
FREE
GOBBLER'S
Turkey Franks

Ingredients: Turkey, Water, Salt, Flavorings, Dextrose, Sodium Phosphate, Sodium Erythorbate, Sodium Nitrite, Extract of Paprika.

Fully Cooked. Heat 5 minutes in simmering water.

Nutrition Information
(Per Portion Size)

Portion Size ....1 Frank	Protein 7g
Portions Per Package 8	Carbohydrates.............1g
Calories 120	Fat 10g

---

GULF STREAM
CHUNK LIGHT TUNA
IN SPRING WATER

NUTRITION INFORMATION PER SERVING

Serving Size (Incl. Liq.) .... 2 oz.	Servings per container...................3.3
Calories 60	Fat ....Less than 1 g
Protein ....13 grams	Sodium ....310 Mg
Carbohydrates.................Less than 1 g	

PERCENTAGE OF U.S. RECOMMENDED DAILY ALLOWANCE
(U.S. RDA)

Protein 25	Riboflavin (B_2) 2	Vitamin E 2
Vitamin A....................*	Niacin 35	Vitamin B_2.....................15
Vitamin C ....*	Calcium...............................*	Vitamin B_{12} 25
Thiamin (B_1) ....*	Iron 4	

* Contains less than 2% of the U.S RDA of these nutrients

INGREDIENTS: Light Tuna, Spring Water, Vegetable Broth, Salt.
For inquiries concerning product, include number shown on lid.

Look at the 2 food labels and compute the percentage of protein and fat in each. Comment on your findings.

Calories	Hot Dog	Tuna
Gm Protein		
% Protein		
Gm Fat		
% Fat		

Comments: _____

_____

_____

_____

Name _____

Chapter
10
Activities

Class/Activity Section _____

Why Do You Eat?

Use the following eating diary to analyze the reasons you eat. Knowing the cues and factors that affect eating can help you manage your eating behavior.

Date _____

Time of Day	Location	Alone or With Whom?	Food Consumed	Quantity	Time Spent Eating	Mood/ Psychological State While Eating	Activity While Eating

Observations:

Strategies For Change:

<table>
<tr><td>Chapter
10
Activities</td></tr>
</table>

Name _____   *Class/Activity Section* _____

How Active Are You?

Finding the time to exercise can be a challenge. However, there are several times during a day that you can "weave" activity into your life (i.e., walking rather than driving; riding a stationary bike while watching TV; taking the stairs rather than the elevator; getting up 45 minutes earlier in the morning to jog; etc.). Use the following log to keep track of your activity during the day. Then, analyze WHEN and HOW you could adapt your lifestyle to include more activity.

Date _____

Time of Day	Activity	Location	How Long?	Positive Outcomes	Any Negatives?

Assess your activity level today:

Describe ways you could fit more activity into your day:

What obstacles do you face in trying to be active?

What are your strategies for combatting these obstacles and for adhering to a lifetime of activity/exercise?

<table>
<tr><td>Name _____</td><td>**Chapter**
10
Activities</td><td>*Class/Activity Section* _____</td></tr>
</table>

Understanding Weight Management

1. Obesity can be described in terms of body fat percentage as: _____ ;

   and in terms of BMI as: _____ .

2. Five health conditions associated with obesity are:

3. Five factors that affect Basal Metabolic Rate are:

4. Four reasons crash dieting does not work as a permanent weight loss plan include:

5. The 3 major components of effective lifetime weight management are:

6. Five ways exercise helps in weight management include:

7. Three ways bulimia and anorexia nervosa are similar:

8. Three ways bulimia and anorexia nervosa are different include:

Substance Abuse

1. Complete each statement according to your feelings:

A. I view substance abuse as . . .

B. The thought that alcohol, tobacco, and caffeine are drugs . . .

C. If my sister continued to smoke while pregnant I would . . .

D. If my 16-year-old brother asked me to get him some beer, I . . .

E. If the police picked me up for driving while intoxicated, I would . . .

F. How serious is substance abuse? (Scale of 1 to 5, 5 being most serious).

• in U.S. _____

• at this university _____

• in my residence hall _____

• in my home _____

• Discussion: Defend your rating (tell why). What substances are being abused; what can/should be done to curb the abuse?

2. A. Does the music listed below reflect society's values? Does it reflect your values? Explain.

• Do cocaine to get over the blues. (" Cocaine," by Eric Clapton)

• Alcohol counteracts loneliness, as a lover does. (" The Piano Man," by Billy Joel)

• Look to drugs for help. (" With a Little Help from My Friends," by the Beatles)

B. What current music depicts substance use? List three examples and tell how it depicts substance use/abuse.

1.

2.

3.

C. How do music/videos influence the use of drugs in our society?

3. Respond to the following:

    A. Leaving a party, you see a girl passed out on the lawn. What should you do? List six actions you should take.

    B. Use five factors that affect alcohol absorption to give a profile of a person who will get drunk fastest.

    C. How does alcohol change people's behavior? Give five examples from your observations.

    D. You want to plan a safe party. List five ways you can help those attempting to reduce or abstain from alcohol (or drugs).

    E. Any pregnant woman has a right to drink alcohol as much as she wants. Argue for/then against.
    For:

      Against:

    F. Describe your strategies to avoid irresponsible use of alcohol. List and describe at least eight.

    G. George can drink 2 six-packs before he feels drunk. Susan feels tipsy after 2 drinks. Should both be considered legally drunk at the same BAC? Discuss the reasons for your response.

Name _____

Chapter
14
Activities

Class/Activity Section _____

Advertisement Assignment

1. List signs of quackery in the advertisement for Shrink-it 5000.

2. What makes this advertisement attractive or seem legitimate to the uninformed consumer?

3. If your sister was ready to send away for this product with the hope of reducing fat thighs, what would you tell her? How would you advise anyone wanting to reduce the fat on their thighs?

Name _____

Chapter

14

Activities

Class/Activity Section _____

Look to the Future

Imagine that you are 10 years older, married, with 2 children, and working in your chosen field.

1. Describe the wellness programs that you would want your employer/company to offer. (If you plan to be self-employed or involved in a small business, describe the wellness programs you would want your hospital or community to offer.)

2. What family activities will be important to you in order to promote family wellness?

3. Describe how you will manage a regular fitness program. (Where? When? What type of activity? etc.)

4. Not including fitness, what other lifestyle and wellness habits will you be committed to for your lifetime? (Your answer may involve the entire wellness spectrum.)

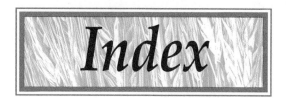

Index

A

B

T,U,–V

W–Y